OTHER BOOKS BY THE AUTHOR

ARCHITECTURAL MEDICINE®
BUILDING THE BRIDGE TO WELLNESS

Are you wanting a better world in which to live, work, and play for both yourself and future generations? The focus of this book is to discuss how these two fields of Architecture and Medicine have a potential to overlap for a better built environment to live within.

(Published December 2020)

INTEGRATIVE ARCHITECTURE

Integrating the processes between green, healthy, and sustainable Architecture methodologies for energy efficient, ecologically aware, and healthier built environments.

(Forthcoming)

SYMBIOSIS GLOBAL
NATURE IS THE MOST ADVANCED TECHNOLOGY
TECHNOLOGY & ECOLOGY : LIVING TOGETHER

How can we navigate the challenges of humanity while also striving for progress in the world of Technology? How can we create a future more aligned to the planet's Ecological systems? Symbiosis Global outlines these topics with a focus on the premise "Nature is the Most Advanced Technology."

(Forthcoming)

THE ARCHITECTURAL DOCTOR®

AN Rx FOR HEALTH & WELLNESS IN BUILDINGS

INTEGRATING THE FIELDS OF ARCHITECTURE & MEDICINE

TIMOTHY D. ROSSI

Copyright © 2022 by Timothy D. Rossi

All rights reserved.

No part of this publication may be reproduced, distributed, or transmitted in any form or by any means, electronic, mechanical, photocopying, recording, or otherwise, without express written permission of the author.

Architectural Medicine®, Architectural Doctor®, and ARxMD® are all trademarks of
Timothy D. Rossi and
Architectural Medicine LLC.

Cover, book design, graphics,
and photography
by Timothy D. Rossi,
except where noted

FIRST EDITION

ISBN NUMBER:
978-1-7347766-2-1

Library of Congress Control Number: 2020915228

This book is dedicated
to my Mother –

Francine E. Rossi

CONTENTS

Acknowledgements .... **xiii**

Introduction .... **xvii**

Part I

Chapter 1: What Is Architectural Medicine? 1

Chapter 2: Who Is This Book For? 30

Chapter 3: Introducing the Architectural Doctor 43

Chapter 4: What is Integrative Architecture? 58

Chapter 5: The Architectural Medicine System (AMS) 101

Chapter 6: ARxMD – The Architectural Medicine Software Solution (Part 1) 147

CONTENTS

Part II

Chapter 7: The Role of the Healthy Building Inspector and Building Informaticist ... **171**

Chapter 8: 8 Steps to Better Health and Wellness in the Built Environment **197**

Chapter 9: The Processes of the Doctor and Health Professionals **213**

Chapter 10: The Processes of the Architect and Building Professionals **233**

Chapter 11: The Role of the Architectural Doctor **248**

Chapter 12: ARxMD – The Architectural Medicine Software Solution (Part 2) **273**

CONTENTS

Part III

Chapter 13: Public Health, Social Determinants of Health (SDoH), & Geomedicine **299**

Chapter 14: ARxMD Standards, Processes, & Protocols **327**

Chapter 15: Bringing It All Together – Integrative Medicine, Integrative Architecture, & Architectural Medicine **346**

Chapter 16: Nurturing Architecture for a Future of Wellness **369**

Chapter 17: What's Next for Architectural Medicine and the Architectural Doctor? **385**

Chapter 18: Some Thoughts on the Future **402**

About the Author **419**

Notes **441**

ACKNOWLEDGMENTS

This is the second book that I've written, and as I mentioned in my first book *Architectural Medicine*, I first have to give thanks to my mother, the late Francine Rossi. She was the biggest supporter of my life's path and believed in my ideas and concepts. She believed in my passion for exploring solutions to problems I've been concerned about, and she provided tremendous support in my journey through life.

This book is dedicated to her.

Without her support throughout my life, I would not have been able to explore these fields, concepts, and ideas with the courage to pursue these dreams of a better future. While many may see these ideas as ideals, I believe they transcend survival toward a world of thriving. I do not believe there is any other ideal more worth exploring than the architecture of thriving for humanity.

I'm also thankful to be able to draw upon the lessons from my father, the late Frank Rossi. He was a tough man often focused on discipline and hard work, and yet his multi-faceted interests, from sports and history to the topics of nature, organic gardening, and his enjoyment of music, gave me a wide range of topics to learn from growing up. This range of topics, in fact, has lasted throughout my adult life. He was a history teacher and a coach of lacrosse and football for over three decades and taught me the value of hard work, education, and the importance of teamwork. In my formative years, he taught me the importance of discipline, without which I am not sure I could have navigated rough seas as they've occurred in my life.

Writing a book has many challenges to traverse, and without the support to achieve this goal, it is extremely difficult to complete. It's important to note that I could not have written this without the support of many people on my journey during many decades on this path.

This support includes some friends and family who have encouraged me, have been supportive, and have shown interest in my ideas that have given me the courage – especially at times when needed the most – to keep going.

A big thank you to all who have been there for me.

A special thank you to Bethany Carson, who has been a constant support for me during the long hours of work, time, and energy that it takes to write a book. I am grateful for her inspiration and amazing encouragement during challenges during this process. I thank her for her wonderful care.

I would like to thank a small group of people whose inspiration and support during my journey have been extremely important to me. Their wisdom and knowledge from which I have learned over the years, set a path for me to explore in an inspiring format. This includes Bosco Büeler, Cedar Rose Guelberth, Christi Graham, James Hubble, Professor Robert Blank, Mary Cordaro, Will Spates, Richard Scarborough, Helmet Ziehe at the International Building Biology Institute, Nancy Sheinbein, and the Yestermorrow Design/Build School in Vermont. A special thanks to Bernadette Soon, whose support during difficult times in my life has been extremely valuable.

A big thank you to my Aunt Valerie and Uncle John. My uncle passed away this year of 2022, he was a wonderful human being that taught me a tremendous amount in his words and his actions. They both planted many important and helpful seeds in my childhood in which, I think, have brought thriving blossoms forth.

I also would like to thank those who I have never met who have been incredibly important to me in my life. This includes the writings, and master teachings of the late Neil Peart of Rush — on the drums as well as in the wisdom of his lyrics and books. While I never met him, his mentorship through his writings and musical expressions, provided many vital topics to ponder during my lifetime.

I am also thankful for the courage and determination of Buckminster Fuller, as well as the inspiring designs of Frank Lloyd Wright. I am grateful for the pioneering perseverance of Rachel Carson, Florence Nightingale, and Henry David Thoreau, who have been inspirational in my life.

A thank you to the Pixar animation company and the inspiring visions of John Lasseter, Ed Catmull, and Apple icon Steve Jobs.

There have also been the spiritual inquiries provided by Joseph Campbell, Alan Watts, Gandhi, and Krishnamurti, whose deeper questions of life have been of great value in my own ventures into the more profound topics and depths of life. I'm also appreciative of the inspiring lives of Dr. Martin Luther King Jr. and the life and lessons of lacrosse legend Oren Lyons of the Iroquois nation.

And finally, I'd like to show my thanks for several architects and designers whose designs and developments have provided examples of a positive, hopeful future for architecture and the built environment. This includes the late Zaha Hadid, with her incredible designs embracing the synergy of nature's wisdom combined with the engineering brilliance and aesthetics for a hopeful future. I am also thankful for the inspiring work of Santiago Calatrava, Sim Van der Ryn, James Hubble, Frei Otto, Eugene Tsui, and Patrik Schumacher, as well as the pioneering work of Janine Benyus, Neri Oxman, and Paul Stamets.

INTRODUCTION

In this day and age, the topics of health and wellness have become increasingly common, with many people, groups, and organizations exploring the questions of what it is to be healthy.

This book has been written over several years and has been revised and edited from the years 2020 to 2022. In this stage of history, we have endured the pandemic of the novel coronavirus as COVID-19, and the state of the world has gone from full stride to almost complete shutdown. It has forced many to spend time indoors at a nearly 100 percent rate, in order to quarantine from the virus.

In doing so, the topic of health in the built environment has become evident. These topics, which, previously, in discussing the impacts on health in buildings, would often be met with perplexity. Yet now, they have become evident for most of the population. The idea that the built environment impacts our health; physically, emotionally, mentally or psychologically has become all the more apparent. The personal experiences of the stay at home initiatives to avoid an airborne virus, has made clear to most the influence that buildings can have on physical health. And to add to this understanding have been the experiences of the impacts that staying in one place can have on both emotional and mental or psychological health. It's become a topic of great concern for many during the pandemic, and these topics have become common in not just the architecture and building circles, yet for the entire public.

Adding to this are the more recent discussions of wellness in this early 21st century, including the increasingly common Social Determinants of Health (SDoH). These topics include the built environment, and the environment in general, into the big themes of the health equations. A large part of these conversations hinge around the built environment, and the impacts buildings have on health.

As I outlined in my first book *Architectural Medicine*®, these topics highlight the questions of "how" these issues can be included in the evaluations for better personal and public health.

My focus on these developments is based on "systems" in evaluating building health issues. Most importantly, the focus on how these topics can be included in a doctor's evaluations and the health care professional's processes, combined with the solutions that an architect and the building professionals can provide. And for such procedures to exist, these important processes require systems.

If you've been paying attention to the responses to the novel coronavirus building issues, many of these concerns have been based on the transmission of the virus as an airborne contaminant. Addressing the building solutions regarding air handling systems to provide safe measures for the public to go back to commercial and public buildings has been a topic since the start of the pandemic. What might be highlighted in this process, is that while there have been great discussions in both the architecture and medical professions, there have been challenges in implementing these solutions. And without systems that bridge different professions, such as architecture and medicine, there are gaps that prevent proper solutions from being executed. This is not to fault either group or any specific professionals. Instead, it can be utilized as an insight into the gaps that exist and how updated integrations between these and other professionals can benefit large issues that the pandemic has underscored.

The main question continues to be how these topics, including social determinants of health, and the built environment in general, can be included in the big picture of human health and well-being.

From my perspective, the answers to these questions originate with systems. If there are no systems in place for the doctors and architects to utilize for evaluation along with proper training for these processes, then how can all of these professions be involved to provide integrated solutions?

If you do not provide training for the medical community, with doctors and health professionals aware of these potential issues and without systems for them to utilize for solutions, how can there be proper support for solutions?

The same for the architecture and building professionals. If they are not taught these topics in school, and then provided with procedures and systems to follow in their professional work, how can they provide solutions in their fields?

And then there is the topic of how these two professionals can work together — not only to be aware of the issues and solutions, but to recognize the benefits of the architecture and medical fields working together to achieve these interconnected goals.

These are just two of the professions involved in this process. There are many other professionals, from epidemiologists, social workers, toxicologists, and public health professionals to inspection and building occupant professionals, that also need to be included in this big picture process.

Complex Integrative Processes Require Sophisticated Systems

These are complex topics and issues, and cannot be resolved without integrative systems developed and supported within each profession, as well as proper integrations provided between these professions in multi-disciplinary formats.

After all, while there has been an increase in research, with many articles and discussions on the importance of health in the built environment, what are the actionables? How can these topics be implemented in the real world?

All of these processes require systems, and with these systems, it also requires professionals to be liaisons in supporting these integrated procedures.

With both the architecture and medical professions being extremely complex, each with their own systems and approaches, the steps required to include the built environment in health evaluations will require not only new systems, yet new professionals for best practices moving forward.

In chapter 1, the outline of topics for health in the built environment will be defined, and then in chapter 3, I will jump right into the discussions of one of these new professionals to support these integrated systems — the *Architectural Doctor®*.

Why Is a Focus on Health in Buildings Important?

This book is a continuation of my first book *Architectural Medicine*, where I provide an overview of the emerging integrations between the fields of architecture and medicine with a focus on health and wellness. These integrated developments are continuing to coalesce for better health in the built environment, with the end result providing support for optimal human health and well-being.

The Architectural Doctor is a new type of professional that is inherently multi-disciplinary, with the goal of bridging the fields of architecture and medicine to support healthier built environments - physically, emotionally, mentally or psychologically — and dare I say, spiritually.

In *Architectural Medicine,* I discuss the integrations possible between architecture and medicine, and in this book, the Architectural Doctor, I will discuss the specific processes and systems required to achieve these goals.

Why Have an Interest in This Book?

If you are wondering why you should read this book, I will offer a reply in the format of a question:

> "Are you wanting a better world in which to live, work, and play for both yourself and future generations? Are you aware of how the built environment impacts your health — physically, emotionally, mentally or psychologically? Are you concerned about the future of your health and the health of your children, grandchildren, and the many other creatures and animals that live on this planet?"

In this book, I will provide a framework for the many topics related to health in the built environment, with the specific intention of providing an

Rx as a blueprint and systems to achieve these goals.

There is an importance in providing the theory of how systems can function, yet there is also the need to put these theories into practice to implement these changes.

I will provide an overview of Architectural Medicine in practice and go into more detail about how these processes can function as full system solutions.

What Can Be Done to Achieve Better Health and Wellness in Architecture?

The modern day world has many benefits, and has provided solutions for the built environment that had not been achieved in recorded history.

And with the benefits of modern materials and methods, there have also been some detriments. In the past fifty years, common topics such as the health issues of lead in paints, asbestos in buildings, and topics related to mold and indoor air quality have become more common for people to be concerned about.

Most modern day buildings include newer synthetic materials and yet are also built airtight, in ways that reduce the exchange of fresh air. These tight buildings can cause problems such as carbon dioxide and carbon monoxide poisoning and high levels of volatile organic compounds (VOCs) that can negatively impact the endocrine system. Some of these chemicals have long term health impacts with small accumulations in the body over time.

And while the medical fields have become more advanced over the past century, there is still a lack of consideration of health impacts from the built environment, and this gap continues to widen as buildings continue to become more complex.

As such, these health issues caused by building situations have the potential to be included in the doctor's evaluations, yet in order to do so there are several steps required and a number of new professionals that need to be included.

This integration of fields and a new process of working together in new formats can provide better solutions for health in buildings, yet it's important to note that these procedures also add more processes to already complex professions.

Therefore, there is the requirement of new professionals to support these integrations, and to support the multitude of professionals involved to achieve these goals.

The intention is to provide an overview and trajectory of solutions from where these developments have been and where it may be going to the important questions of how to get there.

A critical comment to state very early in this book, is to say that the concept of an Architectural Doctor right now, is in its infancy. While there are many involved in both the fields of architecture and medicine who have provided or are currently providing some overlap between these two fields, the idea of this being a known professional is in an early development cycle.

It is my belief that when the Architectural Doctor becomes a regularly defined professional, it will not only help to bridge the gaps between architecture and medicine, yet can provide tremendous benefits to the masses in population health.

The reality is that many of the processes and systems required to achieve the goals of a better future for current and future generations are not yet in place. Humanity has created many complex systems and technologies over the past several hundred years, yet much of this has not scaled in a healthy format, especially when focused on human health.

These bridges to health have not yet been built and require new systems and new professionals to support these developments.

I can't promise I know all of the answers, yet I am asking these questions with great concern, and this book has come to be after many decades of seeking solutions to achieve healthier built environments.

Both this book and the *Architectural Medicine* book came to be after many years of seeking and working toward cohesive, whole system solutions. After years of learning and being involved hands-on with these developments, my experiences, either for work or merely my own explorations towards knowledge, have led to these new systems as potential solutions.

In this book, I will provide a framework for the required new systems and processes relating to health in the built environment, and will provide a blueprint for these complex systems and solutions.

Etiology, the Built Environment, and Public Health

The reality of modern medicine is that, while it is extremely advanced and complex, there are many conditions and illnesses whose cause is often unknown.

Modern medicine has many sophisticated processes and procedures to provide solutions to many of these conditions, yet there is still a lack of knowledge in terms of the root causes of many of these illnesses. In addition, the actual cures for these health problems are often not achieved.

According to the Oxford dictionary, *etiology* is defined as "the causation of (a) disease; a cause or causative agent of disease."[1]

Therefore, there are still many facets in the health and medical fields that can benefit from a root understanding of the cause of diseases, and perhaps there are many facets in the built environment that can help in finding these origins.

The modern world has been built on the foundations of knowledge, and this has occurred due to data and the scientific method. The medical fields depend on evidence-based medicine to provide solid processes to ensure evaluations to best support ailments. The building fields depend on structural engineering and evidence-based design to achieve best practices in the architecture, engineering, and construction (AEC) professions.

And yet, in today's 21st century, there are large gaps in the built environment relative to health and the gathering of data to properly calculate such problems. Most doctors today do not include any topics in the built environment relative to their patient's health, and few architects have proper training in human health. The ability to design structures to ensure optimal health for the occupants is a major goal of Architectural Medicine.

This, of course, is not the fault of these professionals. They already have a tremendous amount of education and training to achieve, and to provide ad hoc processes into their work is neither easy to achieve nor is it a best practice.

As such, an important part of Architectural Medicine and the Architectural Doctor is to provide proper systems for these professionals to achieve these goals.

What can also be said about this topic is the importance of informatics, which in today's data-driven world has become more important for viewing the big picture and providing cohesive solutions. However, the amount of data as informatics that has been collected in the built environment relative to human health is quite small. Throughout this book, I will delve into why this is so, and what can be done about it. Suffice it to say that an increase in this building health data can provide more insights for the building and health professionals.

For health professionals, this means the inclusion of the built environment as part of a patient's evaluation of health, especially relative to the etiology of modern ailments.

Are there issues in the environment and built environments that are negatively impacting health? If so, how can we provide metrics for these issues, which currently are not measured very well and are often not included for health professionals in their evaluation processes?

Is there building data that we can gather for public health professionals to analyze to allow better knowledge for doctors and architects to utilize in their work?

And what about the fields of architecture? Is there data and feedback from health professionals that can guide the architects and designers to ensure that they are using best practices to design and create healthier buildings?

Being that this process is not common for either the medical or the architecture fields, Architectural Medicine strives to provide bridges between these fields to help support this approach toward better health and wellness. And the Architectural Doctor's role is to support these initiatives.

An Rx for Health & Wellness in Buildings

While many are familiar with a doctor's Rx or prescription for testing to provide a restoration towards health, you may be asking, what exactly is an Rx for health in buildings? What does that even mean?

Typically, the current medical approach is to utilize pharmacological solutions, and, as many are now including the realm of integrative medicine, the options for healing include better nutrition, healthy exercise, and mental and emotional approaches utilizing yoga and meditation as examples.

And as these additions can be extremely helpful, there is still a large piece of the puzzle missing from this healthy equation — buildings.

An Rx for health in buildings includes the built environment as part of the medical and health professional's evaluations and can also provide solutions from the architecture fields where there are issues found impacting a patient's health.

As I mentioned above, evidence-based processes in both professions are critical, and right now, there is a lot of building data that is not being reported and evaluated. Moving forward into the future, by gathering, evaluating, and utilizing this type of data, it can provide greater insights for healthier architecture.

8 Steps to Better Health in the Built Environment

A significant part of this book is focused on providing solutions to issues focused on health in the built environment. Throughout this book, I will discuss the main issues that are striving to be solved, and then provide templates of action for solutions. While these topics are large and complex, I will do my best to provide an overview of what is striving to be achieved and the steps that will be involved to get there.

In the first chapter, I'll define the overview of Architectural Medicine, and then in the next few chapters, I will outline an overview of these puzzle pieces to provide context. And then, in chapter 8, I will review these topics in context by providing "8 Steps to Better Health in the Built Environment" as an overview of processes that the Architectural Doctor will provide.

These 8 steps will be both informative and active solutions, including multi-disciplinary processes that cross over between the fields of architecture and medicine. This overlap is critical for whole system solutions. This is vital for true health and wellness in the built environment to be achieved, and moving forward in our current complex, modern day world, it will be required if we as humanity are going to address these topics seriously.

Systems and the Architectural Medicine System (AMS)

In order to provide solutions to achieve these "8 steps," in chapters 5 and 6, I will discuss the importance of systems and how procedures, processes, and software solutions can offer a framework for these professionals to work together.

This includes the topics of the *Architectural Medicine System (AMS)* and *ARxMD® — the Architectural Medicine Software Solution.*

In today's world, we often take for granted the steps of going to the doctor and getting a blood test, which the doctor can utilize to gain insights into ailments for a better understanding of health. This type of laboratory process, and the many professional steps involved, were not always in existence.

Over the past 50 to 60 plus years, these procedures and measurements

As a side note, there are many graphics throughout this book and it may be challenging to see all the details. I have provided a link to many of the core graphics in this book for online viewing. They can be viewed using the QR code or at the following link:
https://architecturalmedicine.com/book

in the medical professions have developed over time and are now commonplace. With the additional implementation of laboratory testing professionals, these roundtrip processes, from a nurse providing a blood sample to the laboratory testing and reporting of the results, have all become common procedures in modern medicine.

However, it was not always that way, and therefore these new additions discussed in this book, utilizing laboratory testing for potential issues in the built environment, can support the doctor's evaluations for their patient's health and can become an inclusive and common practice into the future.

The steps to achieve this process are a big part of this book and a major role of the Architectural Doctor.

Context Is Key

As you read through the topics of each chapter, one critical component that you may recognize is the importance of *context*. In the information age that we are living in, the amount of content has become overwhelming for many, and to provide useful meaning from all of these details, it is vital to have context to all of this information.

In both the architecture and medical fields, the amount of information and data has become extraordinary, and the only way to navigate all of this data is to have context.

In the architecture and construction fields, the utilization of digital files and processes, utilizing Computer Aided Drawing (CAD) and Building Information Modeling (BIM), along with cloud based scheduling and coordination, has provided an increasing amount of datasets and information.

And in the world of health and medicine, data has always been a large part of this profession. Yet since the late 1990s into the 2000s, these fields have increased the number of digital processes, which has expanded the realms of data to an exponential degree. As an example, the term *meaningful use*[2] was utilized in the health profession as an initiative to bring access to electronic, digital data in the USA. The ability to utilize this meaningful use meaningfully is critical for the future of medicine. In fact, U.S. Centers for

Medicare & Medicaid Services (CMS) in 2018 updated their stance on the meaningful use act by stating, "we are proposing to overhaul the Medicare and Medicaid EHR Incentive Programs to focus on interoperability, improve flexibility, relieve burden and place emphasis on measures that require the electronic exchange of health information between providers and patients. To better reflect this new focus, we are re-naming the Meaningful Use program "Promoting Interoperability.""[3]

This interoperability will be a topic that is discussed throughout this book and can both define and represent integrations occurring across many professions.

This is not only a reflection of the changes and updates that exist in the digital world, but also of the forward movement that continues to expand in this evolution. The increase of information, along with the scaling of processes, requires better context. Otherwise, navigating topics lacking context will reduce understanding of these complex scenarios and can increase the gaps in these developments, potentially causing multiple problems in the interest of solving one problem.

In my opinion, context is not only key for the profession of the Architectural Doctor, but is critical for the future of all professionals working together for cohesive solutions.

There cannot be an Architectural Doctor to provide supportive solutions without an integrative mindset and approach between the fields of architecture and medicine. I also believe that once the public becomes more aware of the impacts of the built environment relative to health, there will be more demand for such building solutions.

And in this manner, there will be a need for professionals to provide the supply for these demands. While this is inherently cyclical, I call this process a *spiracycle*, as there is either an upward and positive movement in these cycles, or a downward and negative cycle as a result. If the public demands solutions, yet there are no procedures and systems in place to achieve these goals, then there is a downward spiracycle. Yet providing systems and solutions for such demands can support an upward spiracycle.

Introduction

Once the general public has context for how their built environment impacts their health, they will strive to find solutions. Yet as opposed to changing one's health approaches through diet or adding yoga or meditation to daily life, changes in the built environment will not always be easy to achieve.

These changes will need to be included in regular architectural designs and should inform new designs while providing introspection for those who can provide building changes, retrofits, and upgrades in buildings.

The context of these solutions is not just relevant to one field or profession. As stated, these new systems include the integrations between both fields of architecture and medicine, as well as the demands from the general public.

With a plethora of information on these topics of health in the built environment, solutions will require specific context. And this requires a big picture understanding of these topics enmeshed with detailed solutions provided by both fields in a synergistic format. In chapter 4, I will discuss some of these big picture views in the building fields defined as *Integrative Architecture*.

To achieve these solutions, there is a need for this context to be recognized by each professional and the roles of each field, combined with new professionals to support these integrative solutions. Throughout this book, I will delve into both the big picture views of these topics, as well as detailed procedures to achieve real world solutions.

And because the meaningful use initiative in the USA has provided access to digital data in healthcare, topics of interoperability are now more available than ever, and this opens up the possibilities for more advanced cross-disciplinary processes to be achieved. This will be a main focus of chapters 5 and 6, discussing the Architectural Medicine System (AMS) and ARxMD, respectively, and will be discussed as an important tool for helping to bridge these professionals throughout the latter part of this book.

Personal and Precision Medicine, Digital Twins, Social Determinants of Health (SDoH), Geomedicine, and the Built Environment

Since the start of the second decade of the 21st century, research defined as precision medicine has focused on an individual's personal genetics, including how their exposure to varying environments impacts their health. This focus includes the review of these exposures to provide healthier treatments and protocols for topics such as cancer, yet also to find best solutions for personalized medicine. This precision or personal medicine directive in the USA has been the focus of "The Precision Medicine Initiative." As stated on the U.S. Department of Health and Human Services National Institutes of Health website, the Precision Medicine Initiative is "a long-term research endeavor, involving the National Institutes of Health (NIH) and multiple other research centers, which aims to understand how a person's genetics, environment, and lifestyle can help determine the best approach to prevent or treat disease."[4]

As well, over the past several years, the concept of a Digital Twin has entered the lexicon of both architecture and medicine. This "digital twin" is essentially the digitization of a real-world object, with its origins in the engineering and structures fields. Its purpose is to provide a digital version of a real world structure, to provide analysis for maintenance and testing of systems simulations for upgrades in a digital realm. The end results can be a reduction in costs and provide a better understanding of updates, modifications, and the resulting changes.

A digital twin is defined as a "virtual representation that serves as the real-time digital counterpart of a physical object or process."[5] Initially, this idea was focused on the engineering fields and although "the concept originated earlier (attributed to Michael Grieves, then of the University of Michigan, in 2002) the first practical definition of a digital twin originated from NASA in an attempt to improve physical-model simulation of spacecraft in 2010."[6]

This digital twin concept has expanded to include both buildings and the human body to monitor changes and provide updates that can be evaluated before any modifications in the real world are implemented. In the building world, these twins can provide real world monitoring and simulations of building health, while also ensuring that any changes and updates to the structure are recorded as living documents. In the medical world, combined with the emulated knowledge provided by personalized medicine and a patient's DNA, it can provide simulations of procedures and medications to evaluate the resulting impacts. This can also support best practices for the patient in monitoring their own health. I'll go into more detail on these developments in chapter 12.

Another key takeaway to the above statement from the National Institutes of Health, is the goal to "understand how a person's genetics, *environment*, and lifestyle can help determine the best approach to prevent or treat disease."[7] Relative to this book and the Architectural Medicine processes, this research into a person's "environment" and how this can impact one's health is critical. As more research and awareness on how one's environment, and in particular, the built environment, can impact human health, there are bigger questions about how this data can be recorded and reported.

This includes the increasingly popular topic, especially in the USA, which has been Social Determinants of Health (SDoH). This is defined by the World Health Organization (WHO) as "the conditions in which people are born, grow, work, live, and age, and the wider set of forces and systems shaping the conditions of daily life."[8] This is a wide range of topics, yet these include the environment and the built environments in which people live and work. With the increase in the average person's time spent indoors, spending up to 90 percent of their time inside of buildings, the impacts that these environments have on human health can be significant.

However, the current day medical processes have very limited scope in evaluating the built environment relative to patient health. And this book, along with the *Architectural Medicine* book, strives to bridge these gaps to support better health and wellness in the built environment.

When you explore the topics of social determinants of health specific to locations, you can find the inclusion of geographic data to also be of value. These developments can be included with the geographic information system (GIS) and expanded to include the topic of geomedicine.

Geomedicine is the "branch of medicine that deals with geographic factors in disease."[9] As such, the connection between place and disease can become more important for both personalized medicine and public health.

The Architectural Doctor and the Architectural Medicine System (AMS) are integral components of this research and reporting, to provide better health and wellness for the general public. This is an important theme throughout this book and will be discussed in more detail, especially in chapters 6 through 13.

Meaningful Use, Electronic Health Records, and Interoperability in the Digital Frontier

Whether you are an architect, doctor, or citizen of the general public, in the 21st century, there is certainly one facet of life that has changed dramatically over the past 50 years — and that is the digital realm of life. From a desktop computer and the digitization of health records to the complex systems of electronic design and building processes, advancements in the electronic world have become ubiquitous in the past few decades.

And with the Medicare EHR Incentive Program, also known as *meaningful use* in the USA, establishing the digital, electronic health record (EHR) as part of the common medical system, has availed the potential for data to be shared between healthcare professionals. Obviously, worldwide this has also been occurring, with many countries supporting these digital processes along with the support from the World Health Organization (WHO) on these topics. The advancements in electronic health records have also become more common over the past few decades worldwide.

As stated earlier, both the medical and architecture professions now perform many of their work procedures in a digital format, which provides more opportunities for bridges between these fields to be achieved utilizing interoperability. These evolving digital advancements can be seen in the quote in a previous paragraph from the CMS where they updated the meaningful use definition to "Promoting Interoperability."[10]

Most of the time, interoperability exists within the health care platforms, yet in this book, I will share my views on how this can expand to include the architecture, engineering, and construction (AEC) fields in ways that previously have not existed.

These processes have the potential to improve integrations between professions and provide better solutions for both doctors and architects to achieve better health and wellness in the built environment moving forward into the future.

How This Book Came to Be

After many decades of my research and questioning in the field of architecture, striving to define a better built environment, the term "Architectural Medicine" came to be. The term "better" can be summarized as healthy, green, and sustainable – while also being described as places and spaces that are nurturing and can provide wellness and well-being for quality of life.

During my research and striving for solutions, as I began to unfold the many layers of these topics, I ended up at the core foundations of both *Architecture* and *Medicine*. After years of this questioning, analyzing, and pondering these topics, I would often find myself at these two fields of architecture and medicine as the core of this better built environment. This research, for me, began as a child, even if I was not aware of it at that time. In the late 1980s, as an architecture student in college, I began to contemplate topics of environmental design, energy efficiency, and health in buildings. These are now known as the topics of green, sustainable, and healthy building, respectively. These issues seemed logical and sensible to me to explore, yet were neither taught in school nor practiced in architecture in most parts of the world at that time.

In the 1990s, I found others who had an interest in these issues and began my journey that continues to this day. This includes concerns about health in the built environment, as well as energy efficiency and sustainability, as these definitions expand and evolve.

I've had the great fortune of learning from incredible pioneers and learned from many forward thinking, considerate and caring people and groups for many decades now. This book is a synthesis of this knowledge across many fields and platforms that could not have been done without their foundational work. I'll make references to their work throughout this book and encourage you to dive deeper into these topics that they've developed for us all in striving to create a better life for humanity and the planet.

While my first foray into co-creating a company focused on healthy, green architecture occurred in 1999, the steps of my education along the way were plentiful and enjoyable during the 90s. I've learned many lessons in building and the concepts of healthy, green, and sustainable design along the way, often in piecemeal formats that have taken many years to weave together into a cohesive fabric.

Since I first began "Architectural Medicine" in 2011, I've continued to build upon these concepts, and each time I've built upon and updated these ideas, the core has remained steady. Architectural Medicine has remained as both a foundation and an umbrella term that covers the many multi-faceted aspects of the healthy, green, and sustainable built environment for a future that I dream of.

This includes a wide range of topics in both the architecture and medical fields, from the scientific understanding of the toxicology of materials to building solutions based on data and informatics. And while science is critical to both of these professions, it also includes the less formulaic and more "felt" topics of how spaces feel and how people respond to places emotionally and psychologically.

Both architecture and medicine have aspects of their fields defined by both the "arts" and the "sciences" in their professions, which means that data alone may not be enough to determine best practices.

Throughout this book, in places and topics that include data, I will add relevant information. And in other areas where the senses and arts are a part of the process, this too will be highlighted.

In the book *Architectural Medicine,* I examine this in more detail, discussing the topics of the arts and sciences integrated as a cohesive whole. However, in this book, to provide an overview of these topics, in chapter 4, "Integrative Architecture," I refer to these subjects and also communicate this throughout the book.

A good example of this interconnection between the arts and sciences is the emerging field of *Neuroscience of Architecture,* which can view the brain and body responses to visual design elements showing the design impacts on human physiology.

This includes, for example, the impact that a visual image or design has on the brain center and whether or not the image is seen as a threat and stressor to the body or is viewed as a safe design element. This new capability to "see" how the body responds to design elements in a physiological format through neuroscience is helping to merge the sciences with the arts in the human experience of built environments.

With this level of understanding, future architecture and designs can be better poised to support the sensory aesthetics of places and spaces. They can also provide more insights into the body–mind impact in a physiological format in terms of how humans respond to these design elements of their built environments.

In the book *Architectural Medicine,* I discuss the concept of the "DNA of Cities" and how a single design can scale up from the design of a single rural structure to highly populated cities in either beneficial or detrimental ways. The "DNA of a Building" can be a critical step forward in the future to analyze, evaluate, and literally redesign the architecture on this planet.

However, for these topics to be implemented into the current fields of architecture and medicine, there is a requirement for systems to be in place, including people who can support these integrations. This is where the Architectural Doctor enters into the picture, and this book is focused on guidelines of the roles and processes of this new professional.

While this book builds upon the foundation of Architectural Medicine, the Architectural Doctor is focused on the processes and procedures that each professional will contribute towards achieving these goals. Without proper education, training, and systems in place with these complex fields, the goals of creating whole system solutions are going to be challenging.

My Credentials

In the introduction of my first book, I discussed my background and credentials with a focus on "why" I was writing the book. As I stated in that book, I'm neither an architect nor a doctor, yet through several decades of working in these fields I have found that there are gaps that, if filled or bridged, can provide better solutions in the built environment for health and wellness.

As an architectural engineering student, I began my professional life learning about the appropriate theories and equations that maintain structural integrity to provide buildings as shelters. Yet during my questions about energy efficiency and environmental impacts, these topics were not a part of the curriculums in the late 1980s during my college years. And so, my adventures seeking these questions led me into the big world, where I spent many years learning about these subjects. There were no common classrooms teaching these topics at that time, and barely an internet to provide these answers during these pre-world wide web years. So, my adventures led to learning in the real world from the many pioneers in the USA and around the world exploring these solutions, which today are now known as green, sustainable, and healthy building.

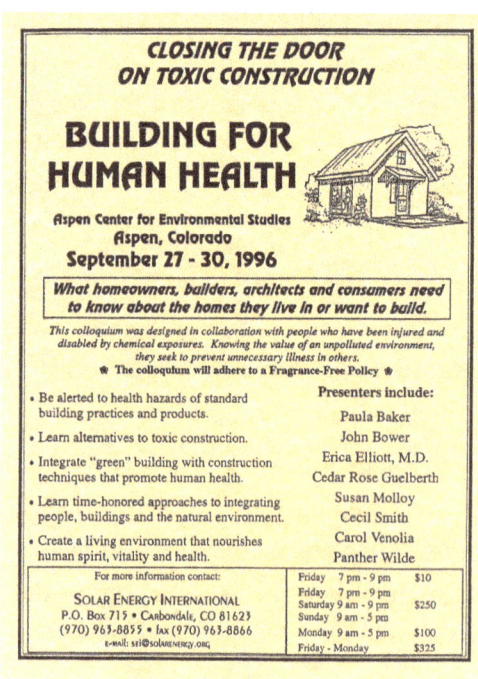

Building For Human Health Conference attended by the author – Aspen, Colorado – 1996

Introduction

I had the great fortune to learn from pioneers in each of these fields, and it is my hope that I can contribute to these on going solutions by providing integrated solutions that I did not have when I first began asking these questions.

In my first book, I stated that – after initial hesitation in writing a book – I decided to continue my writing journey after reading a comment by Richard Branson. In one of his writings, he mentioned that sometimes people on the outside view situations in a different format and see gaps in processes. And with these unique viewpoints, there can be a new approach to providing better solutions.

With this mindset, I continue my journey in writing these books with the intention and hope that my viewpoints and work can contribute to these better solutions, as the world as we know it in the third decade of the 21st century is certainly showing a need for modifications. And these modifications, if focused on health and wellness, can provide a hopeful future for current and future generations.

That said, there are certainly challenges humanity faces right now that, in many ways, have become dire.

Some of these challenges are known by many, and other issues are slowly emerging into awareness. These continue to show up on the radar for not just the professionals, but the general public and all of humanity.

None of these topics, such as built environment issues and environmental problems, are easy to navigate. In my opinion, they require not only integrative solutions, but a multi-disciplinary, collaborative co-creation of solutions moving forward.

The Architectural Doctor is exactly that – a multi-disciplinary professional that strives to provide integrative and collaborative solutions.

What You Can Expect – An Overview of This Book

This book is segmented into three sections. Part I discusses these topics in a big picture viewpoint to provide context for the content in later chapters.

Part II goes into specific details on how these solutions can be implemented. And Part III examines how these can function moving forward into the future. This includes what future possibilities may hold as we venture towards finding solutions focused on well-being and better quality of life.

For example, in chapters 1 through 6, I provide definitions of health in the built environment, including an overview of topics related to energy efficiency and climate change. In chapters 7 to 12, I explore how each professional can work together in a better interconnected format and what the role of the Architectural Doctor can provide. Then in chapters 13 to 18, I discuss how all of these topics can function together and what the future may look like striving to achieve these goals.

And now that I've discussed some of these topics in an introduction, as well as some feedback on how they came into existence, it's time to get into the core topics of this book as we discuss the topics of the Architectural Doctor.

One Last Thing – And a Hopeful View of the Future

One last comment in this introduction that I'd like to leave with you to ponder.

This book has been written in a format that I feel is what I wish I was provided over the past three-plus decades of my learning in contemplating these topics. It is only my view of how processes and procedures would function appropriately, yet please keep in mind that much of this is in its infancy of development.

It is my hope that with a framework defining healthier built environments focused on wellness, this can create an Rx as a blueprint for better health and wellness for humanity. However, in the context of geographical locations around the world, these solutions should also be vernacular. Procedures and processes should be appropriate for the scenario in which you are located, in whatever part of the world in which you are providing solutions. If we all recognize the value of diversity, not only of the diverse life forms on this planet, but of the diversity of people, cultures, and built environments, the future can include a diverse planet for us all to enjoy.

There are certainly challenges in the current world, and the future will be defined by the actions taken now. If we choose to work together to find collaborative, cohesive, whole system solutions, it not only benefits us as individuals, yet it will benefit the entire living world of this planet as well as future generations.

I don't think this should be taken lightly, and it also should not be on the shoulders of the few.

By working together, the heavy load of this lift can be lightened. As my grandmother Rossi always said, "many hands make light work."

To me, there is no architecture as important as the architecture of systems developed for a future that can provide health and wellness to humanity and the many living beings on this planet.

A blueprint for health and wellness in a systems approach can provide processes and procedures that support this initiative – for the individual as well as the masses.

I cannot think of any other architecture that is as important as this for the future.

As we get into the details, it's important to provide context, as I discussed in this introduction. This context is to provide the enormous amount of information in today's world in a usable format appropriate for integrative solutions.

And on that note, I will begin this book with chapter 1, starting with the answer to the question," What is Architectural Medicine?"

"Never doubt that a small group of thoughtful, committed citizens can change the world; indeed, it's the only thing that ever has."

— Margaret Mead

WHAT IS ARCHITECTURAL MEDICINE?

An Overview of this Emerging Development

As I begin to discuss the topics of the Architectural Doctor, it will be important to consider the main topics of Architectural Medicine. The reason is because the Architectural Doctor is involved in bridging these fields of architecture and medicine to support health and wellness in the built environment, which Architectural Medicine defines.

And as the Architectural Doctor's purpose is to implement the goals set by Architectural Medicine, we must first take time to review Architectural Medicine itself.

The subtitle of Architectural Medicine is "building the bridge to wellness." This description is not only the premise of Architectural Medicine, but the purpose of the Architectural Doctor. The main question that remains is," what is this bridge that is being built?"

Building the Bridge Not Yet Built

When viewing the fields of both architecture and medicine, there are large gaps that exist based on the nature of these two fields being focused on different goals. After all, many people would not see a connection between them, and in many ways, the thought process of these fields not having a common thread does have merit.

After all, many people are not focused on evaluating their built environments and the impacts their building has on their health – physically, emotionally, and mentally or psychologically.

Unless, of course, you are focused on the topics of health and wellness, and in this case, the fact that people spend up to 90 percent of their time inside of buildings might bring up questions about the overlap of architecture and medicine relative to the topic of health.[11]

The built environment as architecture is intended to literally protect occupants for better health. Along with the focus of medicine on health and healing, there is theoretically a tremendous amount of overlap between these two fields. For many, this is either a new thought or something that, when read, seems inherently obvious, yet perhaps hasn't been placed into proper terminology.

With populations spending larger amounts of time inside of buildings, the real question should be "how could these built environments *not* impact human health?"

And once you begin to explore these questions, you will often find that the answer is yes, of course, the built environment impacts human health in many facets.

These facets include the physical impacts on the body, yet also the emotional and mental or psychological impacts on human wellness. And the next question might be, "why aren't these two fields already connected in more cohesive formats?"

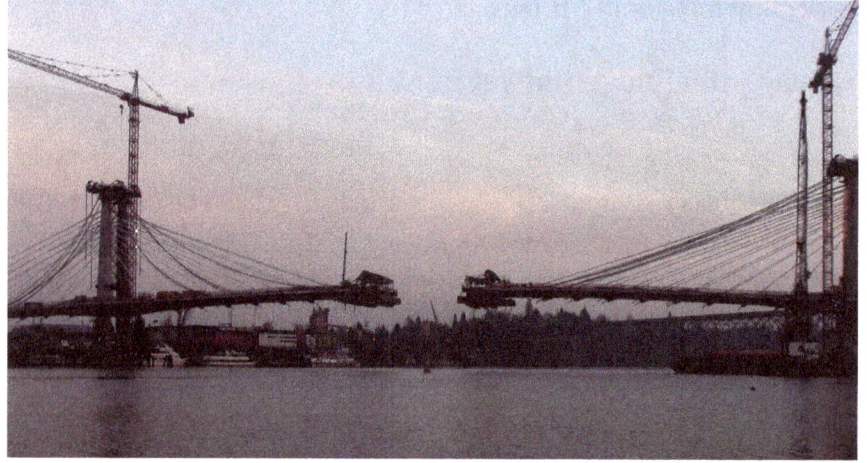

Portland, Oregon – 2014. Photo by author

Currently, in both architecture and medicine, there are very few overlaps between these two fields. This creates a large gap of potential for providing healthier built environments, and as such, is the focus of Architectural Medicine.

Right now, these overlaps between these two fields typically only exists in matters of hospital design. While the origin of hospitals began several centuries ago, the first steps of a central location and place for people to go for medical care go back several millennia.

If you view the ancient texts of the Greeks, as well as ancient India and China, there are references to places of health rooted in their cultures from over 5,000 years ago. This includes the Asklepieion on Kos, the location in which Hippocrates, who is known as the father of medicine, is said to have been born and trained.[12][13]

Hippocrates' book "On Airs, Waters and Places," includes the impacts of places on human health. In this book, the "first systematic attempt was made to set forth a causal relationship between human diseases and the environment."[14]

While Hippocrates is known for including the benefits of healing in certain structures, such as the Asklepieion, there were also those in the fields of architecture who referenced health and healing in the built environment. The architect, Vitruvius, is known for his De architectura (The Ten Books On Architecture), which deals with a range of topics related to architecture and the building process. He also commented on health and medicine, as can be witnessed in the following quote:

> "The architect should also have a knowledge of the study of medicine on account of the questions of climates, air, the healthiness and unhealthiness of sites…for without these considerations the healthiness of a dwelling cannot be assured."[15]

The topics of health, healing, and places have an overlap and can be seen as inclusive from centuries past.

From these ancient times, you can fast forward to the mid-19th century, a mere 150 years ago, and you will find the wisdom of Florence Nightingale. Her concerns about health include her studies of hospital design, much of which began the current day knowledge of epidemiology and public health.[16] [17]

Then from the late 1800s, you can fast forward to the 1950s, and you will find the writings and concerns of Rachel Carson, whose book *Silent Spring* brought to life the concerns of life itself on this planet.[18] Carson's concerns may be most well known for focusing on biology, yet her specific warnings about the impacts of synthetic chemicals on biological systems and organisms include, of course, human health. Too often, humans do not seem to remember that we are part of the biological systems of the planet, and too often forget these connections to biology and health implications from human created developments. As larger populations are spending greater percentages of time inside of buildings and exposed to more synthetic chemicals and materials, there is certainly a correlation. This includes the many potential natural substances that negatively impact human health, as well as synthetic materials and chemicals.

In the past few centuries, another important development is the professional becoming more specialized. This has occurred as each professional's knowledge has advanced, leading to more focus on a single subject or topic to gain deeper insights. This iterative cycle has led to specialists that often have less whole picture viewpoints, and has led to more professional silos.

This brings us to the current day, where a "whole view" of all subjects has become more segmented and less interconnected. Therefore, the view of architecture and medicine being considered in the same sentence relative to each other is a foreign concept for much of the population.

And as I have been writing and editing this book in the second and third decades of the 21st century, the pandemic of the novel coronavirus[19] has brought health in the built environment into focus like never before in recorded history.

At this very time in history in which this book is being published, it's actually a good example of how disconnected these fields of architecture and medicine really are. The coronavirus pandemic has certainly brought concerns about building safety, relative to health, under the microscope. Yet as this should be the case in using a microscope to evaluate these health issues, the fact that the coronavirus and building health has not properly proceeded forward with solutions in tandem with the medical fields, proves the point that there is room for improvement. This demonstrates the gaps that exist between these two fields of architecture and medicine.

The novel coronavirus, while first being reported as spreading through the physical contact on surfaces, has been known months after the world shut down in quarantine that the spread of this disease is mostly as a bioaerosol. An article posted on the Eos website, the science news magazine published by the American Geophysical Union (AGU), titled "Aerosol Scientists Try to Clear the Air About COVID-19 Transmission"[20] was a call to action for the Centers for Disease Control and Prevention (CDC) and the World Health Organization (WHO).

In a letter authored by many esteemed scientists to the White House on February 15, 2021, the first paragraph lists the following concerns:

> "We write as physicians and scientists with expertise in aerosol science, occupational health and infectious disease to commend the Biden Administration's National Strategy for the COVID-19 Response and Pandemic Preparedness and to urge strong immediate action to strengthen measures to limit inhalation exposure to SARSCOV-2 as a cornerstone of this plan."[21]

In another journal article titled "It Is Time to Address Airborne Transmission of Coronavirus Disease 2019 (COVID-19)", a group of 239 scientists worldwide states, "we appeal to the medical community and to the relevant national and international bodies to recognize the potential for airborne spread of coronavirus disease 2019 (COVID-19). There is significant potential for inhalation exposure to viruses in microscopic respiratory droplets (microdroplets) at short to medium distances (up to several meters, or room scale), and we are advocating for the use of preventive measures to mitigate this route of airborne transmission."[22]

The takeaway of this letter and the following processes over the past several years with the pandemic, has highlighted the disconnection between the fields of architecture and medicine. The ability to provide solid, fundamental steps in the built environment to resolve indoor air quality issues for better health has been apparent.

While it may be true that scientists can provide updated information for public policy to utilize for better health in buildings related to this airborne virus, another important facet of this equation is that many architects and building managers don't know how to address these issues and provide solutions.

And the lack of ability for this to be promoted and advertised to create steps that can resolve these indoor air quality issues, is a testament to the fact that many in the health and architecture fields do not know how to work together.

Or perhaps better yet, they are not familiar with working together. It is also a recognition of this "bridge not yet built" in that many in these two professions have never previously worked together in unison.

Yet working together to provide solutions is exactly what is needed right now and into the future. This lack of connectivity means less understanding of how to resolve these issues, and even less confidence from the general public that the spaces and places of the built environment are indeed safe.

The big question with all of this is, "what can be done?"

For this, there actually is a simple answer. However, the simple answer is rooted in complex systems. And these systems, up until now, have never existed before. These new systems would essentially connect the fields of architecture and medicine, and in doing so, will help to bridge the gaps that currently divide these two fields.

This new system is defined as the Architectural Medicine System (AMS).

This system provides bridges between these two fields, connecting the gaps between architecture and medicine. The way in which this is done is by first recognizing that each of these fields already have complex systems required for them to function properly.

The field of medicine has many facets in both education and training, where systems are provided for the doctor and health professionals to do their work. As well, the field of architecture also has many facets of education and training, with systems in place for the architect and the architecture, engineering, and construction (AEC) fields to achieve their work.

In my experience, the topics of health in the built environment have not been popular due to a lack of systems. And this includes an absence of systems both within each profession, as well as a lack of systems connecting these two professions with a focus on health in buildings.

In order for both of these complex professions to achieve their work, there need to be systems of education and training, as well as systems that are inherent in their daily work processes.

For example, the modern day doctor utilizes a system called the Subjective, Objective, Assessment, and Plan (SOAP) note,[23] [24] which provides the doctor with a procedure that can give them insights into the evaluation of their patient's health and a documentation process of providing next steps. Some of these steps may include blood tests, an MRI, or an X-ray, as examples, depending on the evaluation. Yet when it comes to their evaluation procedures, there are currently limited or no systems in place that include the patient's built environment in this health equation.

As well, the architect is not trained on human health issues and therefore has limited scope and knowledge on how materials and methods, as well as how design elements, may negatively impact human health. Except for the more common topics of lead paints, asbestos, and issues related to air particulates and mold, most architects are unsure as to the impacts on health in buildings. As such, they are not poised to provide preventive measures or resolutions when there are issues in built environments impacting occupant health.

The Architectural Medicine System (AMS) discusses this very topic in detail and provides an overview of how this process can function. It provides an overview of each professional functioning with this new system, as well as how different professions can work together in unison.

What Is Architectural Medicine?

And this brings us to focus on the question or definition of Architectural Medicine.

The intent of Architectural Medicine is to help integrate these fields of Architecture and Medicine for the benefit of the general public's health and wellness.

Architectural Medicine is defined as the bridge between architecture and medicine to create health and wellness in the built environment.

The way in which this is achieved is by focusing on the processes required for these two fields to function together in a cohesive manner. And this is achieved by creating procedures as systems to provide evaluations of the built environment, record these measurements as metrics, and enable this data to be analyzed and utilized by medical professionals. The use of this information can then provide direct data for their patient's health, as well as collective knowledge for public health in buildings. This information is also made available to the architecture and building professionals to ensure that solutions can be created for issues found in buildings related to occupant health, and to develop better design approaches to prevent negative health issues from occurring.

A main goal is to help define these various integrations and to participate in creating bridges between these fields in how they might all fit together.

As written above, the impact that the built environment has on human health and wellness is the main focus. And the systems and procedures include both the architecture and medicine fields, both independently and interdependently, providing interconnections between these fields. This is achieved using the *Architectural Medicine System (AMS)*.

Throughout the rest of this book, these topics will define what these systems are and how they will all function together.

The term Architectural Medicine came to be after many decades of my pondering, evaluating, and processing the large amounts of information that each of these professions must address in a very wide range. As I considered all these facets, I began to see a pattern that emerged, showing a core essence that related to health in the built environment. This research resulted in the idea that at the core, and at its heart, were these two topics of "architecture" and "medicine."

Before going further into these integrations, it is important to discuss these two words, architecture and medicine, and how they will be defined and described in this book. It may be evident as to what these terms mean, yet by reviewing them, it may reveal insights that are not often considered. It can also ensure that these terms are clear in definition, which can help in removing obfuscation as I discuss these topics in depth.

The External World is Experienced Internally

When we view the worlds of architecture and medicine, there are two core principles that this focus is based upon. And these core principles are based on the world of architecture and the built environment experienced as the "external world," and the world of medicine and health experienced "internally."

When pondering this concept, while they may at first seem very simple, they can lead to extremely complex subjects. You can easily get existential about these topics, and while that has its place, an important part of this book is to focus on the practical facets of the integrations of these fields. The health impact of buildings has an often unknown, yet large impact on occupants.

If you take time to ponder the idea of architecture as the exterior world and medicine as the interior world, you might find something interesting in terms of the questions of where one begins and the other ends.

For example, in terms of sight, you will quickly notice that what you "see" in the world outside of you is technically "seen" through the processing of this light within your brain. When the light of the exterior world enters your eyes, it is transferred into digital signals, and this electric signal entering your brain is processed and experienced internally. So technically speaking, you "see" and experience the external world internally.

In addition to sight, sound has a similar process. The sound waves from the exterior world encounter your eardrum and inner ear, which in turn converts the analog sound waves into a digital signal. This signal is then processed by your brain and is "heard" internally. Again, the sound in the external world is experienced inside your brain and body.

Your sense of smell, taste, and even touch is also processed in a similar manner, and it can be said that the external world that you see, hear, smell, taste, and touch is actually experienced internally – inside of your body. So, what does this have to do with architecture, and what's more, what does that have to do with health?

In essence, the external world and the built environment are experienced internally, and this internal experience impacts your health in a myriad of ways.

Having a better understanding of how the built environment impacts our internal processes is critical to understanding health, as humans are spending more time indoors. And if these external environments are impacting our internal processes and health, then it would behoove us to ensure that our surroundings are supporting our health and having a positive influence on our well-being.

Architectural Medicine focuses on these impacts and works to create systems to enable solutions to achieve better health.

We dive into how this is achieved throughout the book as we discuss the many facets of these wide ranging topics. I'll discuss how the built environment can impact health and wellness and address solutions to help evaluate buildings for health. And we'll review this potential for new systems in connecting the fields of architecture and medicine to achieve optimal health and wellness in buildings.

This overlap between architecture and medicine can be visually defined in our logo, which consists of the circle of architecture on the left, and the circle of medicine on the right. The overlap of the two circles, as a Venn diagram in the middle, symbolizes the integration between these two fields. As well, the overlap creates a purple segment, and it is this reason why the Architectural Doctor is denoted as purple.

The visual representation of these integrations symbolizes the multi-disciplinary developments of Architectural Medicine and the Architectural Doctor.

Why Do We Need a Focus on Health in Buildings?

This book is focused on the benefits of architecture in supporting health and wellness for optimal living and quality of life. One of the most important parts of this book is to recognize that in today's world – at least the human created world in which we live – our developed world is not always focused on health.

And as we become more data centric and evidence-based in our professions, the problem is not that we can't evaluate the data for best decisions moving forward, yet more so that we don't have enough data.

If you look at the large impacts that the built environment has on human and ecological health, it doesn't take much time to see that there is a lot of missing data that could be reviewed by many professionals showing the impacts built environments have on health.

However, in the built environment, there is a lot of missing data, especially outside of the industrial and commercial settings. And even in those settings, the connection between work environments and occupant health is limited at best.

There are many processes underway that are working to collect facets of this data, yet there is often a lack of understanding in terms of how this data impacts the whole of human health. And that's often because the collected data in the environment is not always correlated directly with human and ecological health.

Yet if we truly are focused on understanding how environments impact health and are serious about learning more about these correlations between environment and health, there needs to be better data and evaluations provided in a cross-functional and multi-disciplinary format. Without these processes in place, a true big picture understanding of these topics is going to be very challenging to discover.

As such, a good portion of this book is focused on how this data can be captured, and the systems that need to be included to provide these evaluations. It is also critical to recognize the importance of different professions working with each other to understand the connections between environment and health.

This collaboration will be required for this big data to be reviewed and established for bioinformatics purposes. In doing so, it can reveal insights into better procedures and education for each profession to implement in their future developments.

"Building" the Bridge to Wellness

The fields of Architecture and Medicine have changed quite a bit in the past century, and with many beneficial developments in each of these extensive fields, gaps relative to health in the built environment exist that can benefit humanity at large. This includes the increasingly important issues of building energy use, and the impacts buildings have on the ecology with a focus on a more sustainable future.

As climate change is on many people's minds, the fact that buildings consume and utilize a substantial percentage of energy and have a large impact on the environment is becoming more of a focal point. A question then becomes, "what can be done about it?"

While there are great developments occurring in both professions, from evidence-based design, green building, environmental psychology, and building science in architecture to integrative medicine and environmental health in medicine, these increasingly complex topics have many facets within each field that increase complexity.

The intent of Architectural Medicine is to help integrate these various fields and create systems to support better building health processes. A key to Architectural Medicine, as opposed to other fields such as Healthy Building, is that it considers all facets of human health – physically, mentally, and emotionally.

A main goal is to help define these integrations between these various fields and create bridges between them to all work together. This is discussed in more detail in later chapters.

In this way, the average person, as the general public can feel empowered to make best decisions in their built environments for the health of themselves, their families, and future generations.

Yet, it's also important to recognize that the professionals in these fields also deserve to have an integrated approach properly defined for them to address client and patient issues, and utilize best practices towards health, healing, and wellness. This book reviews these procedures for each profes-

New Integrated Building Model for Health and Wellness

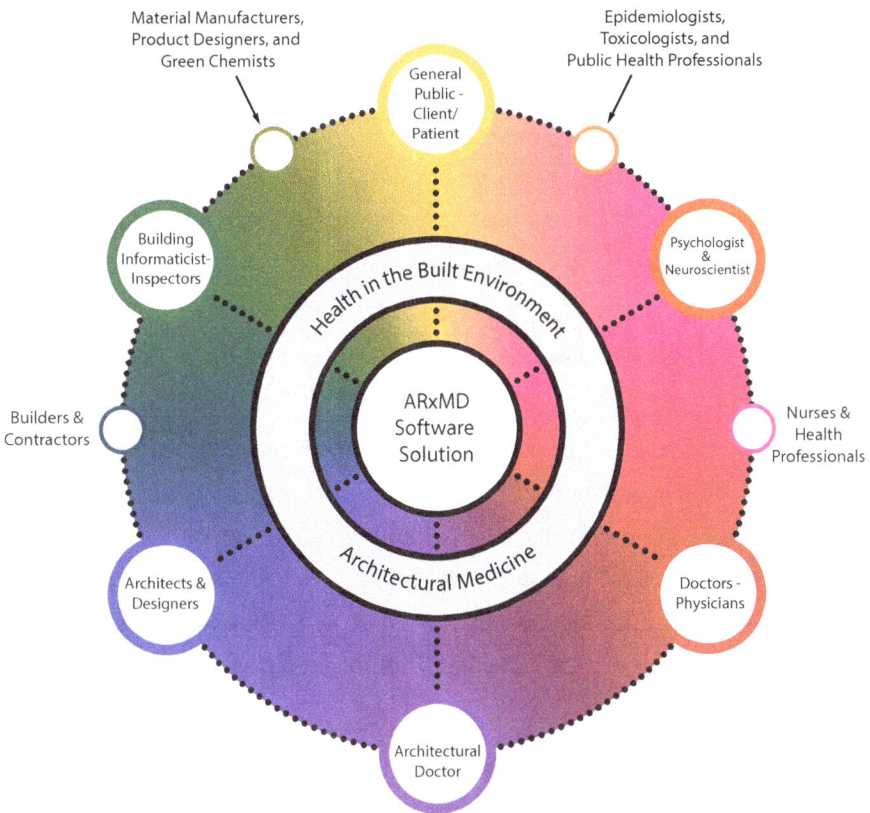

The Architectural Medicine System, the Architectural Doctor, and ARxMD

sional and provides an Rx as a blueprint to achieve these goals.

The diagram above is the result of multiple professionals working together with the new Architectural Doctor, Healthy Building Inspector, and Building Informaticist to support the Architectural Medicine System using the ARxMD software. Right now, the above diagram may not be clear as to its purpose, yet as I discuss each facet of this puzzle, by the end of the book, it will all come together with more clarity.

In chapter 5, I will discuss the Architectural Medicine System, and in chapter 6, I will provide the details of ARxMD, the Architectural Medicine

Software Solution. Then in chapter 7, the Healthy Building Inspector and Building Informaticist will be outlined. And in chapter 11, I will review the role of the Architectural Doctor.

Can Architecture Be Healing?

The impact the built environment has on human health and well-being is becoming a topic of increasing study, interest, and recognition.

And this topic has become even more prevalent in the time of the novel coronavirus and COVID-19.[25] In this year 2022, the world has become more aware of the importance of health in the built environment than since the 1918 influenza *pandemic.*[26]

As the coronavirus has become more known as an airborne virus that can spread throughout building spaces,[27] it has increased awareness of the impact buildings have on health. While this recognition of the physiological impacts has become evident, the fact that populations have had to stay at home to quarantine has also increased awareness of the emotional and mental or psychological impacts that buildings have on health.

Both the medical fields and the architecture and building fields continue to learn of this influence on human health, with recent research combined with the knowledge of this pandemic. As the integration between architecture and medicine continues to develop, there becomes an increasing need for these often independent fields to connect the "dots" of their research to the bigger picture of public health. The collaboration of this research can benefit both the professions involved in the built environment, and the general public who are influenced and affected by these buildings.

Architectural Medicine works to connect these dots to provide updates on the latest information related to these fields and to help create solutions that build bridges for a healthier, greener, and a more sustainable built environment.

In the book Architectural Medicine, I've chosen to discuss this topic with the simple question:

"Can Architecture Be Healing?"

This book is based on Architectural Medicine as a foundation of what is required to achieve a healthy built environment and how these two fields can work together to accomplish this goal. This is no small task, yet at the same time, many facets can be connected to help support this development, which eventually can create built environments that are healthier places in which to live.

Architectural Medicine can be both a foundation on which to build upon, and an umbrella term to include the many different fields and sub-fields that span both professions. There are a considerable number of fields that are involved, and these will be included to show the potential for an interconnectedness in achieving a "whole" picture viewpoint.

Blueprints for Health and Wellness

The concept of a blueprint for many is synonymous with architecture. However, in this realm of design and building, a blueprint is not a formula, and the design process is not an equation. The subtitle of this book, "An Rx for Health and Wellness," infers a potential recipe as a solution and blueprint to connect architecture and medicine that this book examines, while conjuring the image of an actual Rx as a blueprint to achieve these goals.

Throughout this book, the concept of a blueprint relates to several different topics, including the actual building schematic that a blueprint often denotes. However, a blueprint in this book also relates to systems and, as such, highlights the importance of systems in the worlds of architecture and medicine in terms of processes and principles. There may be many facets of the design process that utilize design principles, but these are not always analogous to formulas.

Why am I stating this?

Simple. The blueprint for the future of architecture cannot be formulaic, and while this book will discuss many principles that lead to heathier, greener, and more sustainable built environments, it is critical to understand that one blueprint will not fit all design solutions.

This is incredibly important to comprehend for both those who are designers and those who are seeking designs for themselves. The design process is complex, and this book does not strive to simplify this process, but instead adds more facets to an already complex process. In fact, this book adds many other facets into the design equation that are crucial to include for better health and wellness in buildings moving forward. And due to these solutions being non-formulaic, it will require a knowledge of processes that can be embedded into the whole design to create cohesive solutions. Otherwise, a solution to one approach may create problems in other areas, including the main topics of green, sustainable, and healthy building solutions.

Therefore, understanding the "why" of design implementations that focus on better health to include during the design process in a unified manner, and not just an add-on to the design process, is critical for better, healthier built environments.

Throughout my experiences in the healthy building and architecture fields, a key component of my learning was to recognize that a lack of system processes often caused more harm than good when clients were striving for healthier buildings.

The disparate understanding of interrelated building processes, materials, and methods left the individual building professionals in the dark and confused as to a specific building methodology, and as such, often leaves the professionals unsure of solutions. This can lead to a lack of support from the building professions, and too often, this is passed on to the clients. The result is uncertainty for the client and a lack of full support by the professionals involved. A combination of education for these professionals, along with the building owners and clients, is critical for there to be a supportive professional process. This education results in more developments embracing changes for a positive future for building solutions.

However, if these principles, based on a foundation of health, are included from start to finish, the return on investment in terms of *whealth* cannot be understated. Yes, *whealth*, as in wellness and health as equivalent to wealth. The new currency of the world needs to include wellness as a currency of the future.

What the Pandemic Has Taught Us About Public Health and Building Health

While this book and Architectural Medicine have been a work in progress for many years, after the year 2020 and the worldwide coronavirus pandemic, people have become more aware of three facets of the built environment.

The first is that the virus is an airborne issue, and the indoor air quality, including the functions of the heating, cooling, and ventilation systems (air handlers) in buildings, needs to be seriously re-evaluated moving forward. These new processes need to include the medical and health professionals as active participants in building solutions, and not just the building fields making such decisions.

The second is the amount of time spent indoors has been increasing, with the percentage of time currently up to 60 to 90 percent of time spent inside for the average urban occupant.[28][29] And with the pandemic, many are spending 100 percent of their time indoors across all building types and locations.

This large percentage of time living inside has become so familiar that the impact that building spaces have on our health — physically, emotionally, and mentally or psychologically — has become a topic of increasing awareness for most.

In the past, the topic of health in buildings was not something that many people thought about, yet the novel coronavirus pandemic has changed this. As discussed in a previous section, a huge percentage of people, if not all people, have a better awareness of a building's impact on health and wellness.

And the third topic is that while many have become more aware of these topics of health in buildings, there are still many, from medical and healthcare professionals to public health and epidemiologists, who may not know

The Impact of Stress on Human Health

60% to 80% of primary care doctor visits are related to stress
– JAMA Intern Med. 2013;173(1):76-77

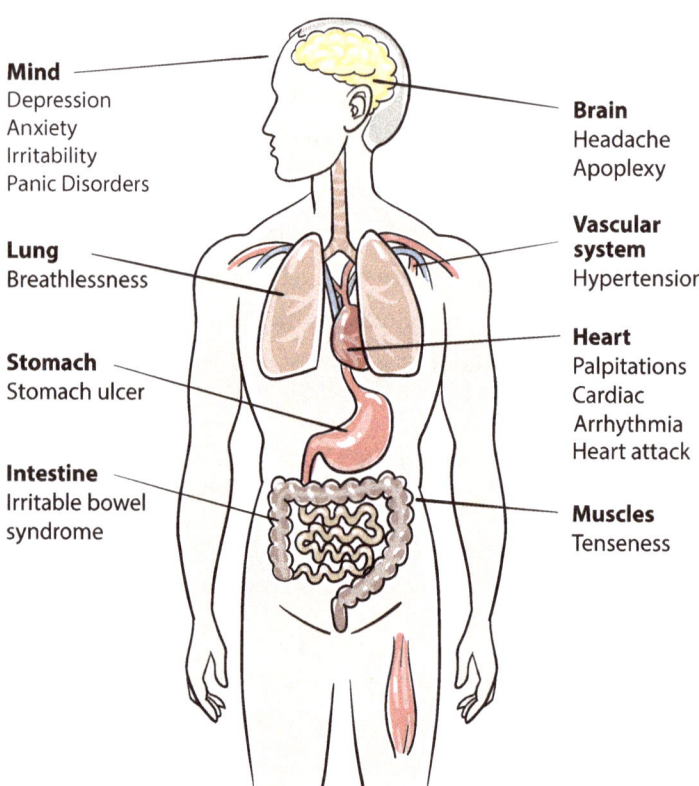

what to do about creating healthy or healthier built environments.

There may be an increase in awareness, which is a critical first step, yet the next steps will require a better understanding of what can be done and how to work with other professionals to achieve these goals.

There are also other topics discussed in this book that add to these issues. They include topics of indoor air quality highlighted by the coronavirus based on airborne viruses and bacteria, along with the fact that many buildings include particulates and building materials that are unhealthy. This is occurring because newer synthetic building materials and more airtight buildings, over the past 40 to 50 years, have increased the potential for toxins to circulate in buildings.

Some of these issues are going to be challenging to navigate, but this is even more reason to have someone to help in navigating these issues — which is the *Architectural Doctor*.

Building Issues and Health Topics

There are many issues in buildings that can cause health problems, from carbon dioxide, carbon monoxide, and other harmful gases to bacteria, particulates, and viruses. This also includes emotional and mental stressors that can increase stress. According to the American Psychological Association[30], chronic stress is the number one source of all deaths. And if you've never thought about the impacts of your built environment on human stress, then you may be surprised to learn of the negative physiological, mental, and emotional impacts that buildings can have on humans.

Below is a small list of topics that can be included as building health issues, with a graphic showing these impacts on the human body.

The Endocrine System and the Impacts of the Built Environment on Health

For many, the question of how the built environment impacts health, to the extent that more complex systems and processes need to be added, may be in question. The modern world has many new obstacles to navigate in both the medical and architecture fields, and this includes new synthetic materials and the negative impacts these can have on the human body.

One such topic of buildings having a negative impact on health is based on the endocrine system. This is the complex system of hormones in your body, and it can also be complicated to analyze as the impacts on the body can occur over longer periods of time.

Many are now familiar with BPa or Bisphenol A as a chemical that causes endocrine system problems, yet how many people are aware that this material exists in many building materials?

As defined by the CDC, "Bisphenol A (BPA) is used to manufacture polycarbonate plastics…this type of plastic is used to make some types of beverage containers, compact disks, plastic dinnerware, impact-resistant safety equipment, automobile parts, and toys."[31]

As stated in a report by the Healthy Building Network, "few, however, are as aware that BPA is a chemical component of epoxy resins used in a wide range of building materials, including high performance coatings (paints, floorsealers, and other protective coatings), adhesives and fillers (caulk, grout, mortar, and putty), fiberglass binders, and cement additives."[32]

Just as lead paint took many years to be included in modern medical analysis, and also took years to remove from use in the building fields along with products such as leaded gasoline, newer chemicals, and their negative impacts may also take some time to acknowledge and remove or alter.

However, many of these chemicals impacting the endocrine system would need to be evaluated by health professionals and data scientists. For example, lead paint is now included in building inspections, and there is a need for other materials and contaminants to be included in building inspections. In chapter 7, I discuss the Healthy Building Inspector and the Building Informaticist as two professionals that can focus on these inspections and data analysis.

And then, there is the advent of removing these components from the building materials and to include education and toolkits for architects and designers to have the knowledge to ensure that lead paint, and other contaminants, will not be specified in building projects. With lead paint, all of this took time to evaluate and then provide education for the building professionals. Time was also needed to provide systems to ensure that each group was working in a collective format.

All these groups, including the medical, architecture, and inspection organizations, would be utilizing the same code base in how this should be addressed and what steps should be taken to evaluate materials that impact health.

In using this material lead as an example of a building material that both the medical and architectural professions recognize as a health issue and include the building inspector in their evaluations, it shows that there are some topics in buildings that do include all of these professions. This can include the occupational professionals to ensure that commercial and industrial building locations are reviewed as well.

This is a good example of one topic that is related to both the medical and architecture fields, and as such, can show an example of interconnections to support better health in the built environment.

On a more positive note, as these topics can become "heavy" in dealing with such negatives, the advent of the Green Chemistry field can provide solutions to some of these issues. Yet this can only occur if materials are seen as problems, and the demand from the public, as well as the professionals, merits new solutions. I will provide more feedback on the positives and benefits of flagging these issues to find solutions later in the book, particularly in chapters 6, 7, 13, and 15.

The Topic of Architecture – What Is Architecture?

As mentioned in a previous paragraph, before we go into more detail about the Architectural Doctor and Architectural Medicine, there needs to be a foundation to build upon in defining this word architecture. As I've defined Architectural Medicine, it is important to define architecture and medicine itself. Instead of assuming there is clarity about these topics, it makes sense to discuss these definitions to ensure a baseline of these terms.

The topic of architecture is sometimes very matter of fact, and other times can be very abstract. Some may define architecture as any building, and others may see architecture as much more — differentiating itself from the simple shed in a backyard to that of the great ancient pyramids or modern-day skyscrapers.

So, what exactly is Architecture?

The Oxford English Dictionary (OED) defines Architecture as the "art or science of building or constructing edifices of any kind for human use."[33] And the OED defines edifice as "a building, usually a large and stately building, as a church, palace, temple, or fortress; a fabric, structure."[34]

While this certainly describes the basics of architecture, a bigger scope expands on this definition from the simple building into architecture. While there are different definitions of architecture, at the core of this topic is shelter, combined with creating a safe and enjoyable space and place to live and work. For centuries, architecture served as basic structures for homes that shielded humans from the elements, whether this meant hot, cold, wet, or dry conditions. In today's 21st century, it can be easy to forget that it's only been in the past century that humans have become adept at building and sheltering in the way known today in achieving these goals.

The Exterior World of Our Lives – The Built Environment

The modern building has the ability to shelter humans from the natural elements, which has previously not been possible. It can provide temperature control, electricity, lighting, and plumbing resources that allow for the comfort and tempered indoor environments that many come to expect in buildings. Before the mid-20th century, it was still common in many developed areas of the world to battle nature's elements, and was a challenging feat for even the best architects. In some parts of the world, we may find it commonplace to find these amenities as a given, while other parts of the world still do not have these modern capabilities.

The etymology of the words "Architecture" and "Architect" can give some insights into these words and help define its purpose:

architecture (n.)

1560s, "the art of building, tasteful application of scientific and traditional rules of good construction to the materials at hand," from Middle French architecture, from Latin architectura, from architectus "master builder, chief workman" (see architect). Meaning "buildings constructed architecturally" is from 1610s.[35]

architect (n.)

"person skilled in the art of building, one who plans and designs buildings and supervises their construction," 1560s, from Middle French architecte, from Latin architectus, from Greek arkhitekton "master builder, director of works," from arkhi- "chief" (see archon) + tekton "builder, carpenter," from PIE root *teks- "to weave," also "to fabricate."[36]

Therefore, architecture can be defined as "structures that are technically and artfully created to support human life and to provide shelter." However, architecture is not just for surviving. At the highest level, its purpose can be focused on human thriving. It can strive to support health and wellness in an optimal format. And this is not just for physical comfort but also for emotional and mental or psychological wellness.

Buildings may exist for basic shelter, yet architecture can support human thriving.

What's important to outline, relative to the topics of Architectural Medicine, is to recognize that architecture is the external world within which we live, work, and spend much of our time within – particularly in the suburban and urban environments. It may sound basic to state, but as we delve into the definitions of *Medicine* in the next segment focusing on our internal world, it becomes relevant to keep this in mind. This is also important to note when we discuss Social Determinants of Health (SDoH), as this definition includes these very terms to define the built environment.

The Topic of Medicine-What Is Medicine?

This brings us to the term *Medicine*. So, what exactly is Medicine? The Oxford English Dictionary (OED) defines Medicine as the "science or practice of the diagnosis, treatment, and prevention of disease."[37]

It can also be defined as a" substance or preparation used in the treatment of illness; a drug; esp. one taken by mouth. Also: such substances generally. To treat or cure (a person, condition, etc.) by means of medicine; to give medicine to."[38]

As the definition of architecture has levels of definitions, the term medicine also has varying definitions and meanings. If we investigate the etymology of the word Medicine, there are a few key features that define the term that is relevant to how the word is used in this book:

medicine (n.)

c. 1200, "medical treatment, cure, remedy," also used figuratively, of spiritual remedies, from Old French *medicine* (Modern French *médicine*) "medicine, art of healing, cure, treatment, potion," from Latin medicina "the healing art, medicine; a remedy," also used figuratively, perhaps originally ars medicina "the medical art," from fem. Of medicinus (adj.) "of a doctor," from medicus "a physician" (from PIE root *med- "take appropriate measures"); though OED finds evidence for this is wanting. Meaning "a medicinal potion or plaster" in English is mid-14c.[39]

healing (n.)

"restoration to health," Old English hæling, verbal noun from heal (v.). Figurative sense of "restoration of wholeness" is from early 13c.; meaning "touch that cures" is from 1670s.[40]

heal (v.)

Old English hælan "cure; save; make whole, sound and well," from Proto-Germanic *hailjan (source also of Old Saxon helian, Old Norse heila, Old Frisian hela, Dutch helen, German heilen, Gothic ga-hailjan "to heal, cure"), literally "to make whole," from PIE *kailo- "whole" (see health). Intransitive sense from late 14c. Related: Healed; healing.[41]

health (n.)

Old English hælþ "wholeness, a being whole, sound or well," from Proto-Germanic *hailitho, from PIE *kailo- "whole, uninjured, of good omen" (source also of Old English hal "hale, whole;" Old Norse heill "healthy;" Old English halig, Old Norse helge "holy, sacred;" Old English hælan "to heal"). With Proto-Germanic abstract noun suffix *-itho (see -th (2)). Of physical health in Middle English, but also "prosperity, happiness, welfare; preservation, safety.[42]

Medicine and Healing

As the above word origins show, the concept and essence of medicine has been based upon "medical treatment, cure, remedy – medicine, art of healing, cure, treatment, potion," and "the healing art, medicine; a remedy."[43] The term medicine references "a remedy," a "treatment, potion," and an "art of healing." And from this, we see that the origins of healing and health are based upon:

healing (n.)

"restoration to health," Old English hæling, verbal noun from heal (v.). Figurative sense of "restoration of wholeness" – heal (v.) Old English hælan "cure; save; make whole, sound and well," health (n.) Old English hælþ "wholeness, a being whole, sound or well,"[44]

If you put the two terms of medicine and healing together, you will find that medicine is the process, treatment, and remedy to a "restoration to health" and a "restoration of wholeness, a being whole, sound or well."

If medicine is seen as your internal world, that which is based on "health," which is focused on a "restoration to health, restoration of wholeness," then the concept of "being whole, sound or well" can relate to the concept of wellness and well-being.

If good health is based on wholeness and being well, then there is another facet of this equation that should be included.

The Interior World of Our Lives

And this is the concept that you experience the exterior world internally. As mentioned earlier in the chapter, the world around you is experienced mostly internally by your senses. Therefore, the environment that is outside of you, including the built environment, is mostly experienced internally.

And if your exposure to the world is experienced internally, such as your vision, hearing, taste, smell, and touch, perhaps it is not as far-fetched to think that the exterior world has an impact and influence on your overall internal health and well-being.

The word medicine is defined as the interior world relative to a "restoration to health, restoration of wholeness, and of being whole, sound or well". Referring to the two terms of medicine and healing together, the term "Medicine" in "Architectural Medicine" is focused on the process, treatment, and remedy to a "restoration to health, restoration of wholeness, a being whole, sound or well."

Medicine's true focus is to help the patient to achieve this "wellness" and "well-being."

In this book, and the work of Architectural Medicine, the term "Architecture" is defined as the exterior built world. It includes "the art of building" and the "tasteful application of scientific and traditional rules of good construction" as a definition.

The Latin architectura, from architectus as "master builder, chief workman," is also a key to the concept of what a master builder is responsible for and how this definition has evolved over time into the modern world of materials and methods.

I will discuss these concepts on a deeper level and explore what the current and future architects will navigate in later chapters. That said, the future of architecture will have to include current day concerns of health in this ever-changing profession.

What these word origins also describe is a "return to wholeness," and so the next question may be, how are we as humans disconnected, causing us a lack of this wholeness? If being ill is a lack of being whole and requires a restoration of wholeness, then the question might be, how are we disconnected or separated? And how can we put these pieces back together to achieve wholeness?

While the discussion of wholeness and how the modern-day world has disconnected us from wholeness, is discussed in more detail in the book Architectural Medicine, the solutions are highlighted in this book in the role of the Architectural Doctor. This book will focus on systems to reconnect the disconnected facets of the built environment to better support health.

Yet before we go into more details to define this Architectural Doctor, let's first discuss who this book is for and what topics will be discussed throughout this book in the next chapter...

COVID 19 and Lessons Learned in the Built Environment

As I have written in other parts of this book, I am writing and editing this book during the novel coronavirus pandemic. This has impacted the world's health in ways that haven't been seen since the 1918 Flu Pandemic. At the time of this editing, the number of deaths has been estimated to be "at least 50 million worldwide with about 675,000 occurring in the United States."[45][46]

As I currently write this, it is 2021 into 2022, and with a vaccine being distributed to the populations, there are still breakouts and high amounts of those impacted by new variants. Since 2020, the pandemic has created isolation for populations, with "stay at home" initiatives designed to prevent the spread of the disease and to provide quarantine measures to help reduce the spread of the virus.

Like the 1918 pandemic, this is an airborne virus and often spread by direct contact between people, yet also spreading through the air handling systems in buildings.[47][48] The combination of the masses spending up to 100 percent of their time inside of the built environment, along with the recognition of how important clean air systems have become to the average person, has brought a level of building awareness unseen for many generations.

Before the pandemic, the topics of health in the built environment might have been known by a very small percentage of the population, and now the topic is known by almost all.

While the topic of indoor air quality has been a main focus, there has also become a great awareness of the impact of one's built spaces. After spending so much time in the same spaces, the average person has become acutely aware of how much their built environment impacts their health — their physical health as well as their mental and emotional well-being.

This, in my opinion, cannot be understated in the importance of the topics of health in buildings, which Architectural Medicine and the Architectural Doctor strive to support.

This increased awareness can provide a larger interest in not only the physical impacts of health from the built environment, yet also the emotional and mental or psychological impacts that buildings have on health. This is a factor in the growing interest from the public to demand solutions and create proper supply from the professionals in the architecture and medical fields. These demands can provide ample movement for professional solutions that Architectural Medicine and the Architectural Doctor are poised to provide.

And before we venture into the core solutions provided in this book, there may still be questions about these topics and who the intended audience really is.

To address this topic, I will discuss this in the next chapter...

"Unless someone like you cares a whole awful lot, nothing is going to get better. It's not."

— Dr. Seuss

WHO IS THIS BOOK FOR AND WHAT TOPICS WILL BE DISCUSSED?

If you've been following the trajectory of health in the built environment, or even human health in a big picture format for the last few decades, many of the topics in this book are not new. And that's because these topics have been discussed for several decades, and each year there are new subjects that are included as potential health issues for human and biological health on this planet.

If you aren't familiar with many of these topics, this is ok too, as many people are becoming aware of these issues and are eventually seeking solutions to these problems.

While the issues may not be unique or new, what is new in this book is the approach toward solutions.

For many decades, I've been following, observing, and participating in the solutions to creating healthier built environments, yet the changes have been very slow in process. The reason why, in my opinion, is that it's not enough to simply observe and be aware of the problems, there need to be solutions available. And many of these problems are extremely complex and therefore require systems that can support solutions.

These systems do not currently exist, yet in my own experiences over the years, I've recognized where these gaps exist. Throughout this book, I will provide a framework for these new systems, which are a large and important part of achievable solutions.

As I mentioned in my first book, *Architectural Medicine*, the topic of health in the built environment has become more common, yet also a recognition of the complexity of these topics to provide solutions has become apparent. It is part of the reason, in my opinion, as to why the topics of green and sustainable building have become more common, with the topic of healthy building lagging behind in development. This reason is based on a lack of systems, and due to health in the built environment spanning the fields of both architecture and medicine, this involves more professionals than is required for green and sustainable building solutions.

In the *Architectural Medicine* book, I examined these topics in a general format and discussed what the many facets are and how they can fit together to create healthier, greener, and more sustainable built environments.

In this book's introduction, I posed the question:

> "Are you wanting a better world in which to live, work, and play for both yourself and future generations? Are you aware of how the built environment impacts your health — physically,

> emotionally, mentally, or psychologically? Are you concerned about the future of your health and the health of your children, grandchildren, and the many other creatures and animals that live on this planet?"

I can't promise I know all the answers, yet I am certainly asking these questions with great concern, and this book came to be after many years of seeking solutions.

After years of being involved with these developments, focused on solutions to greener, more sustainable, and healthier built environments, I can recognize that these topics, while often simple in concept, are extremely complex. This book is a continuation of the first book, with the goal of providing detailed solutions to how this new system functions, and how each professional can collaborate, providing their part of a cohesive whole.

If you read the Architectural Medicine book and want to follow the trajectory of this topic into actionable solutions, then this book is for you.

This new system is defined as the *Architectural Medicine System (AMS)*.

While this book is a deeper dive into the topics of Architectural Medicine, reading the first book is not a requirement, and there will be several references to the topics and concepts of Architectural Medicine, which will provide proper context.

This book will provide a framework for the many topics related to health in the built environment, with the specific intention of providing an Rx as a blueprint, foundation, and system to achieve these goals.

The intention is to provide an overview and trajectory of solutions, from where it has been to where it may likely be going.

In this book, I will examine these topics in more detail and provide specifics on how the Architectural Medicine System (AMS) can be implemented practically and effectively. Based on this approach, this book will be more for the working professionals, yet it will still have context for those who would like to know more about their own health and wellness related to their built environments.

For those interested in these processes, it will provide a big picture view, with detailed steps that are required to fulfill whole system solutions.

It is my hope that these topics will be of interest to the general public, as well as the specific professionals. When enough of the public demands changes with updated systems, then those providing the supply as solutions can provide their work for best results.

A Book for Three Main Groups – The Medical Fields, the Architecture Fields, and the General Public

In the first book, I wrote that it was written for three main groups: the Medical fields, the Architecture fields, and the General Public. And while some seem to think, often rightly so, that having a wide range of topics and audiences is not a great format for book content, there are important reasons for this inclusion.

I've written this book in this manner for two important reasons. One, the solutions being discussed require several professions working together, and two, the main purpose of Architectural Medicine and the Architectural Doctor is to build the bridges between these two main professions. As such, the very nature of this book is inclusivity in order to achieve these goals of health in the built environment.

In my opinion, you cannot achieve these goals without these integrations, hence the nature of this book requiring several professions and not just one group. That said, there is one group that can have the greatest benefit from reading this book, and those are the future Architectural Doctors. This new breed of professional may have many backgrounds, yet the common foundation is the focus on both fields of health and architecture, where these integrations become the main focus.

A Focus on the Professions and the Processes

To achieve this goal of whole system solutions, there needs to be a list of each of the professions and professionals involved and what their roles will be.

Architects, Doctors, Inspectors, and the many professionals involved in the fields of building and health all have their unique roles, and this book will review each role according to this big picture view of the whole system. In chapters 7 to 11, the roles of each professional will be discussed in detail.

While much of the work done to create healthier built environments in the past has been successful for the individual structure, in order to provide more benefits for a larger scale of structures and communities, there need to be systems in place to achieve these goals.

The professions of architecture and medicine are known to have many subfields, and the importance of all these fields working together cannot be overlooked.

This includes all those in the architecture, engineering, and construction (AEC) fields, as well as the mechanical, electrical, and plumbing (MEP) fields, to encompass the entire spectrum of those in the field of architecture and construction.

It's also critical to recognize that there are many other professions and professionals that need to be included in these processes, from public health and epidemiology professionals to those who are building inspectors, material manufacturers, and newer fields such as green chemistry.

In chapter 15, I discuss the importance of working together, and I follow up in chapters 17 and 18 as to possibilities for the future.

Architectural Medicine and the Importance of Context

I will often refer to the *Architectural Medicine* book for context, and in this chapter, I will repeat what I stated in that book as well. While the *Architectural Medicine* book provides a detailed overview of these topics and why they are important, this book focuses on the specifics of how this is achieved.

However, they both include the same three groups of the architect and the doctor, as well as the general public.

This book will delve into more details and is written more for the professionals, yet the general public can glean from these conversations to provide them with insights into their own decision making for better health and wellness. In this manner, the general public, of course, includes the many professionals involved. And if the goal is for professionals to provide a better life for the public, then the recognition of these big picture topics can apply to all of humanity.

8 Steps to Better Health in the Built Environment

In the introduction, I prefaced the fact that throughout this book, there would be critical processes of evaluating the big picture view, and I would provide steps to take to achieve the goals of better health and wellness in buildings.

These steps include the overlap of the architecture and medicine fields in new formats with new systems. These systems include a multi-disciplinary process in order to achieve these goals of better building health.

While all these concepts may define the goals, there need to be actionable procedures, and not just a string of words. To help assist in these steps, the following chart will show each of these 8 steps defined in two segments.

The first segment, steps one through four, is an overview of the four steps that highlight how issues in the built environment can impact human health. The second set, five through eight, focuses on the processes and systems required to achieve and solve the problems.

In the next few chapters, I will delve into these processes with more detail, and provide context for how these steps can be applied by professionals that typically have not worked together.

Later in the book, in chapter 8, I will provide a follow up on these steps discussing how they can be applied in real world applications.

In the next chapter, I begin reviewing these topics to provide a foundation to build upon in defining the Architectural Doctor.

8 STEPS TO BETTER HEALTH IN THE BUILT ENVIRONMENT

1. The development of protocols for ailments potentially caused by built environment issues

2. The training of Doctors to utilize protocols during ailment analysis

3. The training of building inspectors and informaticists to evaluate topics related to health in buildings

4. Systems created to support this process, from the Doctor creating an Rx for a Building Inspection to the interconnected system of evaluation and reports sent back to the doctor for evaluation

5. The training of architects and builders to recognize health issues in the built environment

6. The development of protocols in the built environment that architects and builders are trained to evaluate and resolve

7. The training of doctors, architects, inspectors, and informaticists to work together to resolve health issues in the built environment

8. Software solutions created to support this process, from the Doctor creating an order for a Building Inspection and the inspection procedures to reporting for the doctors and subsequent prescription as building Rx for the architecture and building professionals to solve

Personal and Precision Medicine, Social Determinants of Health (SDoH), Geomedicine, and the Built Environment

As mentioned in the introduction, an important development in the field of medicine is the focus on precision medicine or personal medicine, as it's also known. At least in the USA and other parts of the world, this approach to medicine being more finely tuned for the specific patient, as opposed to general medical practices for the masses, has been in process for several years now.

As stated by the U.S. Department of Health and Human Services National Institutes of Health, "the Precision Medicine Initiative is a long-term research endeavor, involving the National Institutes of Health (NIH) and multiple other research centers, which aims to understand how a person's genetics, environment, and lifestyle can help determine the best approach to prevent or treat disease."[49]

The key here for the topics of this book are "environment and lifestyle," which includes the environment and the built environment.

If the built environment is to be included in this personalized medicine approach, then there must be systems in place for not only the inclusion of the fields of architecture, but for evaluations of these buildings to provide information to achieve these goals. If doctors and health professionals are going to provide succinct, precision medicine solutions for their patients, there is going to be a need for evaluations that include built environments — which currently does not exist.

As an example, geomedicine is a field focused on the location of exposures and how this information can be included in a patient's Electronic Health Record (EHR). How this process can proceed will include the addition of the Building Informaticist and the Healthy Building Inspector, which are discussed in chapter 7.

What You Should Know

These discussions about the built environment, personalized medicine, and environmental impacts such as social determinants of health are emerging developments. The new concepts of an Architectural Doctor, a Building Informaticist, and the Healthy Building Inspector is a new idea for many, yet in some capacity and in different cultures of the past, the goals of this professional overlapping between the architecture and medical fields are not entirely new.

For example, the house call of the doctor of the past included some visual evaluations of places where people lived, and as Florence Nightingale included in her nursing and hospital commentaries, the built environment had a significant impact on health. These evaluations in building quality could be included for the doctor and nurse's recommendations for patient health, such as improving air quality and providing more natural light.[50][51]

> "Badly constructed houses do for the healthy what badly constructed hospitals do for the sick. Once insure that the air in a house is stagnant, and sickness is certain to follow."[52]

However, over time, the house visits from the doctor and the hands on connections that the architect and builder had relative to health have morphed through the years into issues left for others to monitor. Yet the focus on health in buildings has fallen through the cracks, and once again, this needs to be addressed as an important facet in modern society.

As these topics are once again revisited, this book is a work in progress in these emerging developments evaluating building health. At this time, there is still limited interconnectivity between the professions of architecture and medicine, and as such, it will take time for these to become more integrated. It is the intention of this book to help develop these connections, and to provide awareness of these topics of health in buildings, along with professional, supportive systems to achieve these goals.

Through the years, I have benefited from being on both the inside of these fields and yet on the outside to view them from both close-up and afar. And this, in my opinion, has given me some insights that are uniquely my own.

My intention, since I began writing this book, was to continue the development of Architectural Medicine and to contribute my part for proper solutions. The Architectural Doctor can provide support to what seems to me either broken fragments or new systems that haven't yet been considered or implemented.

I also realize that I can't do it all alone. If my contributions can help in the process of healthier, greener, and more sustainable built environments that are nurturing and support better quality of life, then I know I have done my part. It will take a multi-disciplinary effort to supply these solutions and the general public's demands to achieve these goals.

Whether you are an architect, doctor, building inspector, or a professional that is involved in some way with healthcare and the built environment, this book will provide an outline of the many topics involved, as well as information about how these fields can become more connected for better health and wellness.

The Future of Architecture and the Global Citizen

In this third decade of the 21st century, there has been a lot of focus on health and, in particular, building health. This is based on the COVID-19 pandemic, which has impacted the health of all humans around the world. As I write this paragraph, it is December of 2021, and about two years ago is the time when the first epidemiologists and public health professionals started to recognize the novel coronavirus. Then several months later, in the spring of 2020, the virus became an epidemic, and then spread globally, creating the pandemic.

During this time, worldwide, the populations began to quarantine. This process required all of us to stay at home, or at least to stay at one location in how we defined "home" as the building that we live within.

As the virus finally became known as spreading in an airborne process, this staying at home with a focus on air quality, became an enormous recognition of the importance of indoor air quality and building health. Once we began to venture outside of our own built spaces and into other buildings, we began to question the air quality of these buildings relative to our health.

In my lifetime, I've never seen a global recognition of the importance of buildings and health, and this awareness has spurred an appreciation and connection to health in buildings like never before in our lifetimes. This worldwide awareness of the impacts on human health has not just been focused on physical health, but also of mental and emotional health as well. This is another key aspect of reading this book and includes a wide range of professions that may find benefits when reading the procedures I've outlined in this book. It is my hope that all citizens have an interest in these matters, and the demand for better quality indoor living will spur the supply for solutions required, such as the Architectural Medicine System.

An Awareness of Physical, Emotional, and Mental Health in the Built Environment

Being located in the same building for months at a time has impacted not just physical health, but emotional and mental or psychological health. The relevance to either the poor quality of built spaces or of the isolation of so many on a social aspect has increased the awareness of occupant health exponentially. Humans are animals, and social animals at that, and while many professionals are well aware of the importance of these social fabrics, the impacts that built spaces can have on our emotional and psychological health have become magnified. The benefits of better building health will eventually be for all of humanity.

While this book has been a work in progress for the past 25 plus years, many updates in the writing and editing of this book have occurred in the years between 2020 to 2022 during the time of the novel coronavirus pandemic. This worldwide health issue has not only highlighted the importance of a global community relative to health, but it has also highlighted the importance of the global citizen.

Moving forward, the global citizen can help guide humanity towards a better future by having an inclusive mindset and approach to life, which can help to provide both local and global solutions. Without such thinking, decisions made in silos may result in more problems that are created and as such, should not be understated.

As the planet navigates the pandemic, it has been compounded by issues on this planet, such as climate change and other environmental issues that we as a global community must navigate. Just as we all need to work together to address COVID-19 worldwide, many of the decisions in the future for health and wellness must also be made with this global mindset.

Another facet of this complex puzzle is the reality of humans preparing for travel into space and to other planets. The process of humans venturing into space has become a reality with NASA and projects such as Jeff Bezos' Blue Origin and Richard Branson's Virgin Galactic.

The global mindset of the global citizen can also be critical for humanity's exploration of other worlds. It is inappropriate and irresponsible to travel beyond our galaxy to exoplanets without the respect that should be given when traveling to other planets, visiting other life forms, and venturing to worlds that can eventually be explored.

This cannot be stressed enough, and if we cannot properly provide solutions for living on planet Earth, we don't deserve as a species to travel to other places and act irresponsibly in ways that may negatively impact other life forms and locations. Once we begin to see the negative detriments to our current planet and the many life forms that are being impacted, we can then begin to make decisions that are more responsible as stewards of the planet.

With this mindset and approach, the benefits that can be applied here to planet Earth can then allow our explorations beyond our planet, showing a respect that is deserving of meriting space travel.

Whether we are developing built environments on this planet in new locations, reconstructing current and previous locations, or traveling and exploring other planets, the focus on health is paramount. It is this focus on health and wellness that can provide a better quality of life as our growing population of humanity nears 8 billion. Interestingly, the United Nations projects that the world's population will reach 8 billion in November of 2022,[53] the month this book will be published.

Without a focus on these solutions, specifically relative to the "DNA of Cities" and the "DNA of Buildings," the populations will be negatively impacted on an even greater scale. This DNA topic was discussed in the introduction and is discussed in more detail in the *Architectural Medicine* book.

It is imperative for us as humanity to find solutions now that can support current and future generations.

And how we can achieve this begins in the next chapter with the introduction to *the Architectural Doctor*…

"When a flower doesn't bloom,
you fix the environment in which it grows,
not the flower."

– Alexander Den Heijer

INTRODUCING THE ARCHITECTURAL DOCTOR

What is an Architectural Doctor?

As discussed in chapter 1, a critical aspect in defining Architectural Medicine are the processes that are involved in achieving these goals of bridging the gaps between architecture and medicine for better health and wellness in the built environment.

In this manner, the *Architectural Doctor* is introduced into the lexicon of this book.

In order for these methods to be implemented, there is a need for a professional to both support these processes as a liaison between these two professions, and to provide support during the many facets to help weave together the multi-disciplinary topics for whole system solutions.

In many ways, this book is a continuation of the first book I wrote titled *Architectural Medicine*. In the writing of this first book, the focus is on both the big picture view as well as some of the more micro-level viewpoints of how architecture and the built environment impacts health – physically, mentally, and emotionally.

Architectural Medicine is the main foundation and umbrella of the Architectural Doctor, and as such was important to write first, with this book following in a more focused approach on the role of the Architectural Doctor. This includes the key processes involved in working with the architecture and medical fields.

As Architectural Medicine focuses on the integrations between professions and the theoretical processes and systems required to achieve these goals of healthier built environments, the Architectural Doctor focuses on the actual processes and implementation of these systems. It also includes the important work involved in supporting the professionals and the processes of those within the professions of both architecture and medicine.

It is also critical to recognize that the Architectural Doctor provides a bridge between the two main professionals, yet is also an important bridge and liaison between these professionals and the general public. It is critical to ensure that the many other professions involved in this new integrated, multi-disciplinary approach to the healthier built environment are included.

What Is an Architectural Doctor?

The concept of an Architectural Doctor may be confusing for many. What does Architecture have to do with a Doctor? And what does a Doctor have to do with Architecture?

To begin to respond to these questions, which are honestly good and understandable questions, we can take a few moments to discuss the topic and review excerpts from the book Architectural Medicine. As described in chapter 1, the intent of Architectural Medicine is to help integrate these fields of Architecture and Medicine, for the benefit of the general public's health and wellness.

> "Architectural Medicine is defined as the bridge between architecture and medicine to create health and wellness in the built environment."

The way in which this is achieved is by focusing on the processes required for these two fields to function together in a cohesive manner. This is achieved by creating procedures as systems to provide evaluations of the built environment, record these measurements as metrics, and enable this data to be analyzed and utilized by the medical professionals. The use of this information can then provide direct data for their patient's health, as well as collective knowledge for public health in buildings. This information is also made available to the architecture and building professionals to ensure that solutions can be created for issues found in buildings related to occupant health, and to develop better design approaches to prevent negative health issues from occurring.

A main goal is to help define these various integrations and to participate in creating bridges between these fields in how they might all fit together.

As written above, the impact that the built environment has on human health and wellness is the main focus. And the systems and procedures include both the architecture and medicine fields, both independently and interdependently, providing interconnections between these fields. This is achieved using the Architectural Medicine System (AMS) and is supported by the Architectural Doctor.

As the topics of health in architecture continue to emerge and develop, the role of an Architectural Doctor is essential as both a liaison to help interconnect these different processes, and to be a resource to the architecture and medical professionals in bridging these gaps.

When we pause, ponder, and reflect on how our built environment impacts human health and well-being, there becomes a large field of view to analyze, evaluate, and consider in terms of the wholeness of a human being. And not just the impact that physical materials have on the physical body, yet how spaces and places impact our mental and emotional health.

In the past, many of these topics were beyond the scope of the measured world, and in many ways, they are still questioned, yet modern day methods of research and analysis have proved some interesting points that can no longer be ignored if the goal is true health and wellness.

For instance, neuroscience in architecture has brought forth tremendous insights and understanding into this subject. We now know that the brain has a physical response to certain designs, spaces, and materials in ways that do indeed impact our health and overall well-being. The field of environmental psychology and neuroscience in architecture, combined with insights into evidence-based design are all proving that the places we work, live, and play in have more than just a physical impact on our lives. These spaces and places also have an emotional and psychological impact as well. And all these components affect the body's physiological health, as well as emotional and mental wellness.

This concept is new to many people, yet it has actually been around a long time. And the idea that the physical spaces in architecture impact health in negative and positive ways has long been a part of the doctor of the past, including the doctor making house calls. In that process, the doctor could evaluate the built environment of the patient's home and could gather insights into factors in their places of living that may be negatively impacting their health. Of course, there were different factors involved in previous structures, yet this process of evaluating the home and built environment by the doctor for the patient is not new.

In fact, one of the pioneers of our modern world of medicine, focused on statistics and science, is Florence Nightingale, and she sums this up quite perfectly in her quote:

> "The connection between the health and the dwellings of the population is one of the most important that exists."[54]

She also stated in the following two quotes:

> "Badly constructed houses do for the healthy what badly constructed hospitals do for the sick. Once insure that the air in a house is stagnant, and sickness is certain to follow."[55]

> "A dark house is always an unhealthy house, always an ill-aired house, always a dirty house. Want of light stops growth and promotes scrofula, rickets, etc., among the children. People lose their health in a dark house, and if they get ill, they cannot get well again in it."[56]

These quotes exemplify the importance of buildings for occupant health and has been recognized for centuries.

What Problem Does the Architectural Doctor Strive to Resolve?

As Architectural Medicine strives to support these interconnections and multi-disciplinary systems, processes, and solutions, the Architectural Doctor is there to support the application of this knowledge and provide a systems approach to this entire workflow.

And a workflow is exactly what can help describe this process. Listed below is a flow chart that shows a possible process from the patient's initial ailment and doctor visit and the building inspection process to the architectural involvement for solutions.

I will go over these steps in more detail in chapter 5, discussing the Architectural Medicine System (AMS), yet for now, this outlines the basic flow of this system.

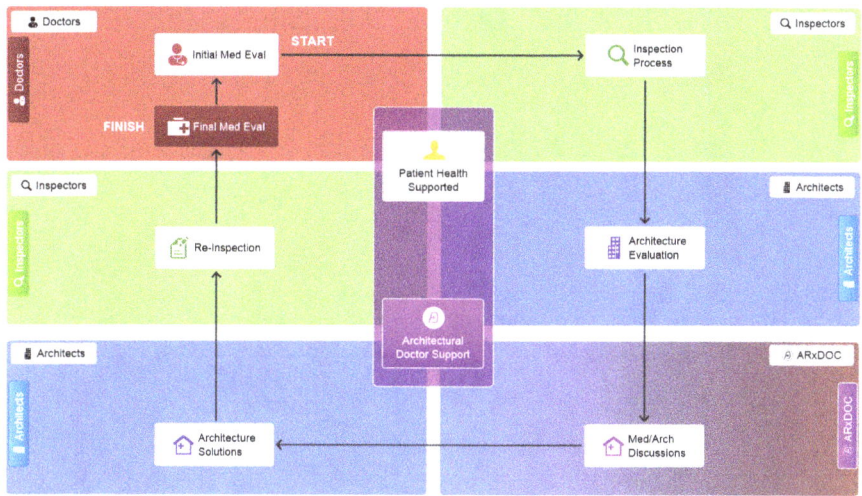

What Is Architectural Medicine and the Architectural Doctor Striving to Achieve?

Before we move forward into the topics discussed throughout this book on the Architectural Medicine System (AMS) and ARxMD – the Architectural Medicine Software Solution, let's start with why we are doing this and what the goals are.

By starting with the end result and goals, we can then reverse engineer the process and walk through the details to achieve these goals.

So, to start, what is the goal and what is the purpose of all of this?

When we view the purpose of Architectural Medicine, we're talking about bridging the fields of architecture and medicine for the purpose of health and wellness in the built environment. So, let's begin with this bridging and define what the purpose is along with the processes.

The built environment can have many issues that are creating health issues. The problem is that the medical profession may not be aware of these building issues and how they are negatively impacting their patient's health. The second issue is that the architecture field might also not be aware of these health issues, and is not trained to design better buildings to eliminate, avoid, and fix any building issues causing health problems.

The Cycle of the Architectural Medicine System (AMS)

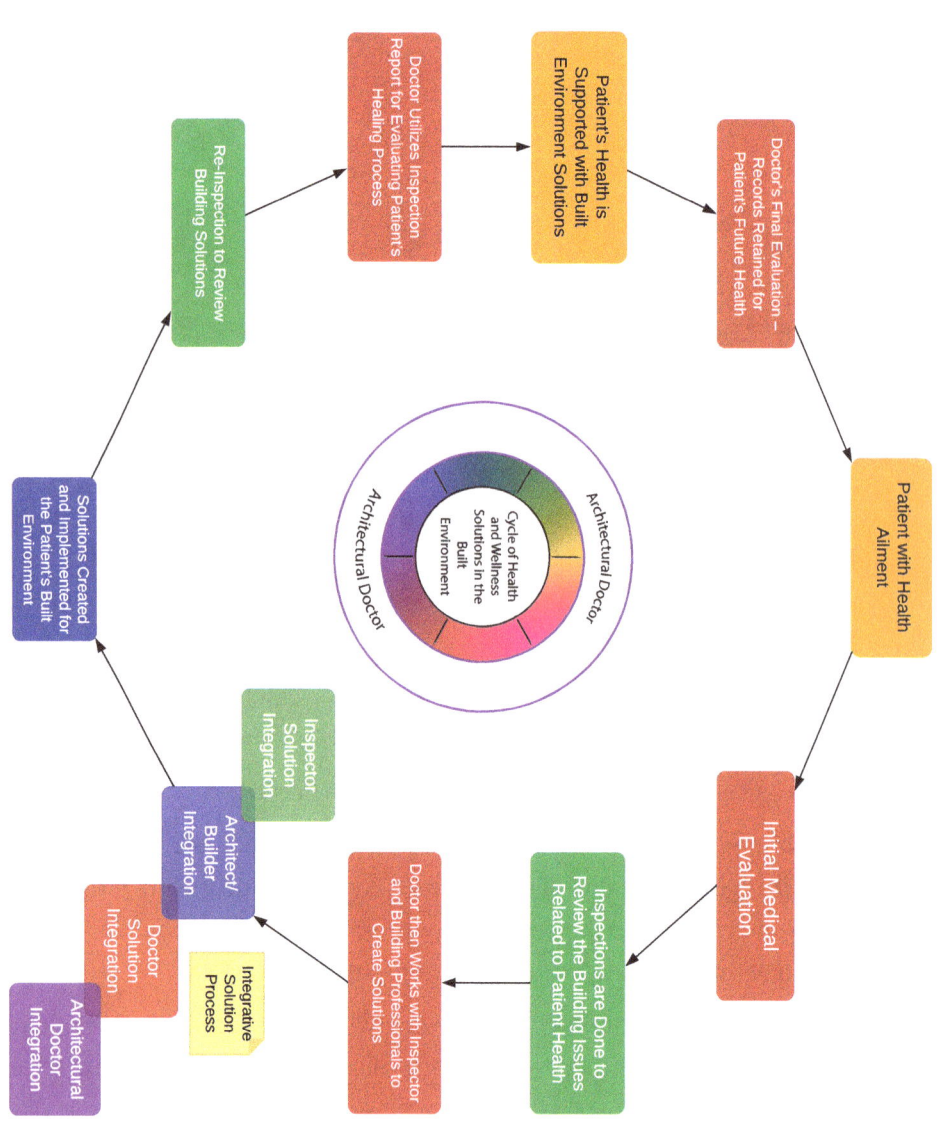

So, both professions may not be aware of building health issues and what to do about them.

This is the purpose of Architectural Medicine and the Architectural Doctor. In this book, I dive into the specific details of how these systems can function to help create better solutions, and include health and wellness in the built environment as part of the focus of these procedures.

Reviewing the diagram listed above, we see a few main processes that are critical to building health, with several that actually do not currently exist.

An example of one version of this process as a flowchart would be that a patient who isn't feeling well goes to the doctor for evaluation. Before we go into any other steps, let's remember that the environment and built environment of the patient is not included in this evaluation process. So, while the doctor can perform all the testing to conclude that the issue is "x," the cause of this might not be determined.

This may be fine for many ailments, yet as an example, if they include topics related to respiratory problems, allergies, skin issues, and even endocrine system problems, the causes of these may be missed. This, of course, is not to blame the doctors. It is simply to state that they are not trained to include this in their evaluations.

Let's include the architect and building professional in this equation. When they are designing and building, how much are they trained to understand human health and are prepared to ensure that the materials and methods utilized are not going to have any negative health impacts on the occupants? For most architects and building professionals, the answer is either none or very little. Unless you are in a cross-training matriculation, or you study in a country or at a university that focuses on these integrative education processes, there are very few building professionals who understand human health topics.

If you simply review the top two paragraphs, you can probably see why this book is being written and why Architectural Medicine exists. As well it may also become more clear about the nature of the Architectural Doctor and their purpose.

So now that we have an example of what the purpose of Architectural Medicine and the Architectural Doctor is, it provides a foundation that the rest of this book can be built upon. This foundation can allow the start of the discussion and begin the steps to ensure that these two complex professions can work together. This includes systems to achieve these goals of health and wellness in the built environment.

Etiology, the Built Environment, and Public Health

As mentioned in the introduction of this book, the causes of many illnesses in today's world are still unknown, and while many diseases are being managed by modern medical treatments, there is still room for improvement to help create better treatments for these conditions.

One of the ways that "better treatments" can be provided is the focus on preventive medicine. To prevent illnesses, there is a need to understand the causation of certain illnesses, and this is where the Architectural Doctor and Architectural Medicine enters the solution picture.

After all, when was the last time your doctor included your built environment in your health evaluations? And when was the last time you discussed with your architect the importance of health and wellness, as well as steps to take to ensure your built environment is not causing health issues?

If you answered rarely or never to the above questions and statements, you are not alone in these answers. And this is because modern day medicine and architecture are extremely complex, and there are many systems required for these professions and professionals to achieve their work.

Let me be very clear with this statement, the work of doctors and architects is among the most complex jobs in the world, and each requires a tremendous amount of education and hard work to achieve these titles. They deserve the respect that such dedication requires to achieve these positions, and throughout this book, these additional steps and bridges created to achieve better integrations are in no way, shape, or form meant to say that they are not working hard enough.

And this is exactly why the Architectural Doctor is being defined in this book, which is to be a liaison between these professionals to ensure that they can be provided the appropriate support in the work that both professionals do on a regular basis. Both of these professions require systems in order for their work to be accomplished.

What Is the Purpose of the Architectural Doctor?

If you view the many professionals that are defined as doctors, you will find many variations in this profession. You will often find the general practitioner, an eye, ear, and throat specialist, a surgeon, an oncologist, and a wide variety of other specialists. This provides the patient with the correct professional that can best support their health condition.

While you might find, depending on where in the world you are located, a difference in the names of these professionals and different segments that define each specialty, there is typically a specialist defined for each of the major functions of the body, along with those who specialize in certain ailments.

The general practitioner can often be the first professional that can help ascertain a patient's issue and can provide recommendations to see specialists. In this manner, the doctors involved will have an overview of the health issues being evaluated, and the appropriate support from a specialist.

In many ways, the general practitioner can help guide the patient in this process, and as such, can provide an evaluation that can help the patient to receive the best medical support possible.

However, in today's modern world of medicine, if there are topics related to Social Determinants of Health, or issues in the environment and built environment that may be causing the health issue to begin with, there is a limited amount of support that the typical general practitioner can provide.

If we look at some of the building health issues that have evolved over the past 40 to 50 years, there is often a similar pattern. The pattern is often a lack of acknowledgment from the medical professionals, until more evidence is gathered that can provide causal relationships between a built environment issue and a health issue.

For instance, the issues of lead, asbestos, and mold are three good examples. The first, lead, has been known that if exposed to ingestion of this material, it can cause a wide range of health issues, especially in young children and their cognitive development. The second, asbestos, is another material that is a known carcinogen. The nature of the material breaking down into small "friable" particulates that enter the lungs and causes scaring of the lung tissue, eventually preventing the exchange of oxygen to the body during respiration. The third topic, mold, has been the most recent of the three, where the mycotoxins created by mold interfere with the immune system and can cause a range of health issues and even death.

What's common about all three of these known health issues?

All three of them were unrecognized for years by the medical profession, and many times, those suffering from these ailments continued to be exposed to these materials over prolonged time exposure.

Today, these are more well known, yet there are still issues of exposure due to the lack of integrations between the architecture and the medical fields, based on missing steps that can be taken to remove these issues.

I'm not inferring that there should not be a scientific determination to ensure causal effects from said materials, but I am stating that to provide more accurate evaluations for medical professionals, there is a need for the common doctor to have proper information regarding these built environments and their potential health issues.

The doctor cannot be expected to provide these building assessments and should also not be responsible for the public health, toxicology, and epidemiology determinants of these topics.

However, who should be responsible for these evaluations and research, and who is doing this type of research currently?

It might be logical to state that the fields of architecture, engineering, and construction (AEC) would be doing this research. But then again, what about public health professionals? And if the AEC fields are doing such research, how is this data shared with public health and medical professionals?

The answer is that the lines are blurry between these topics of research and data gathering, and this is why the Architectural Doctor is important for the future of health in the built environment.

What Does an Architectural Doctor Do?

As we discuss the definition of the Architectural Doctor and highlight the previous paragraphs defining building issues that cause health problems, the lack of a specialist or group to provide building health evaluations and data analysis leads to gaps in potential health issues.

If public health and epidemiology professionals base their research on data, where is this data coming from when it comes to building health issues? Who is collecting this data, and where is the repository of data for analysts to evaluate?

In a more practical format, a building inspection providing inspections would likely be a group that could provide such data, yet most building inspections are focused on structural integrity, and not health topics in their inspections.

This data as informatics could also be valuable in big data analysis, and this is where a Building Informaticist can play a key role in gathering and analyzing such information. As mentioned in a later chapter, the need for a Healthy Building Inspector is also critical to this process, and in chapter 7, I will address these topics in depth.

One of the key components of the Architectural Doctor is to help in providing this data and informatics to doctors and architects, as well as the building professionals, and health professionals. This duty as a liaison is one critical step to help connect these topics, but also to help coordinate the many facets of this big puzzle.

As I will mention in this book many times, the importance of systems cannot be understated. I just mentioned several professionals, all of which have systems in their specific profession that are critical for their workflow. If you do not provide steps that are injected into their systems, the extra work involved will hinder these developments, and will likely cause disruption that will sour the professionals working experience involved in these building health topics.

As such, the Architectural Doctor also needs to support these professionals in their own work, provide integrations and connections between these professionals, and to support the professional development required for education, training, and processes required for each professional involved.

This is a lot of work for one professional to achieve, which is why these processes must be embraced by the education systems of each professional in their schooling process.

As I've seen over the many years being involved in striving for healthier built environments, the main reason why I can see that these topics are not as embedded into the worlds of architecture and medicine is a lack of systems and education to support such developments.

Unfortunately, due to these being complex processes and spanning different professions that are not often familiar with working together, the gaps are too great for the average professional in these discussions to take this upon themselves to develop.

A Reminder of the Times – What the COVID Pandemic Can Teach Us

As I'm writing and editing this paragraph and this book, it is January 2022, and the world has been navigating the novel coronavirus for two years now. That means that many people have died and have suffered from this illness. It also means that most of the world's population has spent their time quarantined and away from others, perhaps even spending most of this time alone.

And hopefully, they have had shelter and been in the comforts of their homes, yet even that is not accurate as many people on this planet don't have a home. That said, for those populations that have spent most of their time indoors, while they all have had different experiences, perhaps the common denominator many people have become aware of are the impacts of one's built environment.

And if there can be positive takeaways from this terrible pandemic, maybe the awareness of the power of architecture can become canon.

One of the key takeaways from this pandemic has been the obvious lack of integrations between the building and medical and health fields, where the Architectural Doctor could have provided integral support. Again, this is not a criticism, yet instead an example of how important these bridges can be to provide interconnected solutions. It is stated to highlight the value of these bridges and the fact that health solutions related to the built environment have room for improvement.

During this pandemic, the impact the built environment has on physical, emotional, and mental wellness is becoming more common for people to notice and question. Topics of how one's space and places of living and working have become more relevant and more important to not only question, but to have higher expectations to be supported for their wellness and well-being.

There are many facets of building health that have become a focus during the pandemic. The reality has been that the virus is often spread through an aerosol format as an airborne pathogen. This means indoor air quality (IAQ) has been critical for society to return to some form of normalcy, if it ever will. And while the topics of IAQ for physical health have become paramount for safety due to the virus, the issues of mental and emotional well-being have also become critical with a focus on the physical spaces where we live and work.

As we venture into the future, this public awareness can be utilized to make our buildings safer from pathogens and can become opportunities supported by demands from the general public. A focus on built environments that also support our mental and emotional wellness can also be highlighted, and more education, research, and literal developments can provide current upgrades in building spaces that can continue into the future.

This is a prime time for many topics to be addressed in the built environment, and the Architectural Doctor, as well as Architectural Medicine, are poised to support this process for human well-being and thriving. The

Architectural Doctor can provide the support for these initiatives, while the professionals involved can find support in the Architectural Medicine System (AMS).

With these building health topics becoming more common, one of the keys to the success of health and wellness in architecture is the inclusion of other topics that the architecture, engineering, and construction (AEC) fields need to navigate. This includes topics such as climate change, environmental degradation, and the requirement for energy efficiency and reduction in building energy use. An important part of this solution process is recognizing that there is a large amount of overlap between these topics, and by understanding more about cohesive solutions, these big topics can be addressed as whole systems solutions.

Just as a building requires a solid foundation to build upon, it is imperative to continue to build our knowledge base and to create solutions that consider the whole picture. There is a requirement for all of these topics to be properly recognized and addressed. While it will be challenging for these issues to be easily solved, they will not be solved unless many are involved, providing their part in contributing to the entire process.

To ensure that the whole picture is included in these solutions, the lexicon of *Integrative Architecture* is introduced in the next chapter providing a big picture overview of these topics. When viewed in this manner, these issues can be included in creating the foundation of the Architectural Doctor's work during the rest of this book.

And so, as humanity navigates these issues of the 21st century, alongside this current day pandemic, the status of buildings and the fields of architecture are at a critical crossroads. If we recognize the problems and can understand what decisions need to be made for solutions, then new developments can be created as whole systems solutions for current and future generations.

"We need to treat the planet as a system, and up until now, we've operated more as if the world were made of separate parts - this part is environment, this part is economy. But everything is connected. You can't fix global warming with a Ph.D. in thermodynamics!"

— Neri Oxman

WHAT IS INTEGRATIVE ARCHITECTURE?

Before moving on to the next chapters discussing the specific procedures that each professional can provide in creating health and wellness in the built environment, it's important to provide some context in the emerging fields of architecture and medicine that impact many of these new goals.

One of the key aspects of Architectural Medicine and the Architectural

Doctor is to provide integrative solutions within each of these professions, as well as the ability to connect with many different professions and professionals. Solutions moving forward require that we function in integrative formats, and this is not restrained to select professional segments. If we don't view health in buildings as inclusive and interdependent with the topics of energy efficiency and sustainability, then there can easily be more problems created by solving one issue, instead of providing goals for the whole picture.

If you have read the Architectural Medicine book, you can choose to skip this chapter as many of these topics have already been discussed. This chapter is a summary of Part II from chapters 6 through 13 of that book.

Over the past 50 years, both architecture and medicine have seen many changes, some in large formats and other developments as smaller, incremental steps. The field of architecture has seen changes in the need to provide greener and more sustainable building materials and methods, with a few changes focused on health. The field of medicine has seen even greater changes, from pharmacological developments to the inclusion of medical procedures and technology providing truly amazing medical capabilities.

However, in the 1980s and '90s, a powerful set of changes entered the medical and health fields to include the integration of more traditional modalities. This development is known as *Integrative Medicine.*

These developments stemmed from both the pressures of the general public demanding the inclusion of other modalities for health, along with the education from respected medical professionals and doctors such as Dr. Andrew Weil. Their promotion to include other methods for better health and healing led the medical profession to make changes to adapt to the needs of their patients' requests for the inclusion of better health approaches.

Integrative Medicine has become common, mainly due to personal health being a choice that is more easily proactive. The individual can make decisions in their diets, exercise habits, and general lifestyle choices that can provide these solutions in a more individuated format.

It is important to note that these changes did not happen easily. As Dr. Weil states in his seminal presentation, "8 weeks to optimum health," the medical profession entered into Integrative Medicine developments "kicking and screaming along the way."[57] The changes were mostly pushed by the demands of the public, not the medical fields pushing for these changes. I note this because the changes in the fields of architecture, especially healthy building topics, have been spurred along by the public, and even other professionals. This includes scientists who have been providing the warnings to the public of the health detriments in which modern day materials and methods are pervading the environment.[58]

Yet to be fair, the building field's slower process of making changes is likely due to two main factors. For one, buildings last much longer than products developed by other fields, and as such, require more time tested procedures. The second is based on greater confusion, in my opinion, as to the choices that can be made for creating greener, more sustainable, and healthier built environments. There are only a few points that all building professionals and groups agree upon, as the options are many, and the focus of each option are vast.

Another reason why healthy building has not been as accessible is the fact that building processes are more complex to change for the individual, whereas personal health choices can be made on a daily basis. Building choices and changes often require more training to complete and sometimes are not as accessible to the public, requiring professionals to make any changes.

These are incredibly complex topics that few professionals are trained on, and even fewer people are able to experiment and explore options as alternatives. Even if there are tried and true building methods used in other parts of the world, using new materials and methods can create pause for many, even if they are experienced builders. Buildings are expensive, and most clients are not willing to explore newer design processes or experiment with different materials and methods.

Integrative Medicine has continued to be a term that is used to define a viewpoint on medicine and health that can be inclusive, particularly for those seeking other options on the path to healing and health.

Many still confuse this term as meaning alternative medicine, which a key pioneer in this field perpetually reflects to others that this is not the case. What I'm stating is that the term "alternative" might seem too far out there when it comes to modalities, yet Integrative Medicine continues to state that it is open to other modalities, especially ones that have shown to be beneficial. This includes acupuncture, Chinese Medicine, and other options such as yoga and meditation. Some of these choices might not have the clinical data to support the exact details of how this might work and what the measurable benefits are, and many gains range from person to person. Yet when people are benefitting from a process that has few detrimental effects, even without clinical studies, more doctors and health professionals have become open to at least providing these as medicinal options.

The purpose of stating this is to say that there are other options that the medical professionals are opening up to, especially those with the potential for less negative impacts, and possible efficacy as an easy to access remedy.

Enter into the Lexicon - Integrative Architecture

Why am I discussing all of these topics, and why do they matter? And why am I taking the time to write a whole chapter to discuss these subjects?

The reason is based on the current and future developments in both of these two fields of architecture and medicine — which requires new developments. With the advent of Integrative Medicine, the fields of health have expanded to be more inclusive of other options, providing the individual with greater choices and control over their personal health. As the medical professionals embrace more of these choices and help to support their patients with these decisions in cohesive, big picture evaluations, it asks the question of what the architecture professionals are providing for their clients in decisions on building options.

In the process of each field progressing, there is the need for overlap between architecture and medicine for many of the big picture issues in the world to be solved, including the topics of building health.

These overlaps require the knowledge base and scope of both architecture and medicine to expand to include new options. It also benefits from a process of working together between these fields to address the issues of wellness in the future.

While health is an obvious topic relative to Architectural Medicine and the Architectural Doctor, the ability to address the health issues in the built environment has not been easy to accomplish. To achieve the changes required for better health, there needs to be more clarity in definitions for these topics to be properly considered. And this requires an overlap between both fields for appropriate discussions.

I reference Integrative Medicine for an important reason. This is to state that the fields of medicine have been actively combining different modalities into their practice for better health. This is being achieved by utilizing traditional practices, such as Chinese medicine and ayurvedic medicine, with approaches to health that are more focused on prevention with a focus on the patient's daily lifestyle. Essentially, it is viewing the whole person and their whole life into how these facets of their life impact their health. And this includes their surroundings and their environments.

This definition is critical to understand to apply to the concepts of Integrative Architecture. As the name states, there is "integration" utilized in these best practices, yet what is being integrated?

An Introduction to Integrative Architecture

In the past few decades, Integrative Medicine has embraced traditional therapies. This has been differentiated in relation to Complementary Medicine's (CM) growing developments – also known as modern medicine. Even though many of these traditional therapies, such as acupuncture and Chinese Medicine, have been around for thousands of years, integrating these modern medicine changes with traditional medicine has not been rapid or easy in many areas in the modern world.

Pioneering doctors such as Dr. Andrew Weil, who is probably one of the most well known in these medical transformations, has stated in his books and lectures that he defines Integrative Medicine as an integration by using "different modalities that utilize best practices from many resources – from both modern and traditional methodologies and treatments."[59]

As the progress of Integrative Medicine continues to benefit many patients, a reflection of this progress in medicine towards these integrations also provides a contrast of progress in the field of architecture relative to similar goals that medicine is striving to achieve — best practices toward optimal health. As health fields have been supporting more traditional therapies for better health, what has been happening in the field of Architecture?

The answer is that while there have been steps to improve architecture, the healthy component has been slow going and mostly focused on Healthy Hospital Designs. Of course, Healthy Hospital Designs are an excellent step in this progress, yet it's also a recognition that there is room for improvement in the many other built environments – from the average home to the modern commercial building.

To provide a more rapid development towards these goals in architecture is to use this example of Integrative Medicine to show a pathway of development for architecture in which to take. By embracing healthier approaches in built environments, while also considering traditional methodologies, many of these goals can be achieved.

This process can be defined as *Integrative Architecture* to support and work in tandem with the positive developments of Integrative Medicine.

The approach of learning from the developments of Integrative Medicine in the field of architecture has many benefits. For one, many people are already familiar with the topics of Integrative Medicine and the positive connotation it has to empower the average person. It also can be utilized as a high standard in discovering and using best practices for better health.

The concept of Integrative Architecture is similar to Integrative Medicine in that it strives to utilize best practices while also merging modern approaches with traditional methodologies. Essentially, it is considering many different approaches to achieve the best results, and these "best results" include a healthier approach for healthier designs.

Why Exactly Is Integrative Architecture Important?

My first job in the working world in my early teens was working as a bricklayer and construction laborer for a mason. During my childhood summers spent at my grandmother's house, I had met this wonderful man named Joe Pitelli. For many years, he spent time raising his home and rebuilding the structure to prevent any flooding issues, as the house was next to an area of water. And being that I had wanted to be an architect since a kid – and let people know this – I would visit him often.

I spent many days visiting him as he worked, as I was young enough to bug him with tons of questions. He was semi-retired and, in retrospect, such a wonderful person to oblige me and encourage me with his answers. As he was semi-retired, in my early teens, he offered me a job to work with him and his son, who had taken over his business. It was extremely hard work, yet hauling bricks and learning the construction specifics were all part of the learning curve in my construction knowledge.

The first building I worked on was a medium-sized business structure, which was clad in brick. One afternoon, as we were all sitting together during lunchtime, Mr. Pitelli Sr. began talking to his son, Mr. Pitelli Jr., about an issue that they were dealing with in the brick laying process. The situation was that the largest of the exterior walls had a dimension problem that required them to cut bricks at each of the rows in staggered layers due to the length of the wall.

After discussing the topic between him and his son, Joe Sr. then turned to me and said, "you see, as you are planning to be an architect, you must understand what we are discussing. Because the architect did not consider the design for the proper length of the specified bricks, this main wall will require each row to have a significant cutting of bricks to ensure that it looks correct. If the architect had construction experience, they would have known to adjust the wall length to an appropriate size for the brick type specified. This would have ensured that the wall would look as good as possible and to support a more efficient brick installation process."

This lesson stated that the aesthetics of the wall would have improved, and the extra work required could have easily been avoided if the architect had designed the size of the wall accordingly.

And this was a key factor for my beginning experience in construction and building to understand the complexities of how buildings are constructed, and I've used this knowledge throughout my life to understand the importance of big picture, integrative planning in any design process. This story and experience have followed me in my life, and the core of this teaching was that there needs to be an understanding of the many facets and systems involved to plan accordingly.

Unfortunately, most architects, especially back several decades ago, have limited experience with construction. This issue was later echoed when I attended the Yestermorrow Design/Build School in Vermont in the US. Several architects created the Yestermorrow school in 1980 who graduated from architecture school with no building experience and have been working ever since to help provide hands-on education for architects and designers in the building fields.[60]

This experience highlighted the importance of integrated systems, which is essentially what Integrative Architecture is all about. Being aware of the many systems involved helps create designs that either anticipate or plan for the multitude of components involved in the design-build process in architecture. And if not factored into the design process, the result can lead to short and long-term problems.

The concept of Integrative Architecture is akin to Integrative Medicine, which strives to see the whole picture and to consider the many facets involved for the best solutions, while being inclusive of other methods that may be helpful. Integrative Medicine, at least in the US and in other places worldwide, has become more than just a buzzword for better health care. It has become a symbol of how integrating different approaches for the goal of best practices can embrace a wide range of modalities to achieve better health and wellness.

As defined by the Arizona Center for Integrative Medicine, "Integrative Medicine (IM) is healing-oriented medicine that takes account of the whole person, including all aspects of lifestyle. It emphasizes the therapeutic relationship between practitioner and patient, is informed by evidence, and makes use of all appropriate therapies."[61]

And Dr. Weil, who is often seen as the father of IM and one of the strongest supporters of Integrative Medicine, defines this as "a healing-oriented medicine that takes account of the whole person (body, mind, and spirit), including all aspects of lifestyle. It emphasizes the therapeutic relationship and makes use of all appropriate therapies, both conventional and alternative."[62]

Reviewing the Many Pieces of the Puzzle

Before I describe the specific definition of Integrative Architecture, it's important to discuss the different subjects in architecture that are striving to be integrated.

An essential component of Architectural Medicine is the integration of many facets of complex professions. When referring to "reviewing of the many pieces of the puzzle," what puzzle pieces are being referenced and why?

What are these different pieces of the puzzle that can be integrated?

They are the topics of *Green*, *Sustainable*, and *Healthy* Building.

The fields of architecture and medicine are wide-ranging, so the facets discussed in this book are a start, yet do not include every aspect. With a focus on health in the built environment, Architectural Medicine includes the fields of green building and sustainable building, as well as healthy building as "pieces" of the puzzle to fit together.

And the reason why these other fields are included is based on biological health. Human beings require clean water, clean air, and clean soil for food to provide and support good health.

Some people forget that you are not only living in the natural world; you *are* a part of the natural world.

The composition of your body consists of about 70 percent of water and is created from natural elements. The calcium of your bones, the silicon of your skin, hair, and nails, as well as your organs and cells are created from many minerals and natural substances.

The architecture of your body is composed of natural elements, and if we pollute the natural environment, eventually, our bodies will be polluted. And when your body is polluted, this causes dis-ease, just as polluting the environment will cause disease for other biological beings that we share this planet with.

Therefore, if we are to focus on human health, there needs to be an emphasis on biological and environmental health as well. You cannot separate the fact that humans are a part of nature. So, if we ensure that we do not pollute our natural world, it can help prevent our bodies from being polluted.

This can be a tremendous support for promoting good health and wellness and cannot be neglected.

As integrative medicine is combining the many facets of traditional and modern methodologies for better health, integrative architecture is also combining different modalities. Yet what are these modalities?

A Brief Overview and Definitions of the Three Main Topics of Healthy, Green, and Sustainable Building

In this segment, I'm going to discuss and define these three topics of *Healthy*, *Green*, and *Sustainable Building*.

> "I approach the world as a whole by taking an integrative approach, not a world of parts, and I like to bring different fields and disciplines together."[63] — Neri Oxman

Neri Oxman is one of the brilliant thinkers in today's world. Her quote above is an example why I state this, and her book *Material Ecology* provides examples of the amazing possibilities of a future in more harmony with this planet. The fact that she continues to establish this work at one of the most prestigious technological universities on the planet, MIT, is a testament that working with nature is not going against technological progress.

I state this because the work of many brilliant minds, such as Neri Oxman, and the renowned genius of Buckminster Fuller, provides humanity with hopefulness and great potential moving forward into this 21st century. In referencing this hopefulness, I will also state that it will take work, and it is my opinion that functioning with more intelligence can be described as working in integrated formats. In the following paragraphs, I intend to describe these cohesive solutions relative to topics that require interdependency to provide smarter solutions into the future.

By providing an overview of how these topics are interrelated, I intend to highlight the goals and end result to provide context into why this is relative to Architectural Medicine.

The reason why I'm starting with the end goal first is simple. If you have context as to why these topics are important, you can recognize how they need to overlap to support each other. And this will be relevant to the work of the Architectural Doctor. As each facet is discussed individually, it can provide a contextual sense of the importance of the interdependence of each of these topics working together.

To start, there is a need to define what these facets are before there can be discussions as to how they can fit together.

So, let's get to these three topics of *Healthy*, *Green*, and *Sustainable Building*.

As we venture into the details of this book, there are graphics that will be used to define these discussions. These images can provide road maps to where these discussions will lead. To start this description of the many pieces involved, below is a graphic of the result of all topics combined.

The following are diagrams that include each of these topics, with overlaps between each segment.

This three-part Venn diagram highlights the independent topics, yet interdependent, with a balanced approach to providing the goal of health in the built environment:

The Intersection of Energy, Ecology, and Health in the Built Environment

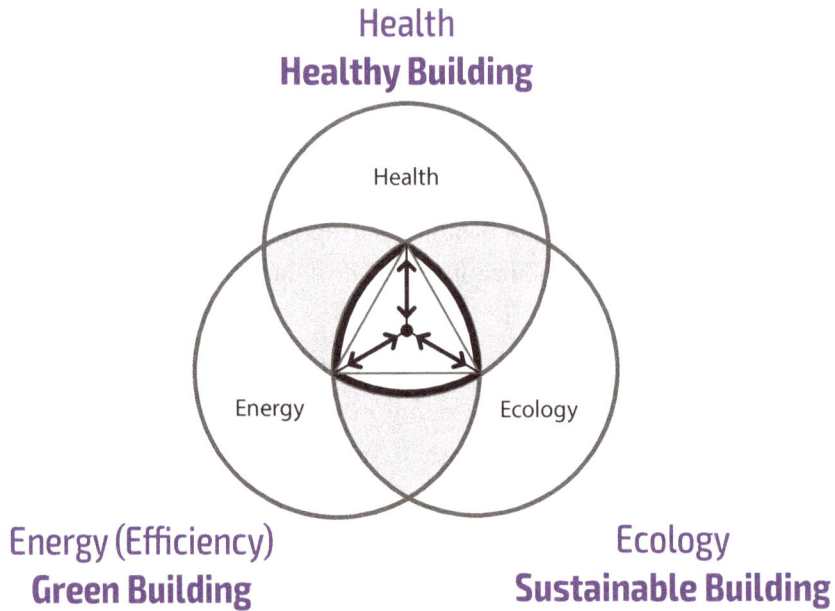

As you can see in the graphic, the overlap between each of these topics is defined as Healthy Building, focusing on Physical Health, Green Building, with a focus on Energy-Efficiency, and Sustainable Building, with a focus on Environmental or Ecological Design.

These three topics, in particular, relate to providing a better future for architecture. This trifecta of *green*, *sustainable*, and *healthy* building will be critical to address if we are to take seriously the future of health in the built environment on a global scale.

The combination of these three topics can merge to form *Integrative Architecture*.

For those new to these topics or perhaps not as well versed, it should be stated there are many definitions of these fields depending on who they are defined by. These definitions will vary from person to person and country to country worldwide. To make sure there is no confusion, I've defined these terms in a format that I've observed over several decades, and which are relative to the content in this book. I discuss why I have chosen these definitions and go into more detail in the *Architectural Medicine* book, yet suffice it to say that the main reason I have outlined these definitions is based on my experience in these fields. This, along with the big picture context of why they matter and what goals these topics are striving to solve.

With that said, we can see in the diagram that these three topics are focused on the topics of *Health*, *Energy*, and *Ecology*. These topics are essential because they highlight the main issues critical to providing current and future generations the possibility of supplying and maintaining biological and ecological health.

Basic Definitions of Healthy, Green, and Sustainable Building

As a quick overview, these three topics will be defined as the following:

Healthy Building: the impact that the building has on the health of the occupants with an emphasis on physical health. This includes topics ranging from Indoor Air Quality (IAQ) to the impacts that materials in buildings can have on the inhabitants.

Green Building: a main focus of green building is to make the structure energy-efficient, with an emphasis on the reduction of energy and fuel consumption. This includes reducing pollution and considering the energy source from its production to its use. Reducing the carbon footprint of the building is also a focus and a goal.

Sustainable Building: a main focus of sustainable building is to consider the impact that the building will have on the environment and ecology of where it's built. This includes reviewing the overall impact that the building materials, production, and end of use (LCA) – Life Cycle Assessment will have on the local and global biology and ecology.

The Intersection of Energy, Ecology, and Health in the Built Environment

Health/**Healthy Building**

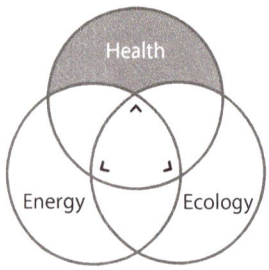

Issues related to physical health, removing toxic materials and improving occupant health.

Groups and organizations with a Health focus in the built environment include:
Healthy Building Network, Bau Biologie and Biophilia

Energy (Efficiency)/**Green Building**

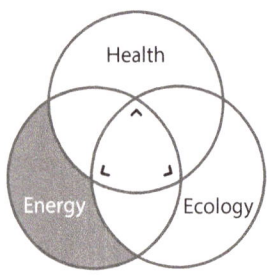

Issues related to optimizing Energy use, sourcing more sustainable energy options, striving to reduce pollution, and working to reduce carbon footprint.

Groups and organizations related to this Energy focus include: Architecture 2030 and the US Green Building Council (USGBC)

Ecology/**Sustainable Building**

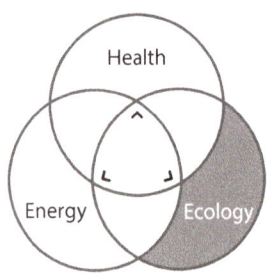

Recognizing and designing for the Ecology, creating more sustainable solutions with materials and methods. Considering Life Cycle Assessment (LCA) in all designs.

Groups and organizations with an Ecological focus in the built environment include:
Biophilic Design and
the Permaculture Institute

While some may recognize and be familiar with these three topics, it's also important to note that many other fields are involved in these developments with a tremendous amount of overlap. While this statement might seem to make things even more complicated, it is intended to provide the entire scope to evaluate properly. This way, all of the facets can be assessed when making decisions.

That said, there are some common attributes that I can pull from many experts in these fields and perhaps sew these together to at least provide a picture of what each is striving to define.

The first topic is *Health* and is defined as Healthy Building. It focuses on the impact of physical health parameters in the built environment. This includes topics such as the materials of the building and the potential for these to cause illness, such as lead paint and asbestos. This can also include indoor air quality (IAQ) topics, such as Carbon Monoxide (CO), Carbon Dioxide (CO2), Nitrogen Dioxide (N2O), and issues such as Volatile Organic Compounds or VOCs. This can also include microbial contaminants, such as bacteria and viruses. All of which can have a negative impact on health and be the cause of morbidities and disease.

The next topic is *Energy*, and this is grouped with Green Building. As many people are aware, science is showing that humans impact the ecological and biological health of the planet, and our choice of energy and sources of energy all contribute to these factors. It's also known that up to 50 percent of all energy used worldwide is utilized in building construction, maintenance, and regular building use.[64]

That is a huge percentage, and if we focus on just the energy efficiency of our buildings, it can have tremendous ecological and health benefits. The reduction in both the use and production of these energy sources means that we can reduce pollution in enormous strides, with outstanding benefits and results.

This brings up the connection to the third topic, which is focused on the *Ecology* and is highlighted as Sustainable Building. Sustainable building and architecture are often described as striving to improve the ecological connections with the built environment while decreasing harmful impacts on the local and global ecology.

With these energy efficiencies and reductions in pollution, this not only means that the benefits support better environmental and human health, yet the health of the entire biology of all sentient beings on the planet.

With the many organisms and creatures that we share this planet with, their good health means that we as humans, can also be provided the potential for good health. When we realize that we are in symbiosis with the planet and all of its many sentient beings, it can help provide context for our choices and actions.

There are many definitions of green and sustainable building, but in order to achieve the end goal of comprehending the core topics of these issues, I've outlined these fields and definitions as such to provide context relative to Integrative Architecture. When you begin to uncover the various layers of creating the healthy, green, and sustainable built environment, you might find that these become overwhelming in scope and depth.

A big part of this book and the *Architectural Medicine* book is defining some of these issues and providing an overview in a less overwhelming and, hopefully, more empowering format. In this process, by defining these topics in a general format, the big picture issues can be addressed, and a focus on solutions can be defined. In the fields of healthy, green, and sustainable building, each has had its own trajectory, and in the next few paragraphs, I will discuss some of the similarities and differences. I will also attempt to continue to define these topics in a loose format, as there are no real, concrete definitions of these fields. The lack of specific definitions can cause confusion in understanding these topics, so while my descriptions may not be an exact standard, I'm doing this to give context to this often overwhelming information.

The big question is, "where to start?" Unfortunately, many people first become aware of these topics when building, renovating, or buying a home or house. People are often unaware of these topics until the deconstruction process has begun on their building projects, creating a rushed time crunch to the already overwhelming number of changes in their lives during building and construction projects.

This becomes a real challenge, as not only are many striving to educate themselves on incredibly complex topics in fields that can often take a lifetime to master, but they now need to learn about all the various components in a condensed amount of time.

To make this more complicated, many of the professionals involved often don't work from commonly integrated standards and definitions. Even if you, as the general public, might have clarity, it doesn't mean that numerous other professionals will have that same clarity and share these specific meanings in discussing these topics.

This is another reason why this book includes the primary professionals of architecture and medicine. It is a hope to bring clarity to all involved and to have enough information to know what conversations to have to bring clarity to the discussions. You may bring your starting point to this process, yet basic topics can be discussed, providing a baseline overview for multiple topics to be considered.

In my opinion, the lack of context has taken the current age of information to the point of overwhelm. Instead of allowing the information age to empower the general public, it has instead led many to become frozen with indecision.

That said, there are some patterns in these fields based on their history and the trajectory of goals they strive to achieve. It's also important to state that the history of these fields plays a vital part in analyzing these three fields, both in how they function by themselves and how they integrate or do not integrate today.

These examples are not defining all of the different professional approaches. However, I'm using these definitions from personal experiences over the past 30 years to highlight some of the main issues.

If you have other ways to define these topics or are personally using these topics in differing definitions, please strive to understand what I am trying to convey, as many people are still not aware of these general, big picture subjects.

The past 50 years show a rich history in each branch of these three topics and developments. Many people may also be familiar with the fields of natural building, sustainable design, organic architecture, healthy building, ecological design, environmental design, and other fields that began development in the past 20th century to make matters even more complex.

While this entire range of fields will not be discussed in this book, we do have more information on our website where you can read about these specific topics and dive deeper into their definitions and history. By going to our website, you can view these topics by clicking the link "Information on the Various Fields of Architecture and Medicine" from our main book page:

https://architecturalmedicine.com/book/

An Overview of These Fields and How They Relate to the Topic of Architectural Medicine

You might think that I'd focus on the discussions of healthy building in terms of these three main topics, yet I'm starting with green and sustainable building for a few reasons that will be clear in a few paragraphs.

Sustainable building and green building are, in many ways striving to create the same or similar solution. They are both approaches to building intended to reduce the building's energy use and decrease the environmental impacts of the building processes on the environment. Providing more fuel efficiency and less fuel use, particularly fossil fuels, leads to fewer carbon emissions and fewer negative impacts on the ecology.

From the manufacturing of materials standpoint, the goal in producing these materials is to use less energy and have a less negative environmental impact from production to application and, of course, the end use of the product. The result leads to less negative ecological impact, less spending in production, and more cost-effectiveness for a better living environment.

However, each field approaches the solution in a different format...

For instance, in sustainable building, some builders will hold steady in their use of mainly natural materials, meaning materials that come from nature, instead of synthetic materials and products manufactured by humans.

In the last 30 years, many Sustainable Builders have used materials such as timber frame, adobe, and the straw bale building approach. Often, these builders will source their materials as local as possible to reduce environmental impact. And when sustainable builders are reviewing these environmental impacts, they are often factoring in the entire life cycle of the product, from the cutting down of trees and milling of the wood to the carbon footprint in the transportation of these products. In terms of the whole cycle, this includes their use and end of service.

Over the entire cycle of the life of the product or Life Cycle Assessment (LCA), these questions are often factored into the decision making process from the very beginning. This includes the important factor of where the building is located and what local resources are most appropriate to provide a decreased impact on the locale.

The life cycle of each product or LCA is also referred to by the comment "cradle to grave" of the products. In the past 30 years, there's been an emphasis on sustainability, focusing on a revised version called "cradle to cradle." This philosophy called cradle to cradle was initially coined by Walter R. Stahel [65], yet is most known by the work and writings of architect William McDonough and chemist Michael Braungart in their book *Cradle to Cradle: Remaking the Way We Make Things*.[66]

In this approach, the production, use, and end use of the products mimic the processes of nature. This means that when the product is no longer used, it can be recycled and repurposed back into the natural system, which of course, is how nature functions. Incidentally, this mimicking of nature is the basis of the term *biomimicry*, which has become an increasingly popular methodology in the design fields.

When plants and organisms die in the natural world, they decompose and return to the soil from which they came. And because there is no degradation of the original materials in this process, it can "sustain" the process repeatedly in perpetuity without a decline in the materials' original quality.

In essence, this is what many in the sustainability fields are striving to achieve – the ability for human-created processes and products to follow this way of nature. Everything that is produced and manufactured can eventually be recycled, reused, and repurposed back into its original form without degradation to the original materials. This allows future generations the opportunity to utilize the materials of the planet in the same manner as previous generations. It provides a return to the original quality of the materials, to begin anew.

However, a difference between sustainable building and green building is often a focus on materials and the way in which energy efficiency is achieved. Green building professionals will often utilize any form of materials, natural or synthetic, to achieve a decrease in energy use and to be more energy efficient. If this includes materials such as synthetic insulation and a focus on mechanic processes to achieve the end goal, then this may be the appropriate selection for green building.

There are overlaps between these two approaches, yet depending on the circumstances, the approach of the solution may be significantly different.

And to revisit my earlier comment, to state that definitions of these three topics are not set in stone as a common description is an understatement. As much as there are writings on defining these three topics, there are as many writings that could be seen as contradictory. Yet the whole point of discussing these topics is to recognize that the built environment impacts human health and the ecology. By reducing the negative impacts on human and biological health, it can support healthier ecosystems of the planet, in which human health is integrally connected.

In terms of the definition of healthy building, there are some basic concepts that can provide a baseline of understanding when discussing this topic. It's quite common sense to think that building should be inherently healthy. After all, a very important part of architecture is to make sure that the building provides shelter and safety for the inhabitants. This would instinctively be defined as a building not falling down and not falling apart. Yet because the building fields have become so sophisticated over the past 50 plus years, it does mean that these issues must be reviewed. The sick building syndrome (SDS) issues of the 1980s first put this term healthy building onto many people's radar, at least in the US.

Over the past 30 plus years, some important pioneers in the healthy building realm have helped define these issues. They should be given credit for their work to provide healthier solutions and hard work that, for many, has been an uphill battle. I feel fortunate that I have met many of these pioneers and will not hesitate to state that my path and their inspiration planted the seeds of what has become Architectural Medicine. Please be sure to review their work and contributions to gain deeper insights into these subjects. Their work through the years and my experiences have led to me thinking about these fields and eventually coming up with the concepts of Architectural Medicine.

In terms of the discussions of these three main topics, the reason why I started with green and sustainable building is based on a particular timeline. A key reason is the importance of occurrences in the 1960s and 1970s leading to the developments of these first two topics of green and sustainable building.

A big reason why many American architects and designers began seeking solutions in their designs to be more energy-efficient with less environmental impact was due to the environmental movements of the time. This includes the energy crisis of the 1970s. I was old enough to remember that in the '70s in the US, the energy crisis significantly impacted daily life. At one point, there were days when gasoline for vehicles was so sparse that you could only get fuel on certain days based on whether your vehicle's license plate ended with an odd or even number. This emphasized the fact that people were dependent on fossil fuels in ways that prevented common functions in daily life, such as the heating and cooling in their buildings and their transportation activities.

These were critical topics on the news, and everyone at that time was immersed in these issues – at least in my life experiences. The main concerns were the lack of fossil fuel energy sources, which for many, spurred the process of seeking alternative energy solutions. And this, combined with the ecological problems in the '60s and '70s, brought up the fact that buildings have a large impact on the ecology – often a negative and detrimental impact.

So, at this time, there were architects and builders who strived to find solutions to these problems. The ability to have energy independence, or at least to have multiple energy sources to depend upon, was a motivating factor for many in these alternative explorations. These solutions included research into passive solar building, the photovoltaic (PV) solar movement, biofuels, and wind and geothermal alternatives.

The approach of having fewer impacts on the environment also led to terms such as "ecological footprint."[67] This term is meant to describe what happens when you walk on areas of the ecology that are sensitive and, therefore, to be aware and cognizant of the detriments to such wear and tear on sites from human involvement.

During this time of energy efficiency and sustainable building advancements, what resulted in many of these design solutions were structures that were more airtight and had less thermal transfer between the outside and inside. Subsequently, this meant less energy and fuel needed to heat and cool a building, which also reduced fuel use and reduced environmental impacts. So, the goal of reducing fuel and saving money was a twofold improvement.

However, it failed to recognize the impacts this would have on the health of the inhabitants, particularly in these buildings that had no functioning windows (or *glazing* as it's called in the architecture field[68]). These are often referred to as tight buildings or tight construction, as in airtight. The result was energy-efficient structures, yet the air quality inside became either toxic or provided a reduction in oxygen for the health of the inhabitants.

In the 1980s, the infamous story of Sick Building Syndrome (SBS) was based on issues that occurred at the US EPA offices. The office upgraded its building interiors, and this included tighter building designs, combined with new synthetic materials installed, such as carpets, furniture, and new paint. This was before the now common topic of low VOCs, and these upgrades led to people in these office spaces becoming ill. Yet, at first, they did not understand why people were getting sick. It was speculated that these new designs, with tighter enclosures for energy efficiency and new materials with high VOC off-gassing, created a toxic interior environment for the people to work within.

This influential case of sick building syndrome occurred at the EPA's Waterside Mall headquarters in southwest D.C.[69] While there was controversy in determining if these building issues did cause sickness for the employees working in these offices, it was undoubtedly a milestone in the topic of building health. And it sparked the interior health aspects, such as fresh air inclusion and the questions of health related to these new synthetic chemicals in newer building materials. In today's building world, the topics of air exchange are common when dealing with tight building designs to provide fresh, clean air for the health of the occupants.

The increase in sick building syndrome was often a factor in striving to reduce energy and decrease the use of energy sources and fuel. From one viewpoint, this is an excellent example of how one problem solved can create other issues when you don't view the whole picture. The idea of decreasing energy is an excellent approach, yet causing health issues for the inhabitants is obviously not a successful outcome.

It's also the reason why I started with green and sustainable building topics, to show the impacts that these new airtight buildings can have on health in an unsuspecting way. The architects, builders, and the general public were striving to find solutions to become more energy efficient and environmentally aware, yet did not anticipate this having a detrimental impact on occupant health.

Another building health issue that placed building health on the map was the advent of Legionnaire's disease, which is due to contamination of cooling towers by legionella organisms. Legionella bacteria can cause a serious type of pneumonia.[70] The name derives from the "1976 state convention of the American Legion, a U.S. military veterans' organization, at a Philadelphia hotel where 182 Legionnaires contracted the disease, 29 of them fatally."[71] And then, there were the topics of lead paint and asbestos in the late 1970s into the 80s, which also brought more awareness to the impacts buildings can have on physical health.

These examples provide insights into building health issues and how this has inspired movements to address these problems and to seek better solutions.

Why Are the Three Topics of Healthy, Green, and Sustainable Building So Important to Include Together?

My writing exploring these topics up to this stage of this book has included the question, "how does the built environment impact human health and wellness?"

And that's a perfect segue to discuss the integration of these three fields to help put the many pieces of the jigsaw puzzle together. In this approach, evaluating "how" the built environment impacts health can lead to "what" can be done about it for better health.

This requires the inclusion of green building, sustainable building, and healthy building topics to be evaluated either at the same time or in similar time frames to see the whole picture of a patient's health. In this manner, new processes and systems are required to achieve these goals, as well as education and information for each group involved. These solutions must anticipate and include all of these topics, or we may fall into the challenges that the sick building syndrome examples showed as a possible unanticipated result. It is critical to have this big picture mindset for whole system solutions.

In chapter 5, I'll discuss how integrations can define new systems and put all of these facets together with the professions of architecture and medicine in an interconnected format. This, of course, will also include the general public as the building occupants.

Whether you are new to these topics in the built environment or have spent decades involved in these fields, an essential part of Architectural Medicine is *integration*.

Now, this word integration has been used quite a lot in the past few decades, so I would rather this not be as much a buzzword and instead, provide a focus on its base definition:

integration (n.)

1610s, "act of bringing together the parts of a whole," from French intégration and directly from Late Latin integrationem (nominative integratio) "renewal, restoration," noun of action from past participle stem of Latin integrare "make whole," also "renew, begin again" (see integrate).[72]

This definition centers on "bringing together parts of the whole," and in the next sections, I will define Integrative Architecture based on the popularly known Integrative Medicine.

The Defining Principles of Integrative Medicine

Returning to the concept of Integrative Medicine, I would like to review the purpose and process of this topic in more detail. The following is a list of principles from the Andrew Weil Center for Integrative Medicine at The University of Arizona:[73]

- A partnership between patient and practitioner in the healing process
- Appropriate use of conventional and alternative methods to facilitate the body's innate healing response
- Consideration of all factors that influence health, wellness and disease, including mind, spirit and community as well as body
- A philosophy that neither rejects conventional medicine nor accepts alternative therapies uncritically
- Recognition that good medicine should be based in good science, be inquiry driven, and be open to new paradigms
- Use of natural, effective, less-invasive interventions whenever possible
- Use of the broader concepts of promotion of health and the preven-

tion of illness as well as the treatment of disease
- Training of practitioners to be models of health and healing, committed to the process of self-exploration and self-development.

There is an interview with Dr. Weil from February of 2010 that is a very concise overview of what Integrative Medicine is and is not, and how its focus is on the health and the healing of the patient. In this interview, he begins by stating the following when asked about Integrative Medicine's definition, "the short answer is it is the intelligent combination of conventional and alternative medicine, but that doesn't capture this movement."[74] And he goes on to say, "I think Integrative Medicine is a real movement, and in essence, it is trying to restore the focus of medicine on health and healing away from disease symptom management. It emphasizes whole-person medicine meaning that we are more than just physical bodies – we are minds, spirits, and community members."

While the interview is a bit longer than two minutes, he follows up with the interviewer by providing this description in more detail. Dr. Weil states, "it looks at all aspects of lifestyle; it emphasizes the importance of the practitioner-patient relationship to the healing practice." And finally, this comment can be applied to the fundamental approach of Integrative Architecture in a similar manner to his statements on Integrative Medicine, "it's willing to look at all methods from whatever tradition they come from that may be of value in treating disease – that is the alternative piece."[75]

Suppose these same approaches to Integrative Medicine are applied to the concept of *Integrative Architecture*? In that case, a few key points can be redefined in terms of how it is applied to architecture.

The ideal in architecture is that all the crucial factors in the built environment, including healthy built environments, green building for energy efficiency, and sustainable architecture, are appropriately defined to ensure proper shelter. This includes the preservation of the ecology and provides inspiring surroundings to live within. These are factors that all biological life depends upon, and it should automatically be a given.

Sadly, these are not always seen as essential as the main focus in today's modern world of building. And in medicine, some modalities do not embrace the best patient health and healing, which then requires integrative medicine. In this manner, integrative architecture is necessary if the path toward green, sustainable, and healthy architecture are goals to achieve. This approach can help achieve optimal health and wellness goals, yet there will be the need for a process for the architecture world to embrace and utilize. Integrative architecture and the developments of integrative medicine can provide best practices for both professions. In essence, the combination of these two can become integrative architectural medicine or, said in a more straightforward term, Architectural Medicine.

The key to Architectural Medicine is the need for progressive thinking and actions to take place within each profession and between each profession. This can allow integrations between each of these fields to help guide and support these initiatives. This, of course, is where the capabilities of the Architectural Doctor become a tremendous support in these interconnections.

Both professions will require the openness to recognize there are issues and problems and are also willing to explore different modalities to achieve better results. If these professions are open enough to embrace and explore these options, the result can allow integration and interconnectivity between these fields. The result of this integrative, multi-disciplinary focus is Architectural Medicine. Integrative Medicine and Integrative Architecture require an open-minded approach for best practices in their fields. And when applied together, it can yield tremendous health benefits in the built environment.

So, in moving forward, how can Integrative Architecture be defined?

Taking the lead from the already successful Integrative Medicine processes, perhaps these principles can be redefined with a focus on the field of architecture in the following formats.

The Defining Principles of Integrative Architecture

Integrative Architecture can be defined using the following principles:

- Client and architect/designer are partners in the creation of green, sustainable, and healing environments
- All building factors that influence human, biological, and ecological health are taken into consideration
- Appropriate use of both conventional and alternative methods and materials facilitates green, sustainable, and healthy buildings
- Effective design solutions that are natural and less invasive should be used whenever possible
- Integrative Architecture neither rejects conventional architecture nor accepts alternative building approaches uncritically
- Good architecture is based on good science. It is inquiry-driven and open to new paradigms. Evidence-Based Design is of critical importance
- Alongside the concept of design solutions, the broader concepts of green, sustainable, and health promotion for human, biological, and ecological health are paramount
- Architects and designers of Integrative Architecture should exemplify its principles and commit themselves to self-exploration and self-development

Yes, these are the verbatim eight principles of Integrative Medicine reworded to fit the field of architecture. Why start from scratch when many, such as Dr. Weil, have already created a solid path and put into practice years of work to achieve approaches and definitions to guide the way?

Taking this one step further, the definition of Integrative Medicine can also be applied to Integrative Architecture in setting a framework for this approach with similar beneficial goals.

As such, the following statement can be referenced:

> "Integrative Medicine is healing-oriented medicine that takes account of the whole person (body, mind, and spirit),

including all aspects of lifestyle. It emphasizes the therapeutic relationship and makes use of all appropriate therapies, both conventional and alternative."[76]

And applying this to the field of architecture, we utilize this wording to define Integrative Architecture as the following:

"Integrative Architecture is an energy-efficient, sustainability-focused, health-oriented approach to architecture that considers human, biological, and ecological health, including all aspects of the built environment and lifestyle. It emphasizes the relationship between occupant and the built environment and makes use of all appropriate building materials and methods, both conventional and alternative."

In many of Dr. Weil's talks and writings, he has encouraged and has been a proponent of places and spaces that promote wellness. Courses at the Andrew Weil Center for Integrative Medicine, such as *Environmental Health*,[77] recognize the importance of the natural and built environments as places where healing can be either supported or unsupported. This also provides the recognition that medicine is not just a general Rx modality of drugs or food, but includes your surroundings and all facets of your life. This includes the built environments that you live and work within. Therefore, if you are to achieve this form of optimal health that is advocated, then the architecture that you live and work within must embrace and support this health and wellness as well.

For the past several decades, the introduction of Integrative Medicine has been an evolving process. From its origins to the current recognition of this topic as a serious and vital part of medicine — at least many whose interests in providing the best health solutions to patients — has been pivotal. Integrative Medicine is known as using the wisdom of traditional medicine in combination with modern medicine for best practices.

In this same way, the concept of Integrative Architecture utilizes the wisdom of traditional building materials and methods, along with modern materials and methodologies. This combination is striving for a result of best practices in architecture and building for best biological and ecological health. It is also working to support climate change issues and better environmental stewardship on this planet.

While these best practices are still being defined in many ways, this book's approach and focus on Architectural Medicine, and the Architectural Doctor strives to support these three fields of healthy, green, and sustainable building to merge and define a better built environment. With more focus on a greener and more energy-efficient building process, and a more sustainable and ecological built environment, the future of buildings will encompass more of these topics over time.

Therefore, how they integrate will be essential to these solutions working together instead of causing more issues. This concept of Integrative Architecture can be seen as a merging of these three topics and integrating the many facets of these approaches into a cohesive whole.

As an example of this critical overlap, many have become aware of the current interest in decreasing dangerous plastics in products, such as BPA and phthalates. This is often driven by toxicologists and epidemiologists, not architects and designers. In this, a new age and day where those in medicine are overlapping with the fields of product manufacturing and the building fields, the emerging interests in health care are creating new pathways.

These new paths can include the built environment as part of health care evaluations for patient health. This is akin to the past, where doctors who provided house calls may have gathered information on the patient's place of living and factored this into their analysis. While some doctors in parts of the world still visit people at their homes, this has not been a common practice for many decades and perhaps even a half-century and longer in most parts of the world practicing modern medicine.

The advent of telemedicine can provide a window into a patient's living spaces, yet the inclusion of an evaluation process of their patient's location is still uncommon at this time.

So perhaps now, revisiting the concept of a doctor visiting and viewing the patient's built environments to help provide information and data about building conditions is not so far-fetched.

Why Architects and Designers Should Include the Trifold of Healthy, Green, and Sustainable Building

There is no doubt that the topics of climate change and health in the built environment have become of greater concern in the past twenty-plus years.

However, I would say we're about 40 years behind what people in the '60s and '70s were warning us about. In this section, I'm going to talk about the cause-effect relationship of the built environment on both of these topics, as well as the reasons why you can't separate the issues of green, sustainable, and healthy building moving forward into the future.

The main reason you cannot separate these topics is that if we foresee a future that supports better health and wellness for humans and the entire planet, these topics will all have to be recognized as integrally connected. You cannot separate biological health from ecological health, and each of these topics relates to each other.

In discussing these reasons, I think history can have a role as a learning process and show potential patterns. The trajectory of this history can be utilized to plan for more strategic solutions. With that said, this history is not that far from the past and can be referenced from a mere 50 - 60 years ago. In the world of architecture, this is a mere speck on the timeline of history.

However, what's important to note is that never in recorded history have we seen human developments have such a massive impact on the planet's ecosystems and humanity's health.

Since the 1960s and 1970s, there have been plenty of warning signs to heed, and perhaps none is as prevalent and epic as the Cuyahoga river spontaneously catching fire. For those unfamiliar with this story, the Cuyahoga river became a dumping location in Ohio's industrial section from the

Industrial Revolution onward. It became so toxic from the chemicals being dumped into the river that the river spontaneously caught on fire. And not just once, but multiple times.[78]

For all creatures on this planet, such as humans, who consist of around 70 percent water, the idea that water spontaneously combusts should be terrifying.

This issue of massive industrial pollutants being siphoned into the Cuyahoga river significantly impacted the industry's environmental rules and contributed to creating the Environmental Protection Agency (EPA).[79] It should also show us that these issues should be monitored to prevent such environmental and biological tragedies.

And then, as mentioned previously, in the 1970s, the shortage of petroleum as the primary energy source brought up a more prominent topic to evaluate, which is the dependency on fossil fuels. In the 1981 Special Edition of National Geographic titled "Energy," this critical topic garnered the attention to such a point that the magazine's entire issue was focused on these topics of fuel, energy, and the potential of alternative options in the future.[80] The magazine issue not only focused on energy but also on the many facets of energy, including human and biological health.

If you have the chance to read this, it can provide meaningful recognition of a pattern emerging from the 1960s into the 80s, which can be traced to pioneers such as Rachel Carson and her book *Silent Spring*. While the mainstream and science community of her time ignored her work and warnings, advocates of environmental concerns in the 60s and 70s brought up these same issues. Even prominent magazines such as National Geographic seemed to be ignored by the masses when they created this special edition on this matter. This 1981 National Geographic publication was in contrast to an emerging change of mindsets from the energy and environmental concerns of the 1960s and '70s. In the USA, this was perhaps best summed up by the 1987 movie character Gordon Gecko, who stated, "Greed is Good"[81] in the movie *Wall Street*. It was the mantra of many corporations and of the people who benefited from such developments.

However, this spurred many grassroots movements of the time. From the 1990s onward, many individuals and groups have turned away from the assumption that companies and government would enforce healthy policies and have taken it upon themselves to devote their lives towards solutions.

Those such as Amory Lovins of the Rocky Mountain Institute (RMI) have been advocates for change and a voice of reason, even previous to his quoted words in the National Geographic magazine from 1981.[82]

As a result of many of these concerns of both energy and ecology, many groups began to seek alternate solutions to the mainstream energy sources of fossil fuels. These "alternative" sources have become more well known today as solar, wind, and geothermal power, to name just a few of the alternatives.

I'd say, based on the trajectory of their developments, they have occurred in the following chronological order – *Green Building* and *Sustainable Building* in similar timeframes, followed by the emerging field of *Healthy Building*.

As mentioned earlier, green building is often focused on the science of researching the energy impacts and the reduction of energy use in buildings. Whether this is focused on the insulation of old and new buildings or the use of higher efficiency heating and cooling systems, the focal point is often "energy efficiency." And by reducing fossil fuel dependency and increasing the energy efficiency of buildings' electricity demands, this can help decrease the 40 percent of the world's energy expenditure used in building creation and use.

Global Warming and Climate Change – Different Name, Same Purpose & Important Progress

Around the same time, sustainable building became a hot topic, quite literally. This is based on one of many topics focused on global warming concerns. Sustainable building is often focused on the environmental considerations or impact that the built environment has on the ecology, both the local and global impacts.

This approach often strives to reduce the use of manufactured materials to reduce the excess materials from the building waste cycle. These design approaches typically range from the initial landscaping in building the structure to the materials and methods of how they impact the environment. And, of course, the long term effects that the building has on the location, the planet, and the occupants in the building.

Essentially, many core tenets of sustainable building have the mantra of using fewer materials, having less impact on the environment, and removing the "cradle to grave" concept. This coincides with the common terms today of the *Circular Economy*. This view is often striving to transcend the mindset of how products are made, used, and deposited when they are finished being utilized. The common modern perspective is that these products will go to the landfill or be sent away when they are finished being used. As many will state striving to achieve these goals, there is no "away."

The Circular Economy, Sustainability, and the Cycles of Life as Spiracycles

What is meant by the phrase "cradle to grave" is that, too often, there is a linear viewpoint of products and building processes. This linear idea starts with the manufacturing or birth of a product (cradle) to the end use of the product that is discarded and sent to the landfill (grave). From the production and use of the product, this linear path becomes garbage or trash after use. This linear mindset is in juxtaposition with how the systems of nature function.

And this term is used in opposition to "cradle to cradle," a term discussed earlier made common by William McDonough and Michael Braungart in their book *Cradle to Cradle*.[83] Cradle to cradle denotes a circular process. Circular means that when the product is no longer being used at its end of life, it can then be recycled or repurposed into something else. As opposed to the linear process of cradle to grave, the circular process can continue repeatedly.

If this repurposing of a product can only be done a few times or cycles, then this is referred to as "downcycling." This means that each time it is recycled or reused, it degrades or downgrades in quality to the point where eventually, it will become waste or garbage.

If it can be "upcycled," then each time it is reused, it does not degrade and can be used in perpetuity. This is how nature's ecological systems function. Each time a living creature is born, from a plant to an animal, it uses the materials of nature to become a living organism. At the end of life, the physical body dies and then returns to its original material components through decomposition. In this process, it returns to the soil to its initial material components. And as nutrients, it then becomes materials for other organisms in which to live and grow. Each time these natural materials are utilized, they return to nature and are not degraded. In this manner, they can exist as the same components in perpetuity.

This life cycle evaluation process is referred to as Life Cycle Assessment (LCA).

The concept of a circular economy, or cradle to cradle, is essentially based on a product's end of life becoming the beginning of life for another product. Ideally, this occurs without any degradation to the quality of the materials.

I utilize the term spiracycle to define these processes as they circle around and either degrade in quality and spiral downward, or maintain quality and the cycle spirals upward.

Integrative Architecture and Next Steps in the World of Architecture and Building

If we focus on human health, especially in preventing illness, we should be looking at the built environment and recognizing that people in the modern-day are spending up to 90 percent of their time indoors.[84]

What new design approaches can be taken to prevent illness and support wellness as a proactive process?

As to the design process, what can be recognized is that the single home or building is critical in addressing these issues. This is because a general blueprint in approaching these building solutions is that the single building often leads to multiple buildings, eventually leading to our cities.

As such, the single structure's DNA is actually the blueprint for the entire city or a major influence on cities. If each building is designed in a functionally similar manner, then this single design "DNA" will eventually influence a whole city as the "DNA of the city."

So it matters that the individual structure has a solid blueprint and DNA to address these trifold topics to provide green, sustainable, and healthy buildings. Fundamentally, the focus on all three will impact the individuals who reside in that single building, but the multiplication of such buildings forming a city eventually defines the DNA of the city itself.

And this is an important reason why I have listed these three topics in this order. It provides a bit of background about how these issues came to be, including the motivating factors and the resulting methods in researching better solutions.

While, historically, some of these individual solutions and developments have caused issues, the initial intention of finding and seeking solutions provided a framework for today's energy-efficient and sustainable design solutions. Fortunately for us, in the 21st century, the pioneering research and experimentation from decades past have provided many solutions and more in-depth knowledge of these issues for current day results.

While sick building syndrome brought great awareness to these topics in the mid to late 80s, it wasn't until the 1990s that healthy building became a topic that more designers and architects began pursuing.

All of these developments have room for improvement, yet if we are aware of these challenges, we can build upon this knowledge for best practices and helpful solutions.

Nurturing Architecture - Including Emotional and Mental Wellness

While the above topics discuss the many facets of green, sustainable, and healthy building, these are focused on the physical health of the occupants

An Overview of Mental, Physical, and Emotional Wellness in the Built Environment

Physical Wellness

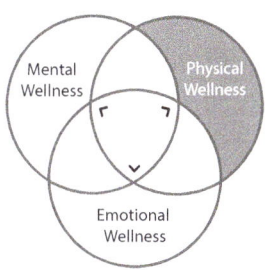

Are you surrounded by stagnant, polluted air? Are there chemicals and chemical smells in your space all day? Are getting enough sunlight? Is your body being cared for and allowing for topics such as ergonomic functionality? Are you around constant stress? What is this impact on your physical wellness and your immune system?

Mental Wellness

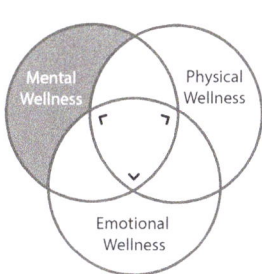

Do you have the ability to think clearly? Is the space you're in comforting for your mind or chaotic in sights, sounds, and thinking as well as sensory stress? How does this affect your mindset? What impact does this have on your ability to concentrate, on your mental wellness, and on your immune system?

Emotional Wellness

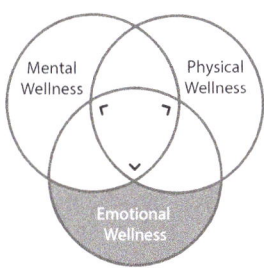

Are you surrounded by loud noises and a chaotic emotional environment? How does this affect your nervous system? Are the sights, sounds, smells, and sensory inputs impacting your emotional wellness? What impact does this have on your stress levels, your emotional wellness, and on your immune system?

and the ecology. What should also be included in great architecture is the inclusion of emotional and mental or psychological wellness.

In defining Architectural Medicine, I discuss the reason why I do not use the term healthy building to define these topics and, instead, utilize Architectural Medicine as the defining term. This is due to healthy building most often being used to define the physical impacts the building has on the occupants.

However, Architectural Medicine includes all facets of human health — physically, emotionally, and mentally or psychologically. In this manner, Architectural Medicine considers all of these topics and not just physical health.

For many, the concept of architecture impacting your emotional and mental health may sound abstract. Yet, the more time you spend reflecting on how your environment influences your health in these realms, the easier it is to see how much the built environment impacts your overall health.

These topics of physical, emotional, and mental wellness can be defined as another triad of graphics in the following diagram:

The Intersection of Mental, Physical, and Emotional Wellness in the Built Environment

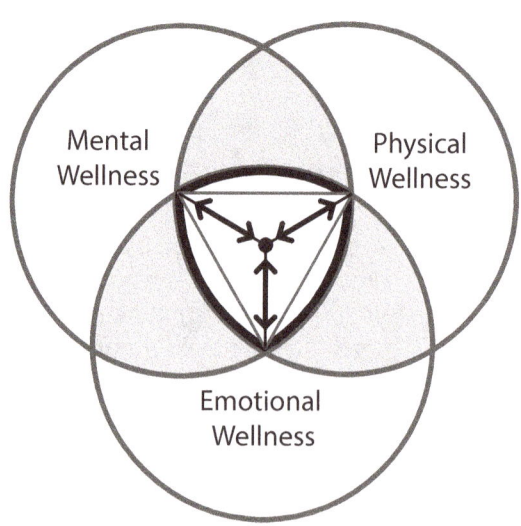

The Topics of Mental, Physical, and Emotional Wellness in the Built Environment

Are you performing at your optimal potential? Or are you feeling gray, foggy, and lacking energy?

The Result: Spaces that are geared towards the mental development and utilization, yet also considering the physical health and wellness of the occupants.

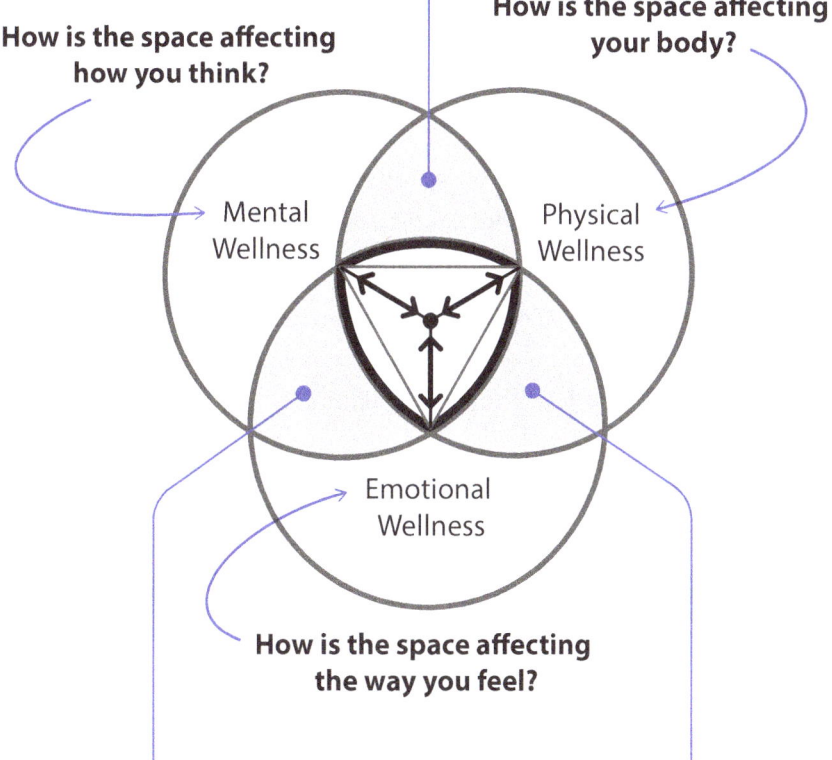

How is the space affecting how you think?

How is the space affecting your body?

Mental Wellness

Physical Wellness

Emotional Wellness

How is the space affecting the way you feel?

The Result: Spaces that are geared towards the mental development and utilization, while also considering the emotional well being of the person.

The Result: Spaces that are geared towards the physical health and wellness of the occupants, while also attending to the emotional needs of the occupants.

The ideal focus of Integrative Architecture is to combine the best of many approaches, materials, and methods for best practices in a similar format that Integrative Medicine achieves this combination of medical modalities for best practices. I originally came up with Integrative Architecture as I was inspired by Dr. Andrew Weil's processes and those who have championed Integrative Medicine.

This is critical to state, and while much of this book does focus on building health processes, evaluations, and considerations from the perspective of the physical body, you cannot separate these building impacts on the physical body alone. In order to view these topics of building health, you have to consider the whole person, and this includes the emotional and mental impacts that the built environment has on human health.

These subjects will be included in later chapters with processes that can be included in the evaluation process, yet as they are complex topics within themselves, they do require more details that cannot be properly addressed in this book.

I write more about each of these subjects in the book *Architectural Medicine* and will also discuss these topics of architecture and building in the forthcoming book — *Integrative Architecture.*

A Summary of Integrative Architecture and the Future of Architecture

This is just one example of the importance of Integrative Architecture and the importance of providing building solutions that consist of systems, and not just pieces that are placed together without much rhyme or reason. Moving forward into the future, it will become vital that this approach to architecture is achieved in a way that supports integrative solutions using intelligence, caring, and wisdom.

By understanding how all the pieces fit together and not just taking several design elements and placing them together without a systems approach, it can be the difference between a future that embraces necessary changes for a less detrimental impact on people and the planet versus a dystopic future.

As I mentioned previously, healthy building is often focused on physical health, whereas Architectural Medicine includes the facets of physical, emotional, and mental wellness. The interconnection of the topics of Integrative Architecture and Integrative Medicine highlights the processes of Architectural Medicine as outlined in the following diagrams:

The Double Triad of Architectural Medicine – Health and Wellness in the Built Environment

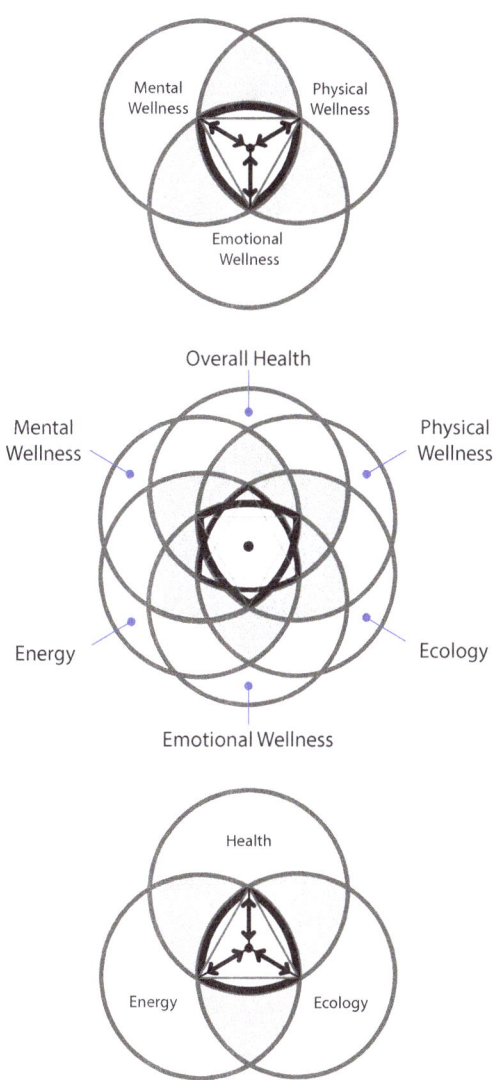

The Double Triad of Architectural Medicine: Health and Wellness in the Built Environment

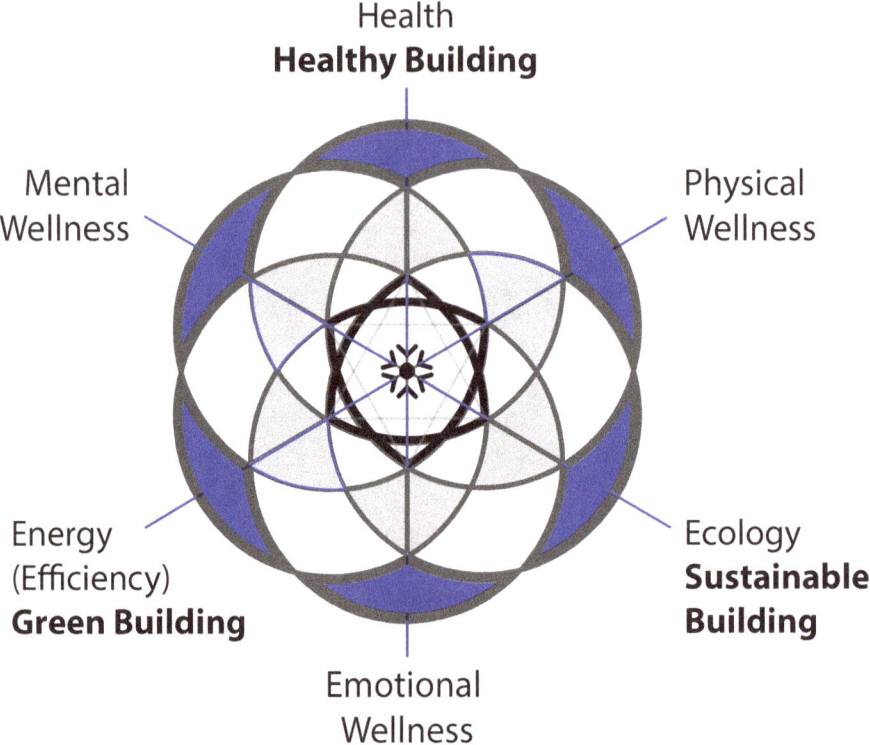

It's critical to understand how these facets fit and work together in the field of architecture, and not just for the structural integrity, energy efficiency, and sustainability of the building. Yet also to ensure that the health of the occupants is cared for and designed into the blueprint of the building plans.

This can be seen in the issues discussed earlier caused by the creation of airtight buildings. Providing a solution for one issue, that of energy efficiency, yet causing another problem resulting in negative impacts on the health of the occupants.

In this manner, there is a big picture Rx as a prescription or recipe that can be integrated into the building blueprints. The result is the support of optimum health and wellness for the inhabitants and planetary health.

As I mentioned in a previous paragraph, in the near future, I will be publishing a book titled *Integrative Architecture*, which will have more details with examples of these integrated systems and the benefits they can provide for future architecture. In chapter 15, I continue to discuss this overlap of Integrative Architecture and Integrative Medicine and how these approaches overlap to form Architectural Medicine. For now, this provides a baseline foundation for discussions on Architectural Medicine and the Architectural Doctor.

Moving Forward - Integrative Architecture and Architectural Medicine

In this chapter, I strived to provide the context of Integrative Architecture relative to Architectural Medicine, and in doing so, provided a baseline for the rest of the topics of this book to be built upon. Each of the topics in this book requires strategic solutions for each profession, yet it's critical that these solutions include the many facets that overlap. Otherwise, many important steps will exclude important components leading to further problems. Solving one problem can often create more problems if the entire scenario is not evaluated. And this requires that professionals work together in ways that previously have not existed. This is where the Architectural Doctor can help bridge such gaps and provide overlap in unfamiliar territory for many professionals working together for the first time.

These steps require new systems for each group to work together, ensuring that each facet of the whole is considered and factored into the big equation for solutions. And now that we have some context and a foundation of these topics, we can delve into more details of how these two fields can become more integrated.

And speaking of systems, in the next chapter, we'll delve right into these whole system benefits as I discuss the *Architectural Medicine System (AMS)*...

"You never change things by fighting the existing reality.
To change something, build a new model that
makes the existing model obsolete."

– R. Buckminster Fuller

THE ARCHITECTURAL MEDICINE SYSTEM (AMS)

In previous chapters, I've discussed the importance of systems to achieve better health in the built environment. In this chapter, I will provide the details of these specifics. To start, the trajectory of this path has taken time to develop, and while there is much written about the topic of health in the built environment, there are still large gaps in providing solutions. This is where a system can support the integration of many professions, which can utilize new knowledge and apply research in practical and usable formats.

The key is to have systems in place where each professional can implement this knowledge into their workflows and have solutions that coordinate with other professionals as a cohesive whole. To achieve this, several important components have to be in place.

The Pulse of the Healthy Built Environment

The first is each professional's ability to understand these facets and be trained and familiar with processes in achieving these goals. The second is to have standards in place and to be aware of potential issues that each professional will need to navigate. And the third is to have a system in place for each professional, with functioning procedures providing integrations between professions.

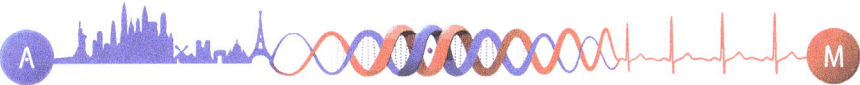

With this in place, a system can be utilized to provide better building solutions focused on health. Having this foundation upon which standards are developed and processes and procedures can be built upon, can achieve the goal of healthier built environments.

Uncharted Territory for Architecture and Medicine

In this chapter, I will have to admit that I am going into details where some basic protocols are utilized in the real world and many that are in their infancy. This will be a chapter that is interwoven with experimental and practical processes with much room for development.

This is also a main goal of the Architectural Doctor – to support the development and procedures for health in the built environment moving forward.

In the previous chapter, we discussed some of the histories of these developments. While we have much to learn from this history, there are more nuances and developments to address in the current day. This chapter will provide an outline that can be used with new steps to achieve these goals.

With that stated, what exactly is the *Architectural Medicine System (AMS)*? Let's dive into this topic, as it is an essential core of Architectural Medicine.

An Overview of the Architectural Medicine System (AMS)

In chapter 3, in discussing the Architectural Doctor, I provided a graphic to highlight the processes of Architectural Medicine that currently do not exist. Yet if the built environment is to be evaluated for better human health, this needs to be included. This graphic brought attention to the fact that the current models of a physician's analysis of their patient's health often do not include the built environment.

The Architectural Medicine System (AMS) is an integrated set of procedures that allows the built environment to be included in patient health and the health of the general public at large. And so, how does this integration occur? How do we put these concepts into reality and practice?

As we delve into these topics of systems, let's first discuss systems and their purpose.

A Systems Approach – Connections Between Architecture and Medicine

While there have been great strides in the emerging fields of health in the built environment, a big part of what makes this book different is the focus on systems. In my honest opinion, a cohesive systems approach in a multi-disciplinary format is key to providing healthier built environments for current and future architecture.

And by systems, I am referring to the fact that there are few evaluations provided between the worlds of building and architecture and the worlds of medicine and health. With people spending from 60 to 90 percent of their lives inside architecture, the fact that we are rarely factoring building health into the equation of wellness, is to me, strange.

The fact that so much time is spent indoors with so many potential pollutants and impacts that buildings can have on health, the lack of methodologies in place to examine these issues is often a perplexing scenario for me to understand. The question of why there is an absence of better systems in place to evaluate these topics, along with few standard processes evaluating building health in diagnosing ailments, seems odd to me. If you follow the latest research on health in the built environment, you will find there is an increasing depth of information defining issues that can provide positive benefits for health professionals in supporting the best health for their patients.

Why haven't these topics become more common, and why haven't the professions integrated this knowledge into their work sooner?

At times, I am both perplexed and not surprised based on my personal experience working in construction and the architecture fields. What I've learned over the years is that it's often not a lack of interest or concern, it's usually a question of how to achieve these goals.

How are doctors and health professionals supposed to include the built environment in their evaluations? They aren't trained to go into buildings to inspect and find potential health culprits. And even if they did find these issues, perhaps akin to the previous doctor's home visit, what would a doctor do about a possible health issue they have found? Would they write an Rx as a prescription for a healthier building solution for architecture professionals to solve?

The answer right now to this is an obvious no, yet a follow up to this question is "why not?"

My answer to why these solutions do not yet exist is that there have not been systems for these two professionals to work together to provide such evaluations, and a lack of systems to follow up on health issues in buildings. The methods of how this research can be applied in a practical format for the medical and architecture fields have been unclear.

What's missing are systems for each of these professions to work together to manifest these solutions. And what's missing is an Rx or a prescription for health and wellness in the built environment to be achieved.

What's meant by this is that in terms of doctors and architects having a system in place akin to, say, the process of ordering a blood test or MRI is practically non-existent. Even if a doctor were to evaluate a patient's condition and see possible connections to the built environment, what would a doctor do about this? And even if there were health issues found in the built environment, how would the doctor request inspections or building solutions if needed?

An Rx for better building health does not yet exist, yet perhaps moving forward, it should, and, hint, this is an interoperability topic I discuss in the next chapter defined as ARxMD.

As an example of systems that are in place and the successful procedures that this can achieve, you can view an architect working with an engineer to establish design specifications. In this case, a process and system is in place that allows the architect to proceed with proper analysis and receive the requested results from the engineers. In this manner, the architect is familiar with the systems to work with the engineer and vice versa. These systems are in place for both professions to know the procedures and to proceed with the creation of solutions.

Another example is the procedures of a doctor and a nurse, where systems are in place to provide health evaluations for the patient. This includes the diagnosis of the doctor, and when a blood test is required, the doctor communicates with the nurse to provide this procedure to be completed. This includes laboratory testing processes and documentation, such as an electronic health record (EHR) updated with the results. As all professionals involved are familiar with the steps and protocols to accomplish this course of action, a complex system can be navigated with proper solutions.

From lab testing to engineering evaluations for the doctor and architect, respectively, these procedures, along with the education on these topics, have allowed developments to evolve in the fields of both architecture and medicine.

However, when it comes to health topics related to the built environment, most doctors are not trained or educated on what to look for. This includes potential red flags and procedures to take if the built environment might be the cause of symptoms or conditions.

As well, the architecture field is not trained nor educated about health topics and may not be aware of building processes and materials that may cause health issues and how to resolve such problems.

In the current building and health fields, there may be a focus on physical building materials and topics such as lead, mold, and general indoor air quality, yet many other issues related to health, such as building toxins, particulates, and a lack of natural lighting and noise levels are generally not taught.

When you add building topics related to environmental psychology and neuroscience in architecture, you can find that many facets of health and wellness are not included in patient and public health. All of these topics have impacts on physical, mental, and emotional health and well being.

An architect must be aware of these topics and include them in the overall design process, just as ergonomics and anthropometrics are factored into the design equation. And a doctor should have knowledge of these topics as potential issues related to their patient's diagnosis and overall health.

Many gaps exist for each profession, and the most significant gap is probably the lack of systems in place where a doctor can work with an architect, and an architect can work with a doctor. The lack of systems, lack of education, and lack of training have led to these topics being more conceptual than actionable.

To revisit this comment on systems, these two professions of architecture and medicine are arguably two of the most demanding careers in terms of training and education. They already have tremendously complex systems to navigate to achieve their high level of capabilities. And so, adding additional steps to their already systemized processes without proper procedures is not exactly fair to these professionals.

When you begin to think about all of the steps and procedures required for this process to happen as outlined in this book, you will soon see that many processes do not currently exist. These new processes also require several new types of professionals – the Architectural Doctor, the Building

Informaticist, and the Healthy Building Inspector.

An essential part of Architectural Medicine and the Architectural Doctor is to support these integrations, both in terms of education, teaching, and knowledge, as well as providing interconnected systems. This can support the doctor and architect to work together and utilize this knowledge for both of their professions. These integrated systems can provide bridges allowing for collaboration.

It is also critical that the many other professionals involved become part of the system, such as the above mentioned building informaticist and healthy building inspector. Each can be trained to look for structural issues in the building and issues related to health. This information can be critical in working with the doctors and architects to evaluate and resolve building health issues.

The Architectural Doctor, which in many ways can help build these bridges between professions to support the multi-disciplinary process required, is a central focus and an important part of achieving the goal of better health in buildings.

While this may sound extensive, it is also critical to consider it as an investment toward human health. Taking steps to provide integrated solutions as systems can offer better health and wellness for humanity at large.

What is meant by system solutions? To begin, let's review the comments above about the doctor needing to evaluate one's built environment to gain insights into potential health issues. These steps can begin the process required to focus on issues that can be resolved. And that is step one – an Rx as a prescription for a healthier built environment.

This alone requires a few steps. The first is to include the doctor's evaluation of ailments in their analysis, so they are aware of potential health issues related to the built environment. Once that is achieved, there is a need for connections between the doctor and a building informaticist, and a healthy building inspector so that a building evaluation can be reviewed. This is akin to a doctor ordering lab testing for blood work or an X-ray or MRI to provide analysis and insights. This may sound strange right now, yet a hundred years ago, a doctor requesting an MRI or blood test would have also sounded strange.

This process would also require a Building Informaticist and a Healthy Building Inspector trained in such evaluations of buildings related to health issues. Currently, the typical building inspector does not look for health issues unless they are related to building issues in an indirect manner. For example, mold problems might trigger water infiltration issues related to the integrity of the building materials. However, the average building inspector would not be reviewing most of the building for problems related to health. And they would need to be trained on these protocols and trained in working directly with doctors and health professionals. The discovery of lead paint and asbestos, as examples, can flag issues that are directly related to health. And so, there are a few inspections that do focus on occupant health that can be used as examples to build upon.

What can be seen in the above sentences are more systems required to make these evaluations and overlap between professions in the building and health field to occur.

Then, of course, if there are issues found, the architecture and building professionals would need to help provide the required building solutions. This would mean that architects and the construction fields would need to be trained on these issues, in both preventing them from occurring in the future and resolving them when they are found.

And there is also another facet of training and education these integrations require in connecting the inspectors to the builders with the doctors. Ideally, this is where the Architectural Doctor can help bridge these different fields and act as a liaison between the many professionals involved along the way. And of course, the patient as the client is also essential to keep in the loop, and the role of the Architectural Doctor can assist with this as well.

The process of creating healthier built environments requires systems to be in place, including training and education. This includes working with different professionals, who are often outside of the scope with which each professional is typically working with. The overlap between doctors and architects working together is rare, yet in order for these systems to function, this must change.

What Are Systems?

If you've been reading to this point in the book, you may have noticed an extensive use of word origins and the etymology of words. It is true that I do love these word origins, yet the reasons why are based on insights and the clarity this brings forth to terminologies. And this includes the origins of the word "system" in providing deeper insights into why systems are critical in bridging these fields:

system (n.)

1610s, "the whole creation, the universe," from Late Latin systema "an arrangement, system," from Greek systema "organized whole, a whole compounded of parts," from stem of synistanai "to place together, organize, form in order," from syn- "together" (see syn-) + root of histanai "cause to stand," from PIE root *sta- "to stand, make or be firm."[85]

The Oxford Dictionary defines a system as:

- An organized or connected group of things.
- A group or set of related or associated things perceived or thought of as a unity or complex whole.
- A collection of natural objects, features, or phenomena considered as or forming a connected or complex whole.[86]

The idea of a large group of professions working together to evaluate, analyze, define, discuss, and then provide solutions for the patient's health is a perfect example of a complex, functional system. This concept of a system as an integrated whole of parts that are placed together for organization fits into the overall goals of Architectural Medicine.

It also requires many facets to fit together with precision, along with the sharing of data and training that crosses disciplines for quality results. If you view this as a whole, these are very complicated processes. Yet if you take each part and focus on the evaluations of each group involved, it can allow for manageable segments for synergistic benefits.

The key is to provide each group with the segment appropriate for their profession. This part of the puzzle is then connected to the other segments in a meaningful and useful format. And this is where the system itself can provide steps for each profession, yet connect these steps in sharing data and reporting as a cohesive solution.

Systems and Ecosystems

Since the early 21st century, the term ecosystem has been used as a buzzword to discuss and define many types of "whole systems." What's fascinating about this, at least in my worldview, is the actual definition of an ecosystem:

eco-

word-forming element referring to the environment and man's relation to it, abstracted from ecology, ecological; attested from 1969.[87]

ecology (n.)

1873, oecology, "branch of science dealing with the relationship of living things to their environments," coined in German by German zoologist Ernst Haeckel as Ökologie, from Greek oikos "house, dwelling place, habitation" (from PIE root *weik- (1) "clan") + -logia "study of" (see -logy).[88]

The origins of the word eco is based on the Greek word oikos, which is defined as "house, dwelling place, habitation."[89] What can be gleaned from this is the use of common terms used today prefaced with eco, as that which refers to our places of habitation – our homes and places of dwelling.

Ponder this for a moment and recognize the power of how a word prefix – often used by many as an off the cuff generalization for whole systems – is defined as a study of our place of habitation, our homes, and places of dwelling.

This word "system" is based on the word origin "syn," which means together, combined with "cause to stand, from PIE root *sta- to stand, make or be firm."[90] If systems are a combination of many parts put together to stand firm, then this can illuminate the many processes which the Architectural Medicine System (AMS) is putting together.

This process is achieved by creating steps that can be taken to address the many potential building health issues. And because these different parts include many different professions, this ventures into new territory for both the building and health professions.

What Systems Would Be Required for These Integrations?

In the following flowchart, the first step involves the doctor's evaluation of the patient's condition. In this process, it is recognized that a potential cause of the patient's health issue is related to their built environment.

For there to be a proper evaluation, the next step is for an evaluation of the building to be provided by the healthy building inspector or a building informaticist. This also requires a process for the inspection to take place and the data to be recorded. These results, along with any appropriate laboratory tests, can provide a better picture of the building health issues to be included in the evaluation process. These steps include the informaticist and the inspector's procedures and protocols, which are also new to both the doctor and the typical building inspector.

With this building data, the doctor and health professionals can better evaluate the health for their patient. And if and when there are building issues found that are negatively impacting the patient's health, then the next step is to involve the building professionals. This is done by exchanging appropriate building data discovered by the inspection and informaticist and provided for the architect to review for solutions.

As a side note, there are many graphics throughout this book and it may be challenging to see all the details. I have provided a link to many of the core graphics in this book for online viewing. They can be viewed using the QR code or at the following link:

https://architecturalmedicine.com/book

This unique process can be a collaboration between all professionals involved, from doctor, inspector, and informaticist to the architect and the Architectural Doctor. The insights that each professional can convey can help with ensuring that all facets of the solutions are supporting the patient and occupant's health. These solutions are the building Rx as prescriptions for better health and wellness in the patient's building.

And to ensure that all facets are included, the patient is also a critical component to add into these discussions, so that they are properly informed and updated as to next steps and the procedures that will be required to solve the building issues.

This process results in building procedures to fix the issues and a follow up inspection and evaluation of these solutions. This results in a final report for the doctor, Architectural Doctor, and health professionals to review, and the data of these processes recorded in the EHR.

The Architectural Medicine System (AMS) Flowchart

The first flowchart is the entire diagram as an overview of the complete Architectural Medicine System (AMS). While the following text on the whole chart is very small, on the following pages, the graphics provide larger views of the flowchart.

The flowchart has a number of segments that have more details, including an expanded version for each of the main processes. On the left of the whole graphic is the main flowchart, and on the right are the expanded components. These expanded components are signified as "AM" with the subsequent number denoting the location of each step. I will also note that the flowchart key has "training" listed, and these extended details are included in chapter 11, when discussing the training steps providing the professionals with more information on each procedure.

Over the next several pages, the flowchart will be shown in more detail with larger views. The main steps are listed as the Architectural Medicine System (AMS) flowchart, parts 1 through 4. These sections are comprised of five detailed expansions listed as "AM-1" through "AM-5."

The Architectural Doctor – An Rx for Health & Wellness in Buildings Part I

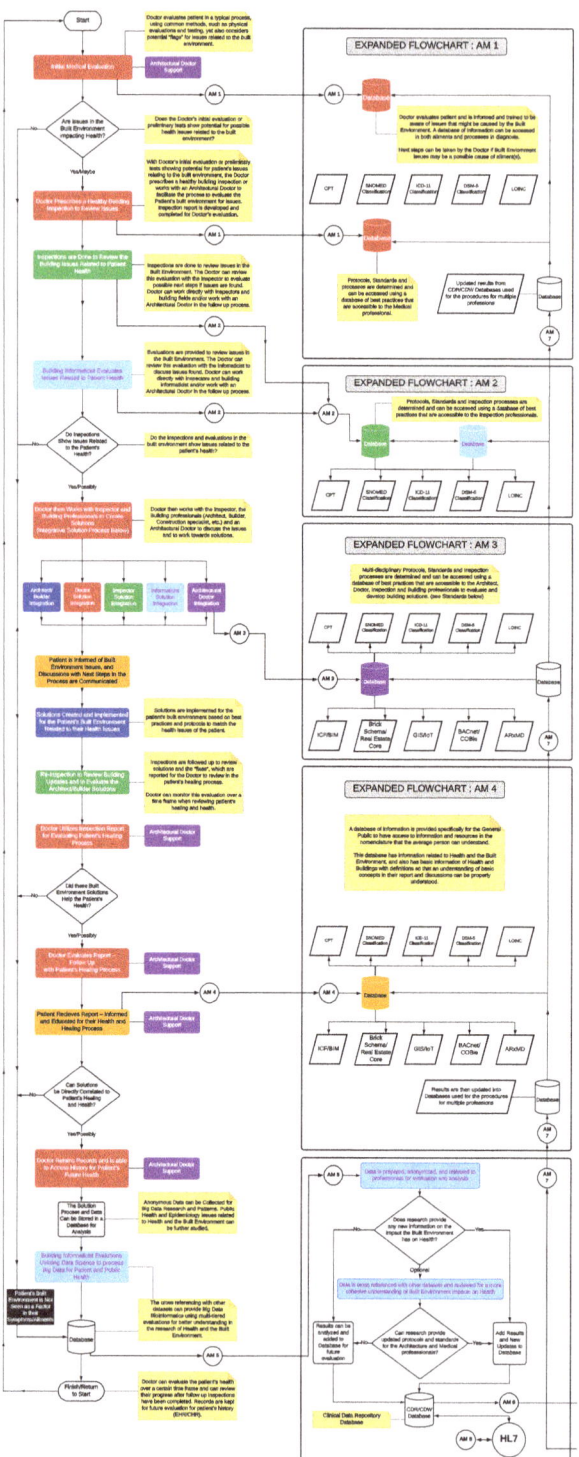

Key to Diagrams

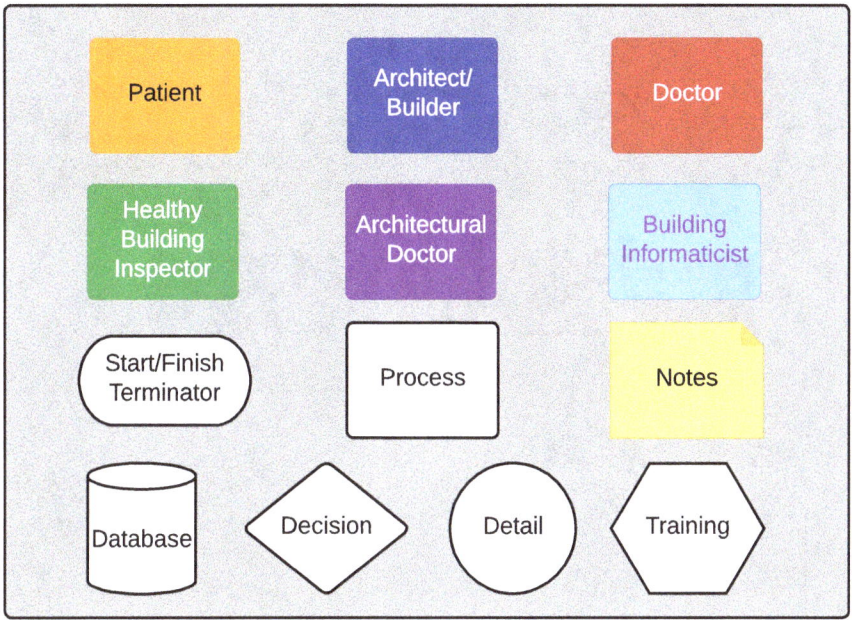

Please note that segment AM-5 consists of multiple connectors from AM-5 to AM-8. As you view these graphics, you will note that AM-7 and AM-8 consist of big data and data science details that provide an iterative system supplying updates to each of the professions involved. As you view the expanded flowchart sections, note the database providing updates are from these extended informatics listed from AM-5 to AM-8.

These procedures provide beneficial improvements from datasets attained through these inspections, evaluations, and results, which are then provided for further analysis by informatics and data science professionals. By including many other professionals, such as epidemiologists, toxicologists, and public health experts, the resulting datasets provided, after ensuring anonymity, can result in an extensive field of data that is often not included in health informatics.

It is this inclusion of datasets, provided by the inspector and building informaticist, that can yield a tremendous increase in data for built environment issues to be included with the overlap of patient health.

The Architectural Medicine System (AMS) Flowchart

Part 1 of 4

Start → **Initial Medical Evaluation** — *Architectural Doctor Support*

> Doctor evaluates patient in a typical process, using common SOAP note methods, such as physical evaluations and testing, yet also considers potential "flags" for issues related to the built environment.

→ **AM 1**

Are issues in the Built Environment impacting Health?

> Does the Doctor's initial evaluation or preliminary tests show potential for possible health issues related to the built environment?

- No → (loops back to Start)
- Yes/Maybe ↓

Doctor Prescribes a Healthy Building Inspection to Review Issues

> With Doctor's initial evaluation or preliminary tests showing potential for patient's issues relating to the built environment, the Doctor prescribes a healthy building inspection as Rx or works with an Architectural Doctor to facilitate the process to evaluate the Patient's built environment for issues. Inspection report is developed and completed for Doctor's evaluation.

→ **AM 1**

Inspections are Done to Review the Building Issues Related to Patient Health

> Inspections are done to review issues in the Built Environment. The Doctor can review this evaluation with the Inspector to evaluate possible next steps if issues are found. Doctor can work directly with inspectors and building fields and/or work with an Architectural Doctor in the follow up process.

→ **AM 2**

115

Chapter: 5   The Architectural Medicine System (AMS)

The Architectural Medicine System (AMS) Expanded Section

Part 1 of 4

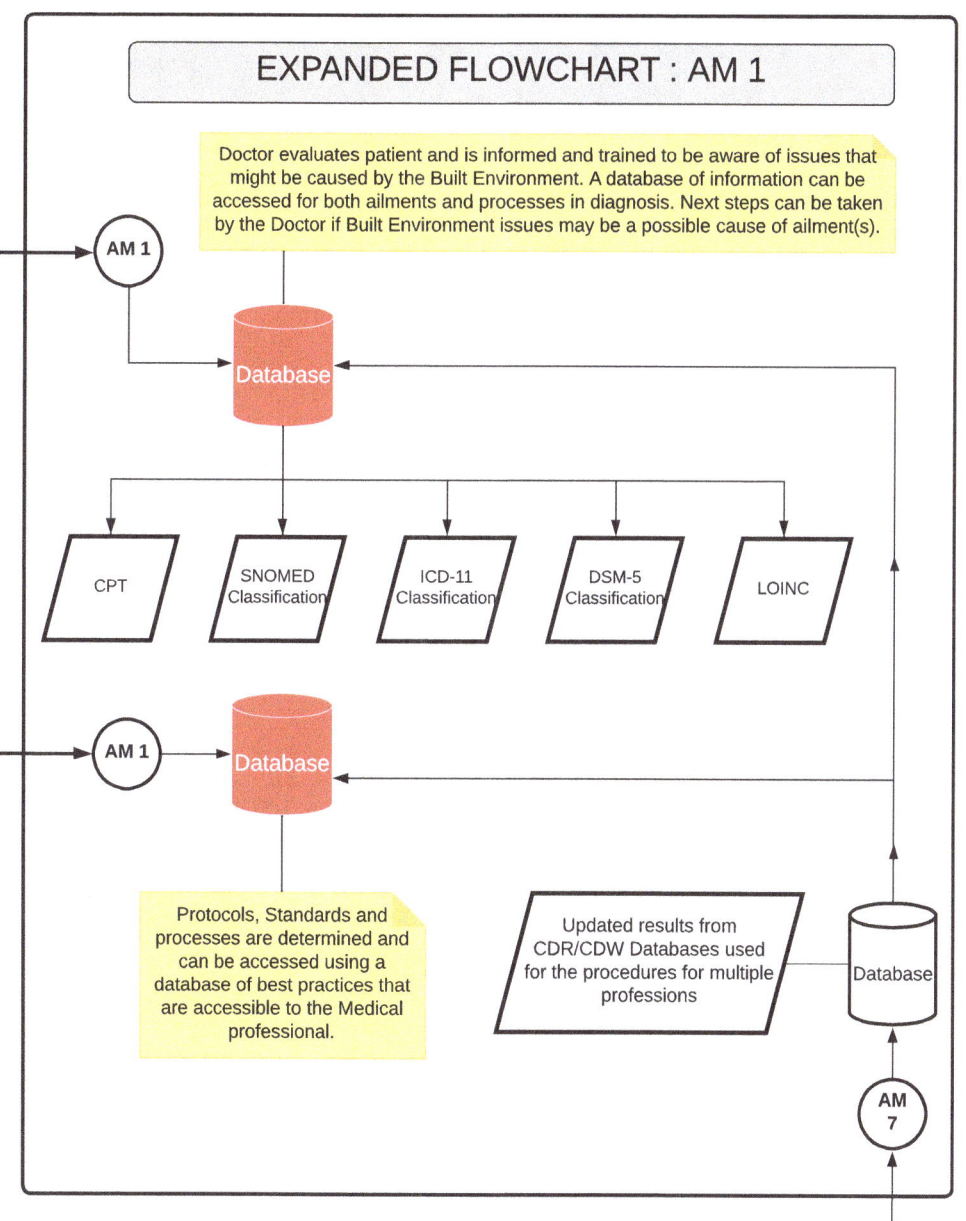

The Architectural Medicine System (AMS) Flowchart
Part 2 of 4

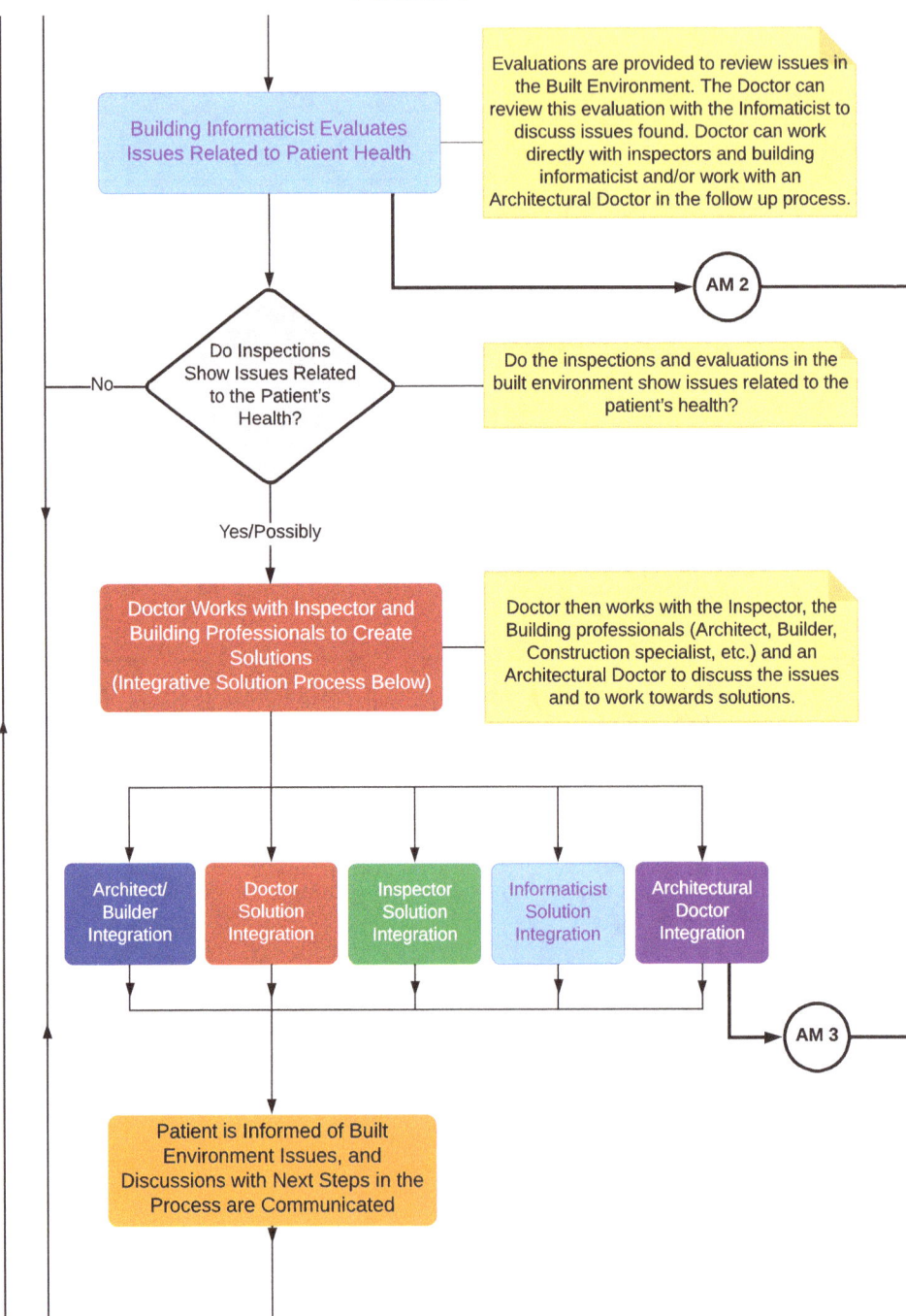

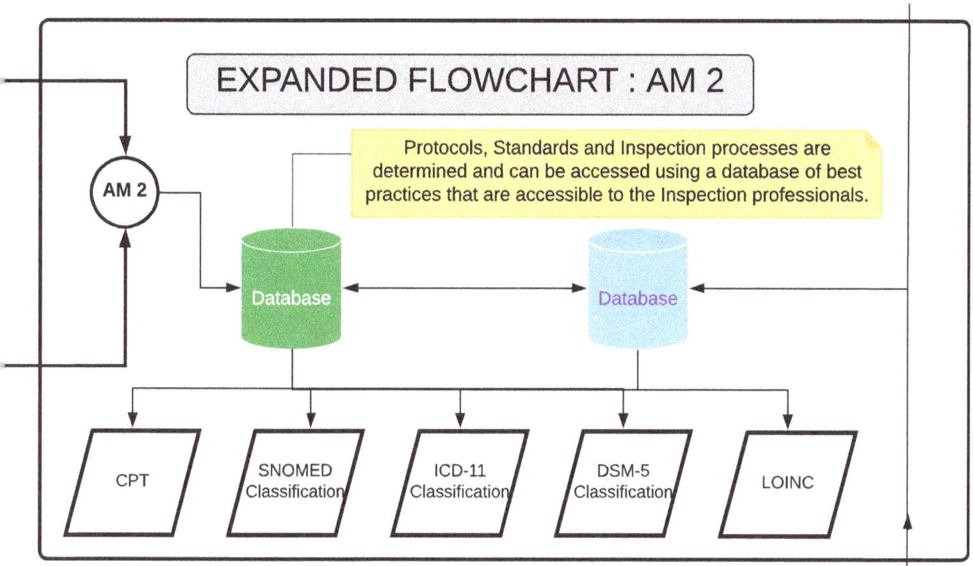

EXPANDED FLOWCHART : AM 2

AM 2

Protocols, Standards and Inspection processes are determined and can be accessed using a database of best practices that are accessible to the Inspection professionals.

Database → Database

- CPT
- SNOMED Classification
- ICD-11 Classification
- DSM-5 Classification
- LOINC

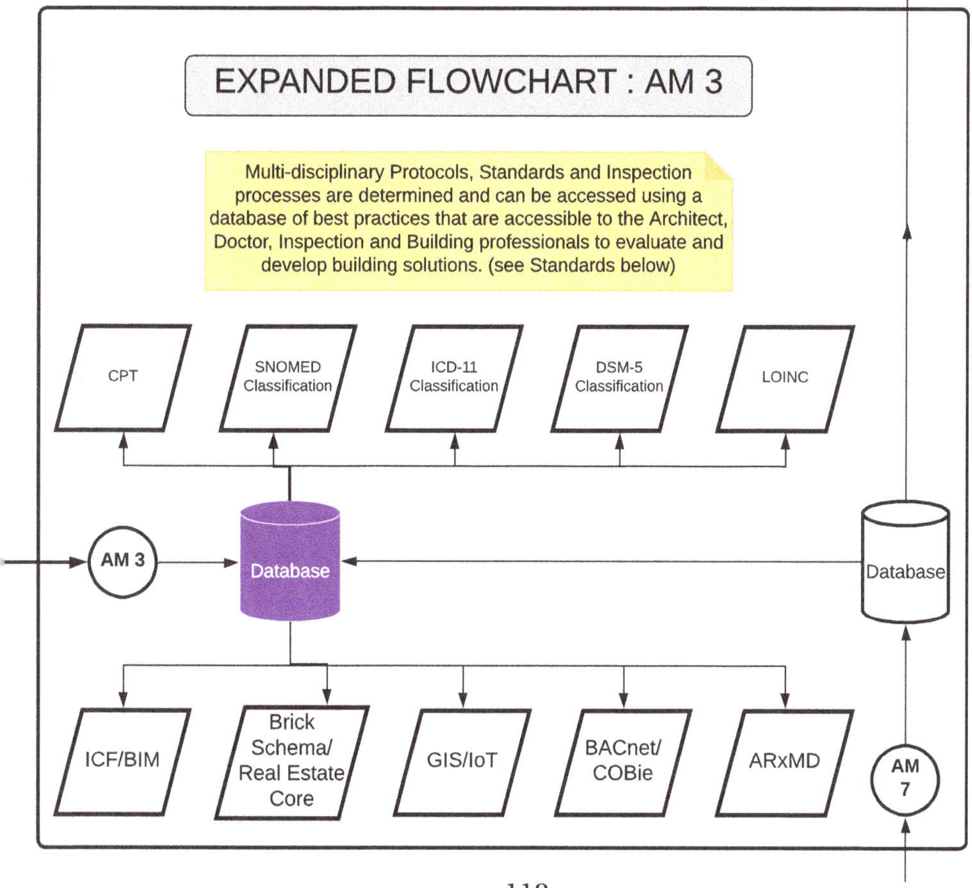

EXPANDED FLOWCHART : AM 3

Multi-disciplinary Protocols, Standards and Inspection processes are determined and can be accessed using a database of best practices that are accessible to the Architect, Doctor, Inspection and Building professionals to evaluate and develop building solutions. (see Standards below)

- CPT
- SNOMED Classification
- ICD-11 Classification
- DSM-5 Classification
- LOINC

AM 3 → Database ← Database

- ICF/BIM
- Brick Schema/Real Estate Core
- GIS/IoT
- BACnet/COBie
- ARxMD
- **AM 7**

The Architectural Doctor – An Rx for Health & Wellness in Buildings   Part I

The Architectural Medicine System (AMS) Flowchart
Part 3 of 4

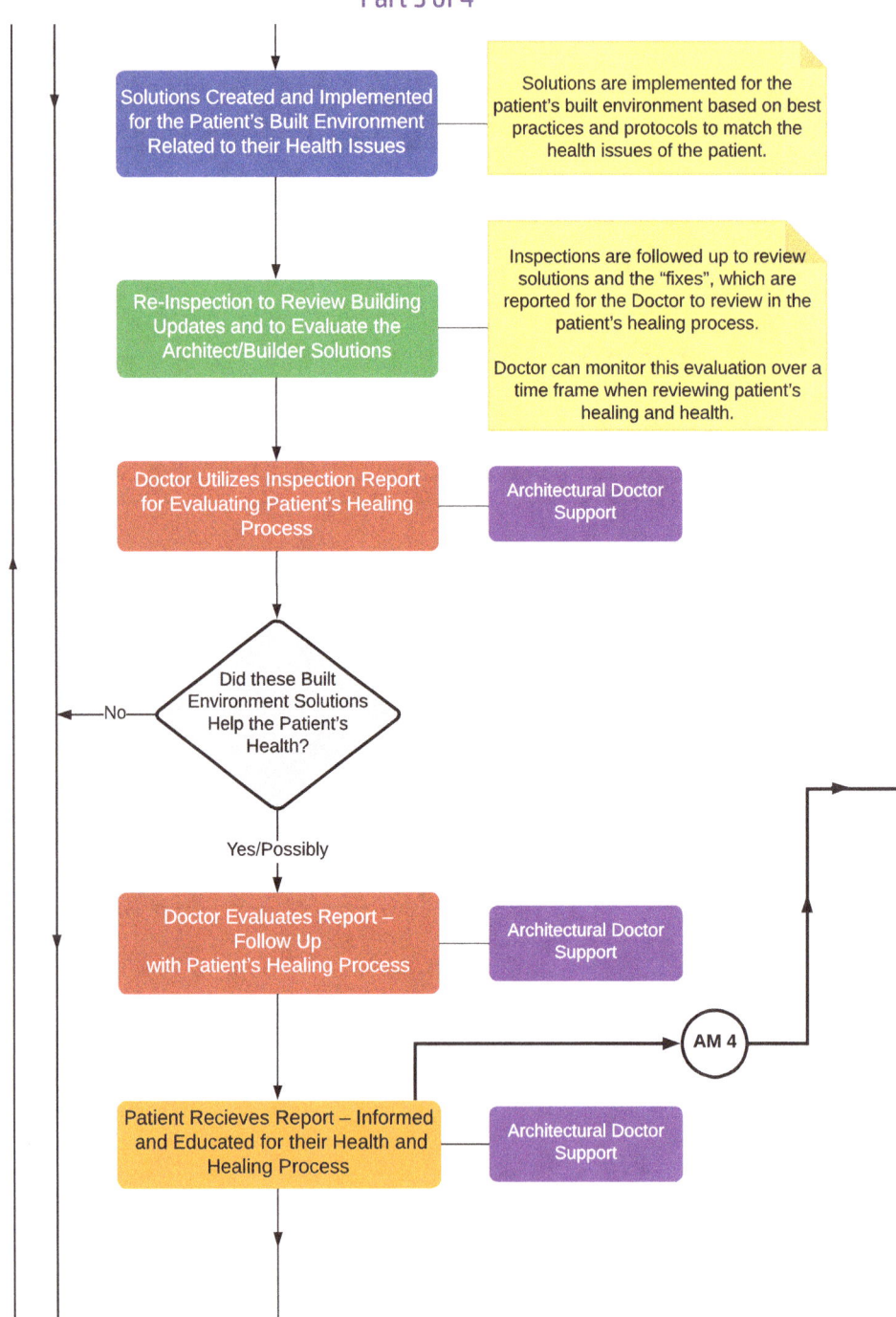

Chapter: 5   The Architectural Medicine System (AMS)

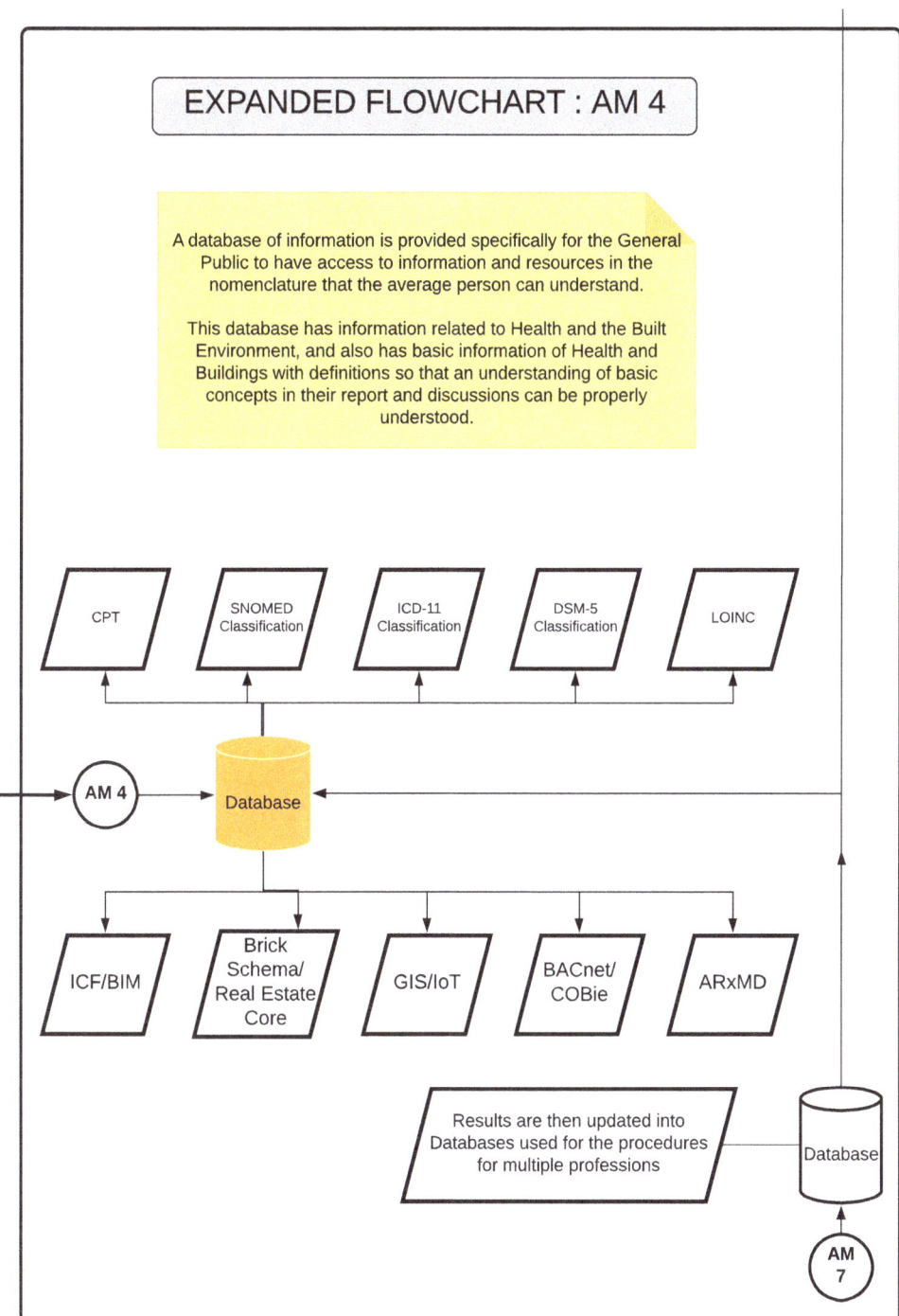

The Architectural Medicine System (AMS) Flowchart
Part 4 of 4

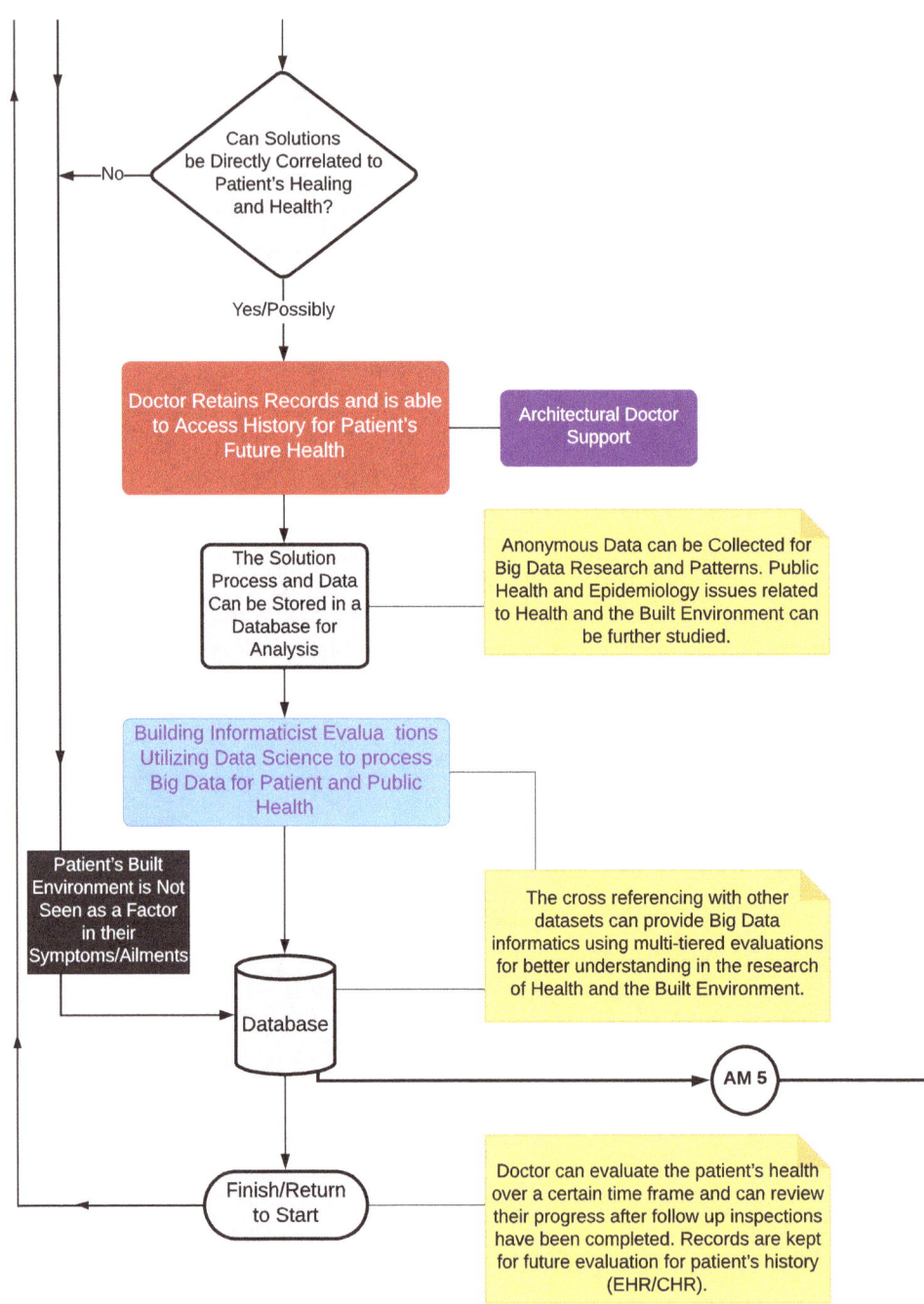

You will also see the connector listed as HL7, which is the Health Level Seven standard utilized for interoperability between medical platforms. I will discuss this in the next few chapters, as it will also provide interconnectivity between the architecture, engineering, and construction (AEC) platforms to achieve the goals of the Architectural Doctor.

Why Is the Finish Listed as a "Return to Start"?

Health is a lifelong process, and as such, the Doctor-Patient connection is about evaluating health over a lifetime. By adding into the "health equation" the built environment aspects that can impact illness or wellness, there can be a better understanding and, subsequently, control in achieving better health over a lifetime.

In addition to the focus on the individual's health, by providing metrics and evaluating data relative to health in the built environment, there can also be a better understanding for epidemiological and public health. Using big data procedures and collecting larger datasets in an anonymous format can provide insights into how the built environment can impact and influence health.

As a reminder, here is a link to the Architectural Medicine website to view the entire flowchart online to ensure that this process can be easily viewed.

https://architecturalmedicine.com/book

Why is this listed as "Return to Start"?

Health is a life long process, and as such, the Doctor/Patient connection is about evaluating Health over a lifetime. By adding into the "Health equation" how the Built Environment impacts illness or wellness, there can be a better understanding and, subsequently, control over better Health over a lifetime.

In addition to the focus on the individual's Health, by providing metrics and evaluating data relative to Health and the Built Environment, there can also be an epidemiological and overall Public Health understanding using big data in collecting larger data in an anonymous format to gain insights into how the Built Environment can impact and influence Health.

The Architectural Doctor – An Rx for Health & Wellness in Buildings   Part I

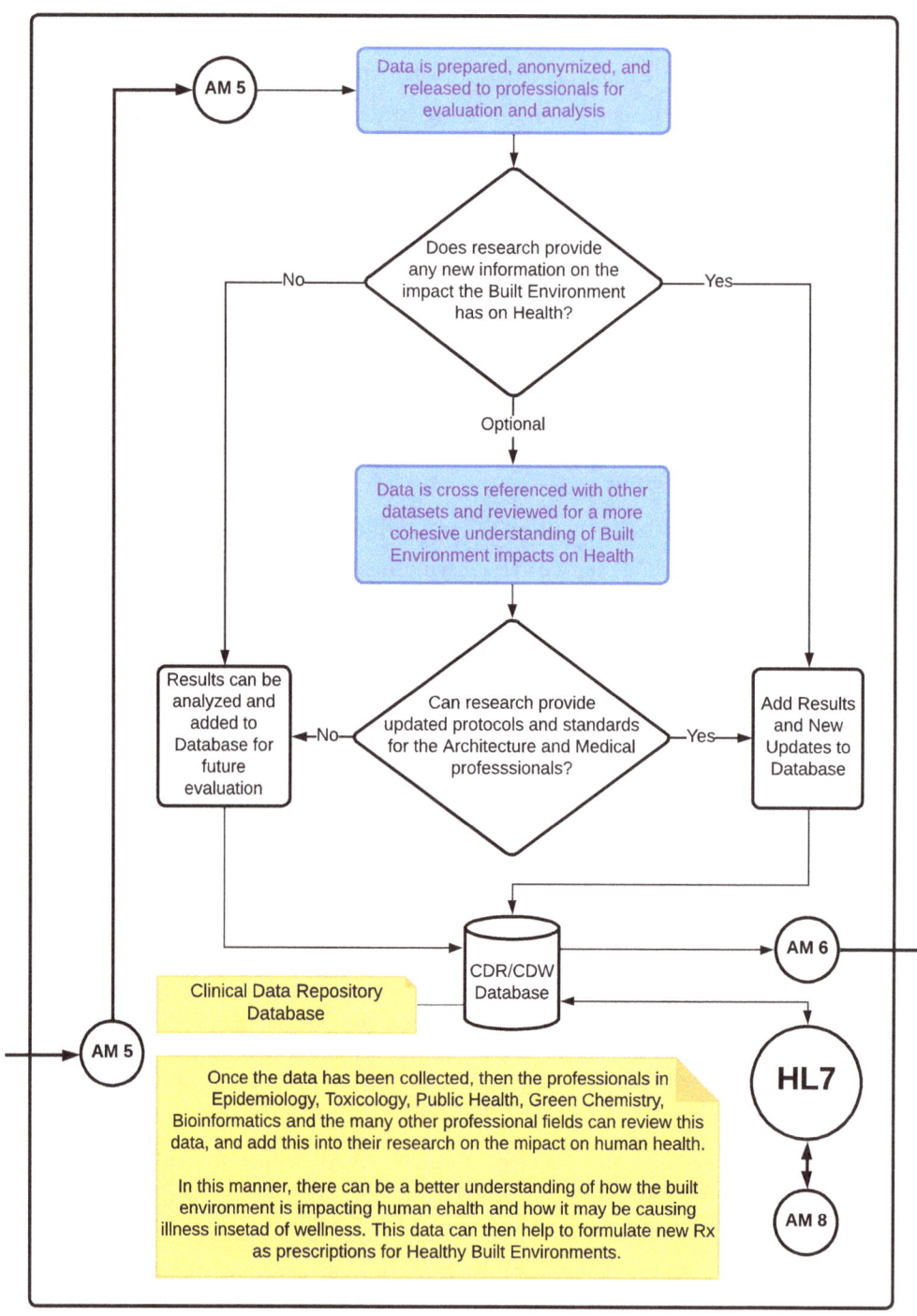

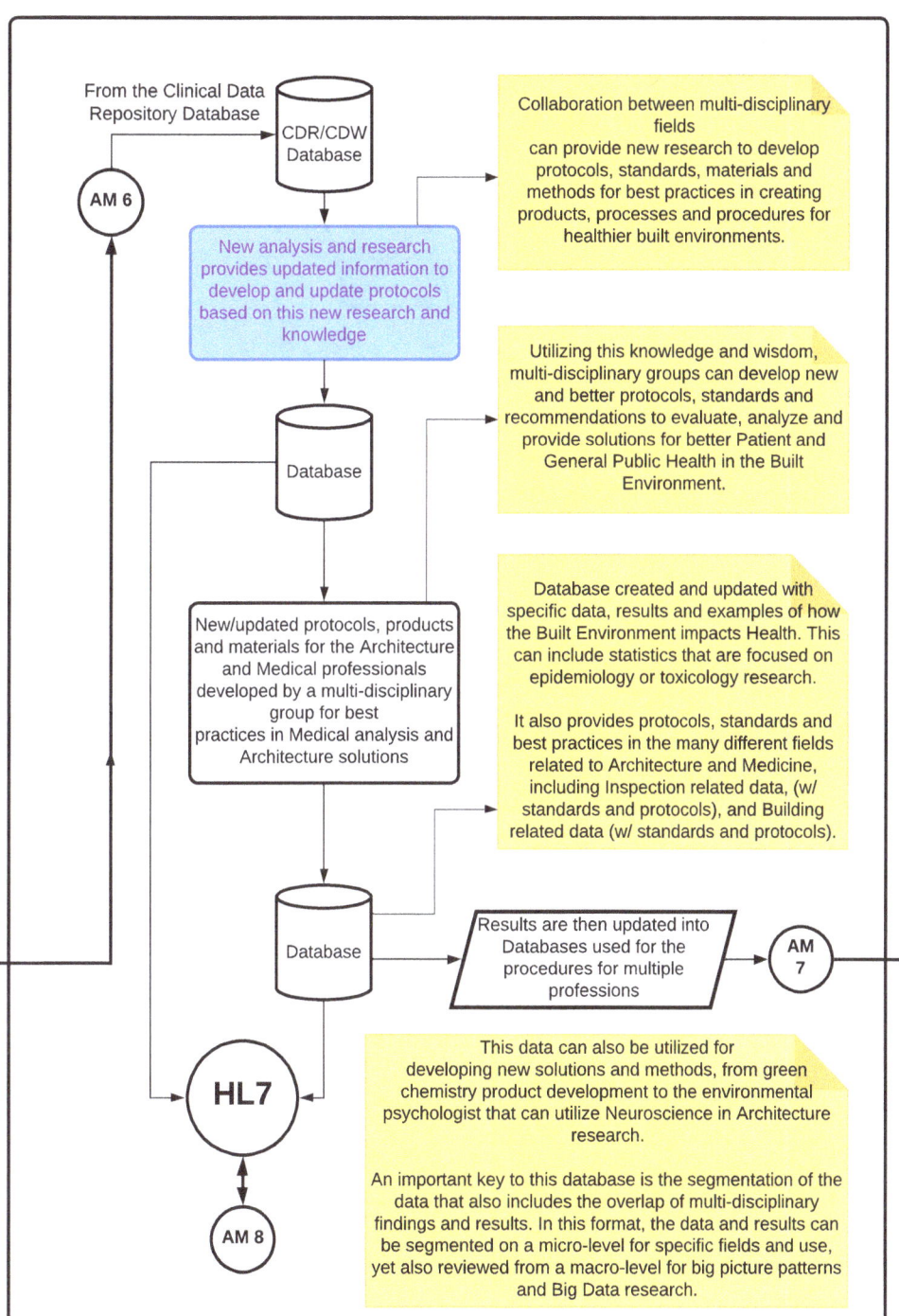

INTERNATIONAL STANDARDS, CLASSIFICATIONS & INTEGRATIONS FOR ARCHITECTURE, ENGINEERING, AND CONSTRUCTION (AEC) FIELDS

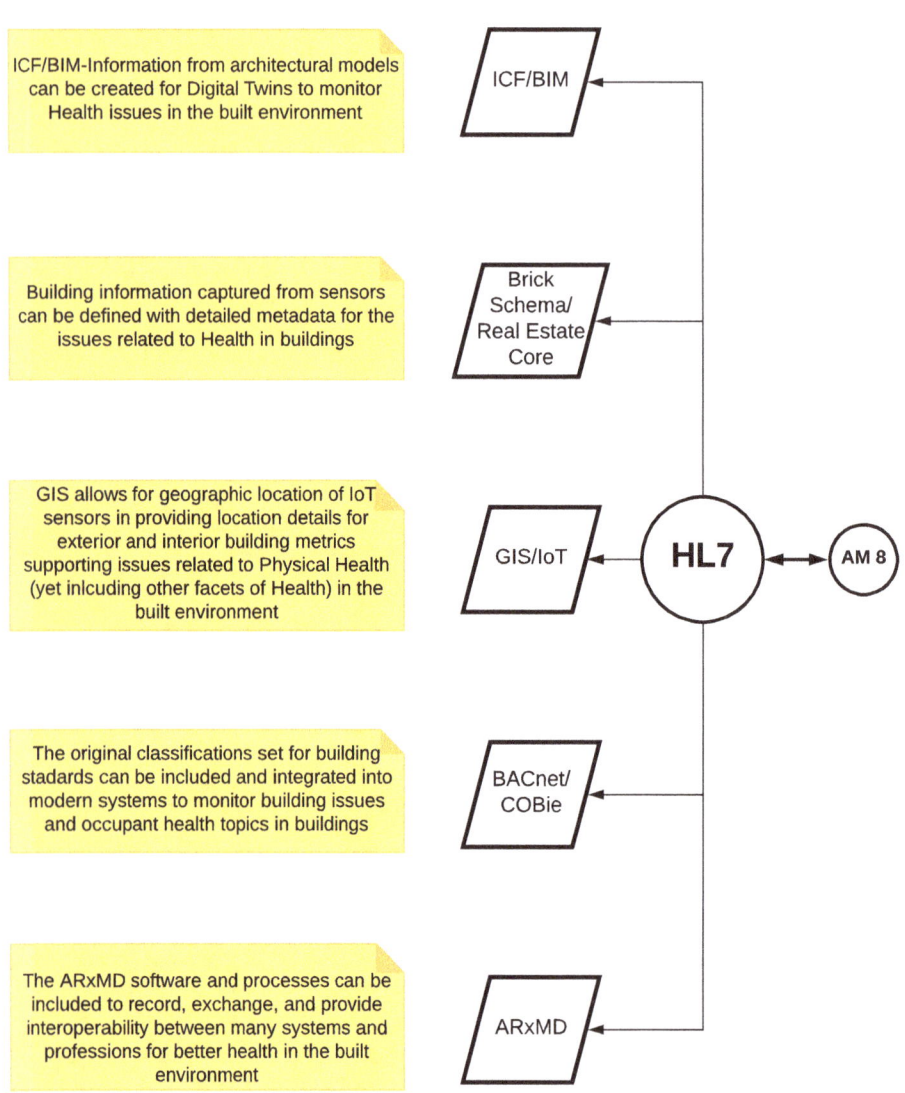

Chapter: 5 The Architectural Medicine System (AMS)

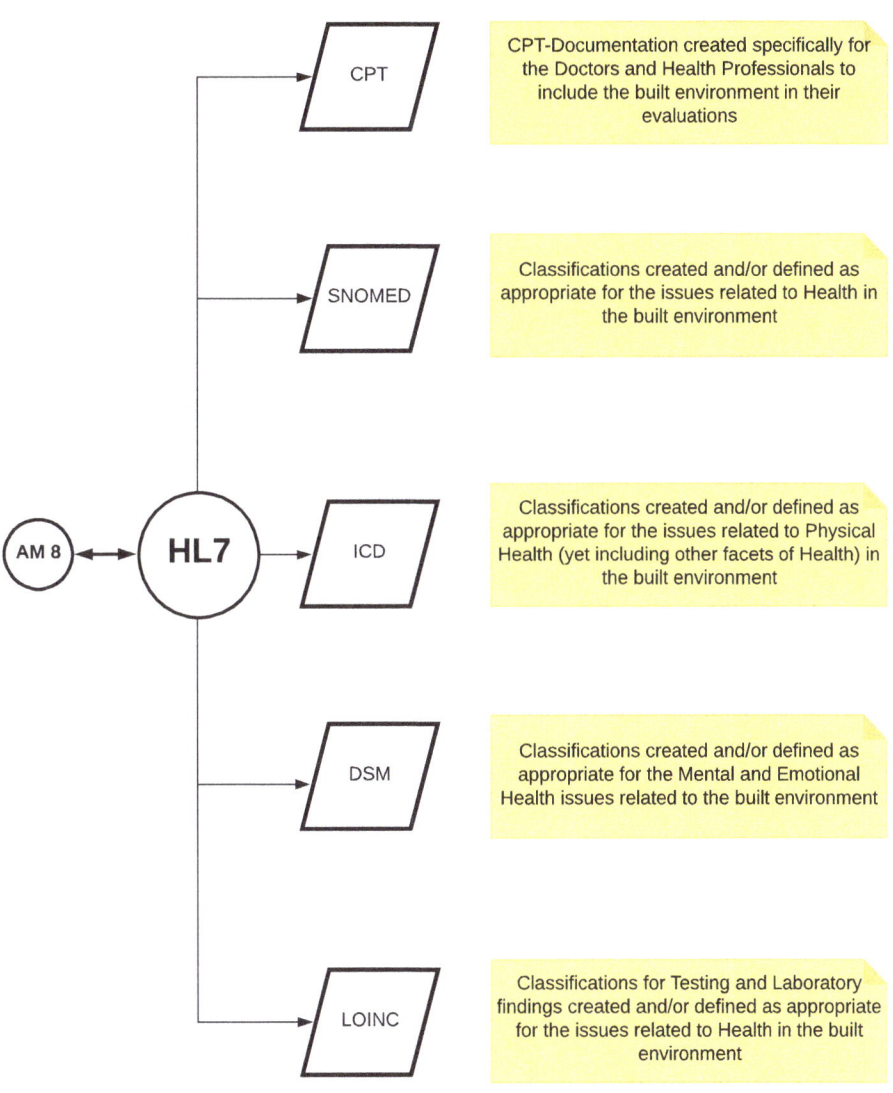

Architectural Medicine and the Architectural Doctor

The above flowchart shows the doctors' processes evaluating ailments, the inspection when the built environment needs to be evaluated and tested, the connection with architects and builders in evaluating problems, and the prescriptions or an Rx as recipes for healthier architecture solutions. The overall structure of this process recognizes the importance of whole systems solutions.

During this entire process, the Architectural Doctor can help support the system itself and can also provide support for each professional. By having these integrated steps, the doctor can include building issues in their patient evaluations and work with the inspector, building informaticist, and building professionals to provide solutions. As these are complex processes, there is an additional facet to support this workflow. The Architectural Medicine Software Solution – ARxMD offers the opportunity to facilitate these goals. In the next chapter, I will go into more detail on the topic of interoperability.

The Architectural Doctor can also help define ailments connected to the built environment and the doctor's evaluations in their analysis. This process will also be new for each professional and profession. These new systems can fill a gap to provide a bridge between multiple professions that typically do not have an overlap or work together. This new system of integrations between architects and doctors with inspectors and building professionals to create healthier built environments can ensure that each facet of these developments is interconnected for positive results.

Both architects and doctors have a substantial role in working independently to support the best health and wellness through buildings and medical support. Yet perhaps the overview of this flowchart can bring clarity to how these two professions and groups can work together to create healthier built environments.

This also brings up the topic of system processes. Typically, these professions have a form of hierarchical structure, and a change in procedures will include new methods requiring nodal systems for best solutions. A nodal system is one in which collaboration is more integrated, where different nodes as groups can work together in tandem. Instead of there being an authority group that makes all decisions, the collective group of professionals can work together to provide best solutions for the patient and the public at large. This encourages group participation, and while it doesn't remove required processes, it instead is more inclusive to ensure that the multiple professions can contribute for the best results. It is an important topic to discuss, as the Architectural Doctor's role and this new Architectural Medicine System (AMS) requires new methods and new mindsets with these professions collaborating together.

The Architectural Medicine Flowchart – Steps Involved in Bringing It All Together

The above flowchart provides new systems and new workflows involving multiple groups. While flowcharts are often an if-then procedure of decisions that are based on linear paths, the successful iteration of these steps will need to be more cyclical. I define this as a spiracycle, leading towards successful iterations that can continue to develop and improve over time in an upward, positive movement. The steps below outline the basic workflow of this flow chart process:

- Doctor evaluation
- Inspection prescribed
- Inspection/Informatics report provided to Doctor
- Discussions of building issues with Architecture/Building professionals
- Building issues and solutions discussed with the Patient
- Building solutions created
- Building solutions implemented
- Re-Inspection performed and recorded
- Re-evaluation of health issues for Patient included over time

It's important to note that the Architectural Doctor can be involved to support each of these steps appropriately. In chapters 7 to 11, I will discuss more details on the roles of each professional, including the role of the Architectural Doctor.

The Architectural Doctor and New Processes for Integrative Solutions

The role of each professional will have its own set of procedures, and this is critical to ensure that the entire system is functioning in a collaborative format. The steps of the flowchart and the diagram above can be outlined in the following processes:

- Doctor's process (with Building Informaticist and the Healthy Building Inspector)
- Architect's process (with Building Informaticist and the Healthy Building Inspector)
- Architectural Doctor's involvement
- Building Informaticist and the Healthy Building Inspector procedures
- Laboratory involvement and processes
- Protocols, standards, and procedures for interoperability
- ARxMD – Architectural Medicine Software Solution
- ARxMD standards, processes, and protocols

The above steps are not always in this order, yet the processes will be cyclical and require an integrative, multi-disciplinary approach in order for the entire system to function in a positive and effective manner. These round trip or spiracycle processes for better built environment solutions can be achieved using the Architectural Medicine System (AMS) and ARxMD, the Architectural Medicine Software Solution.

Chapter: 5 The Architectural Medicine System (AMS)

The graphic below shows the initial flowchart process that has been reconfigured in a circular diagram:

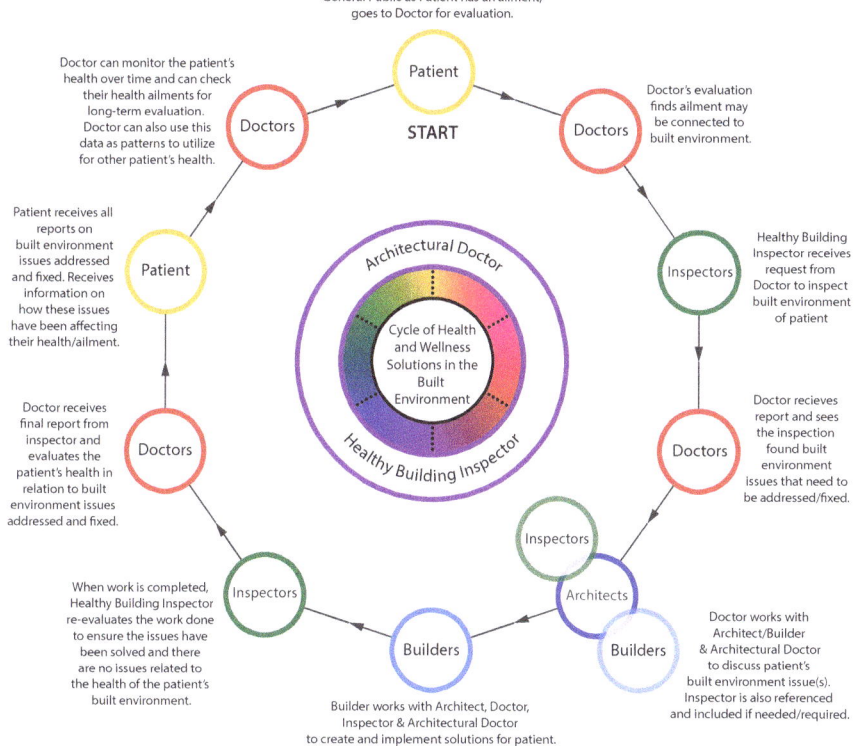

These steps can then be shown in a more simplified process, as shown in the diagram below:

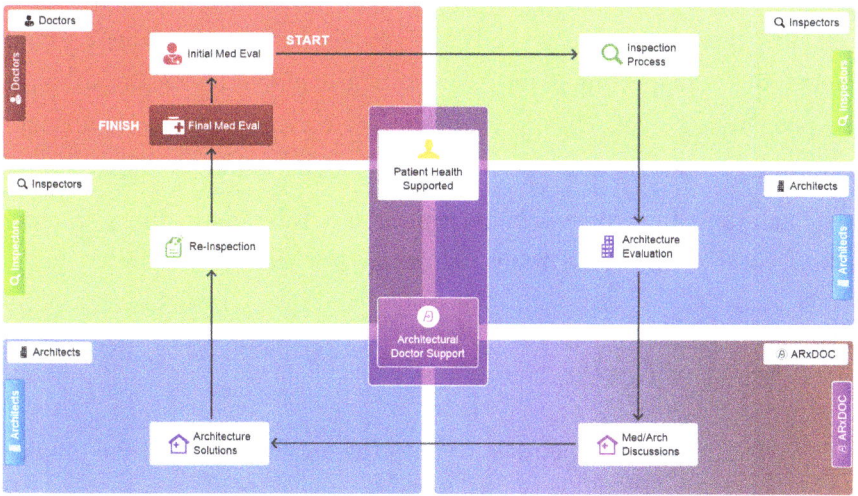

This graphic shows the system's simple process from start to finish, beginning with the doctor's initial evaluations. This system provides the synthesis or the system's creation towards connecting the two primary professions of architecture and medicine focused on health.

These initial steps lead to the Healthy Building Inspection process, which can also include the Building Informaticist. When issues are found in the built environment, these reports are then sent to the doctor and the Architectural Doctor for evaluation. This leads to the next steps of discussions with an architect, the building professionals, and the Architectural Doctor for cohesive support with plans for solutions. It's important to note that the Architectural Doctor can be involved in supporting each of these steps appropriately, as can be seen in the graphic as this role is placed in the center of the diagram alongside the patient.

What also should be highlighted is the importance of including the patient in each step and communicating in a supportive and non-jargon format. This way, they have an understanding of their health processes and the building solutions that can support their good health in an empowering format. It's critical to remember that health issues and topics related to one's home and place where one lives are among the most vulnerable human scenarios that one can experience in life. It's imperative that each step along the way can be properly communicated with the patient, and the Architectural Doctor can also play an important role in this process.

Once the solutions are agreed upon, and the building remedies are completed, the re-inspection of the issues can be evaluated to ensure solutions are properly achieved. The resulting reports are then provided for the doctor and Architectural Doctor to review and provided for their medical records.

Each step along the way of these processes will require integrative, collaborative processes. And many of these are not yet in existence.

The Architectural Doctor – Working Together With the Architect and Doctor

When there is the openness of both the architecture and the medical professionals, who choose to utilize best practices in each of their respective fields, their focus can be on their patients' and clients' best and optimal health. And when there are professionals who have this mindset and approach, they will seek ideal solutions for their patients and clients.

When it comes to medicine and health, the doctor may begin to recognize that external factors such as the built environment, where the average person spends a large percent of their time each day indoors, which may significantly impact their health and well-being.

When the architect begins to recognize the impact of architecture and their designs on occupant health and wellness, they may conclude that their approach to health-focused designs requires knowledge from the health and medical fields.

Each of these professionals may be wise enough to realize that they cannot achieve these goals alone and, therefore, may conclude that they can work together to accomplish these large goals.

This can be achieved by combining the knowledge, wisdom, and best practices of the many other fields involved, from building inspectors, nurses, and epidemiologists to those in the areas of green chemistry, evidence-based design, biophilia, and environmental psychology.

This workflow can be constructed of toxicologists, epidemiologists, and public health professionals utilizing big data and medical research to define issues. This knowledge can then be combined by working together with the fields of green chemists, material manufacturers, and product designers to explore new solutions. And then, when these products are developed and implemented into the building material world, the resulting impacts can be evaluated over time using the same process of data retrieval and analysis in an iterative format. These processes can be supported by the research of the building informaticist and healthy building inspector, along with building sensor data.

The extended range of these professionals does not necessarily mean that they have to be well versed in all of these topics, yet to know how they can all work together and have these connections is perhaps the most important factor. In practical terms, this means that both the sharing of knowledge and the ability to work together in different ways, which may be new and unprecedented, can yield synergistic and beneficial results.

New systems can be introduced to support these integrated processes, and along the way, these new integrations can lead to more robust systems that provide better solutions over time.

The following diagrams visually show how these fields can be connected with better communication and overlap for cohesive solutions.

Current Building Model – Limited Integrations

Limited Communication and often no direct review of building health related issues between the building fields, the health fields, and the occupants (general public).

Occupants/General Public

Communication

?

Architects & the Building Community   **Doctors & Health Practitioners**

Limited Communication
Between Fields of Architecture
and Fields of Medicine

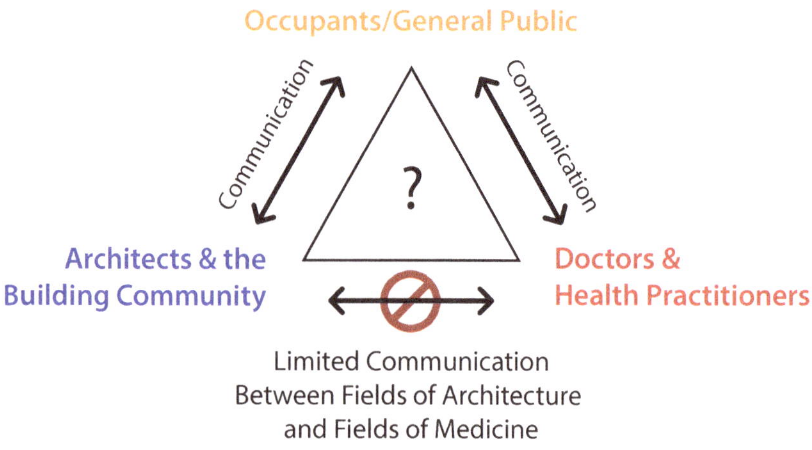

As you can see in the graphic above, the communication status between the fields of architecture and medicine is limited. There can be better integrations and new systems created to support these integrations, which can result in better health and wellness in the built environment.

The following diagrams show these new integrations with the support of the Architectural Doctor. We'll discuss the role of the Architectural Doctor in chapter 11.

Chapter: 5 — The Architectural Medicine System (AMS)

New Integration Between the Occupant, the Building Fields, and the Doctors and Health Professionals

Direct Communication and review of building health related issues with the building fields, the health fields, and the occupants (general public) through interconnections among all groups and the Consultant-Architectural Doctor.

Occupants/General Public

Consultant-
Architectural Doctor

Architects & the
Building Community

Doctors &
Health Practitioners

Occupants/General Public

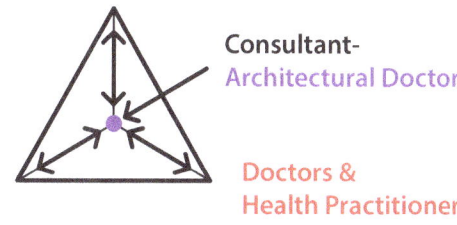

Consultant-
Architectural Doctor

Architects & the
Building Community

Doctors &
Health Practitioners

The flowchart and these graphics can show the details of the Architectural Medicine System (AMS), showing how these professionals can work together in more unified formats, providing procedures and processes to achieve these healthier goals.

As we revisit the initial diagrams that show a lack of integration between the fields of architecture and medicine, including the general public, the following diagrams show the progressive movement in the direction of integration.

Starting with the first triangle diagram, we have the general public at the top, then the architecture field in the lower left, and the lower right is the medical field. Building upon this integration, with the Architectural Doctor's support, we begin to add these connections into the diagrams where the fields start working with each other.

This communication also includes the general public as the occupant and leads to more clarity about the built environment's health for all involved.

The next step is to include the Healthy Building Inspector, the Building Informaticist, and the building professionals, along with the health practitioners. This can consist of nurses and psychologists, and the many other professionals involved in healthcare.

New and Revised Building Model for Health and Wellness

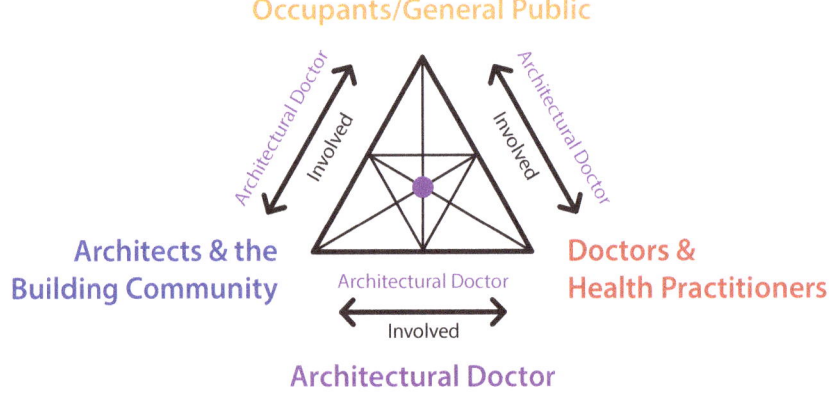

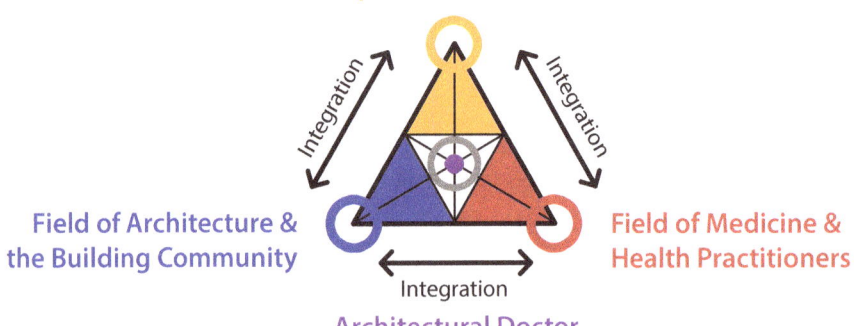

Once we have these integrations in place, there can be better support systems to achieve integrative solutions between all groups to benefit the patient and the general public.

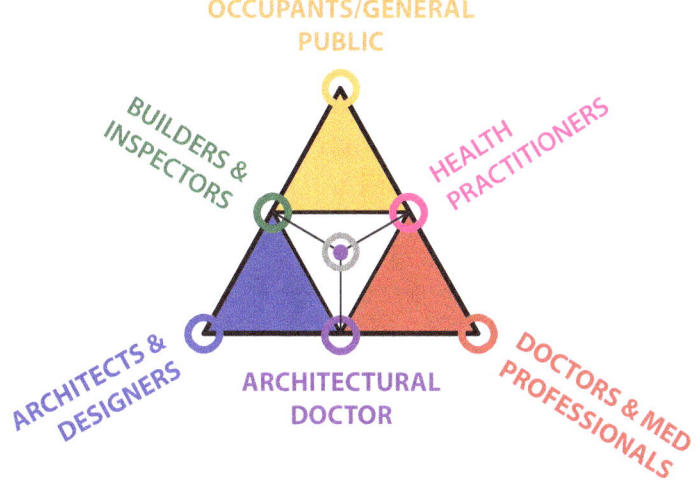

As shown in the graphics, this process consists of connections between each field and all of the many facets involved. These diagrams outline the many pieces and the processes to connect them.

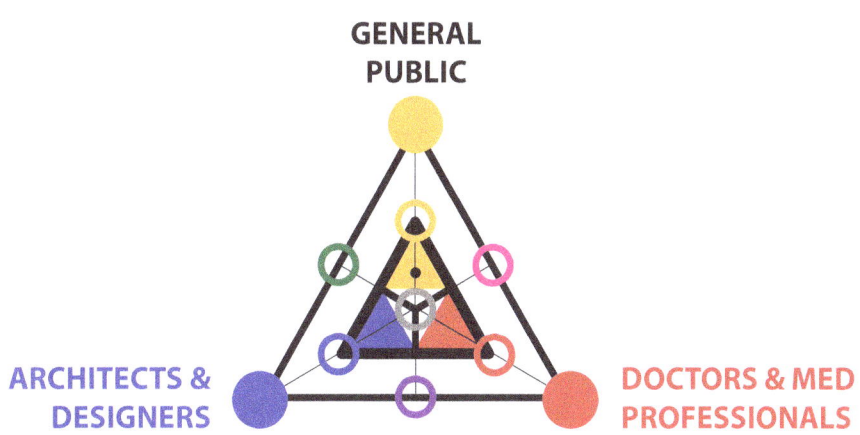

Having these integrations can provide pathways for various fields to work together and provide more cohesive solutions by viewing the many parts of the puzzle together.

New and Revised Building Model for Health and Wellness

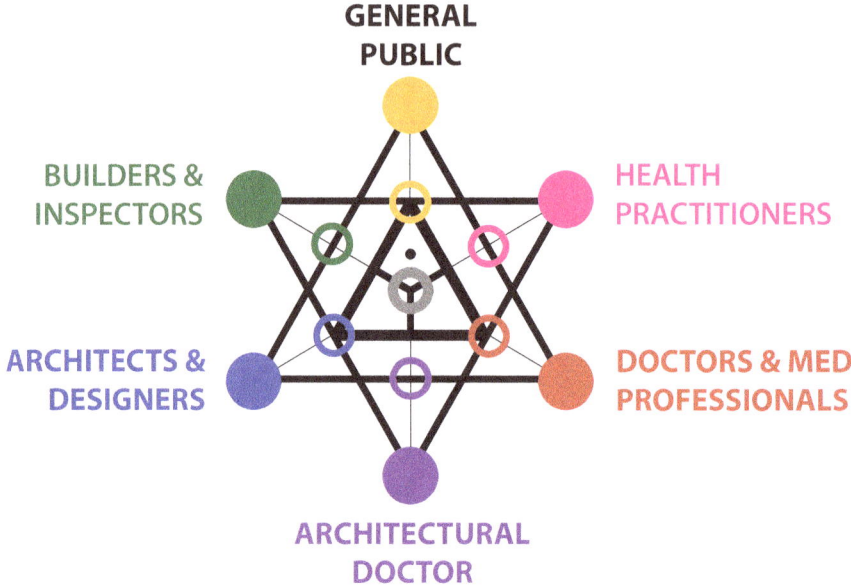

With a view of all of the different facets, there can be planning and considerations to provide whole system solutions. Instead of piecemeal solutions that can create more problems, these connections can ensure all aspects are factored into the equation.

The following diagrams show more details, along with a key for each of the diagrams. The final diagram shows all of the facets of these topics as a cohesive whole.

Key to Diagrams

The final graphic embraces the collaborative integrations between many professions in a multi-disciplinary format and as a result, can yield better solutions for each of the many professionals involved in an exponential way.

The steps to achieving the goals of this new flowchart process providing support for these new integrations will require new approaches, yet also new mindsets in how these professionals all work together.

New Integrated Building Model for Health and Wellness

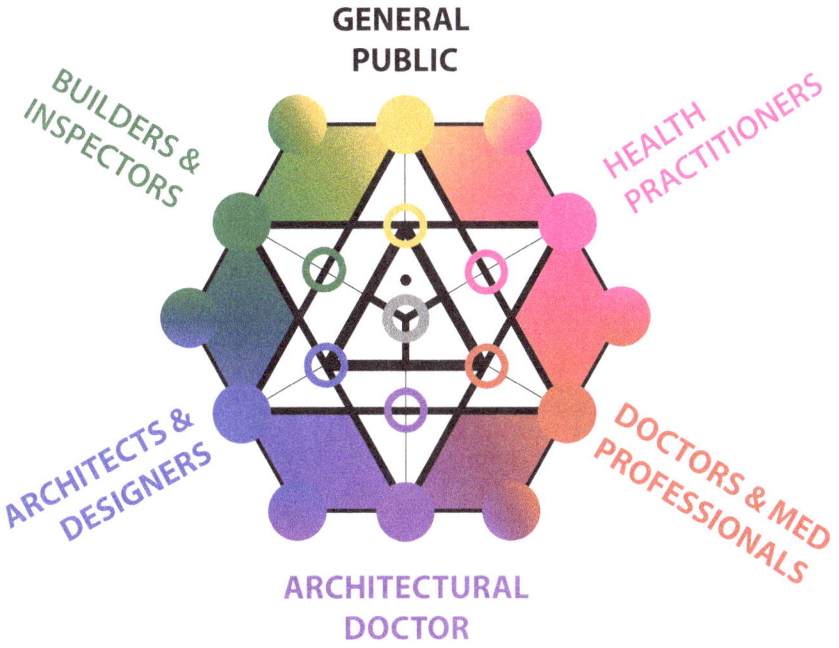

This requires the need for new steps to be taken by each profession, as well as different professions working together that have never done so previously.

Re-Evaluating the Built Environment and the Many Facets of Health and Wellness

It's important to note that while these comments can be viewed as criticisms in evaluating these issues in the built environment that are causing health issues, it's not to state that it's the fault of those professions and professionals involved in designing, building, and constructing these built environments. Many are simply not aware of these issues, and in other ways, some problems are created by the eventual breakdown of building materials or the use of chemicals and biocides that have found their way inside of these buildings.

The Architectural Doctor – An Rx for Health & Wellness in Buildings — Part I

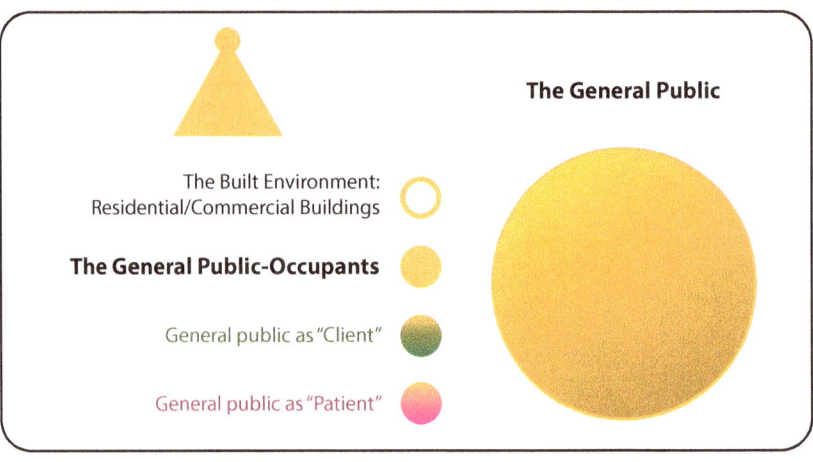

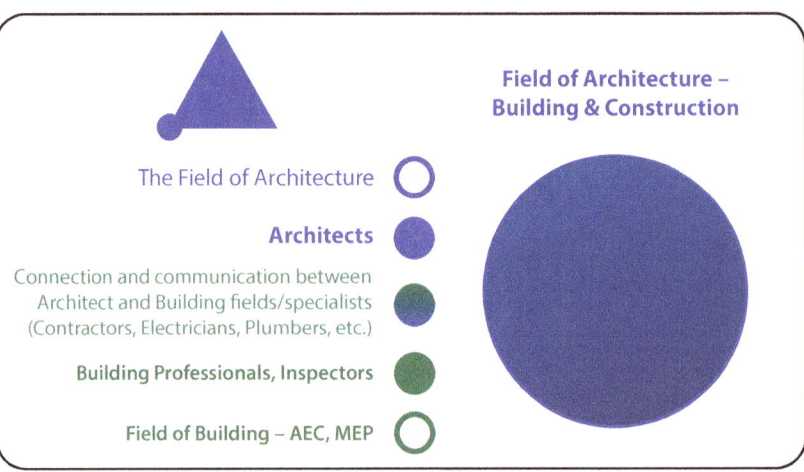

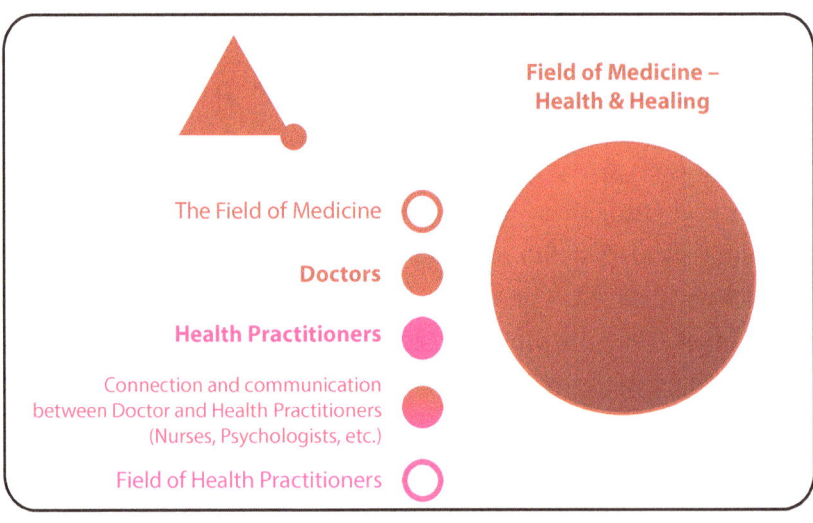

Chapter: 5 — The Architectural Medicine System (AMS)

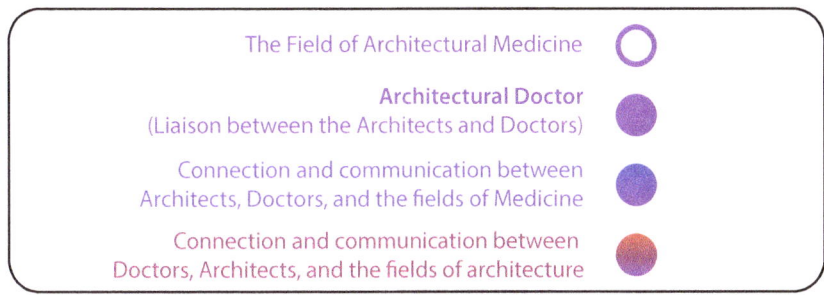

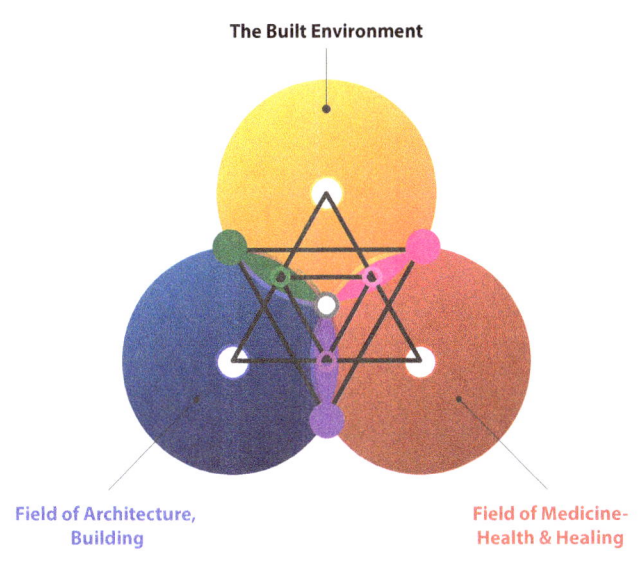

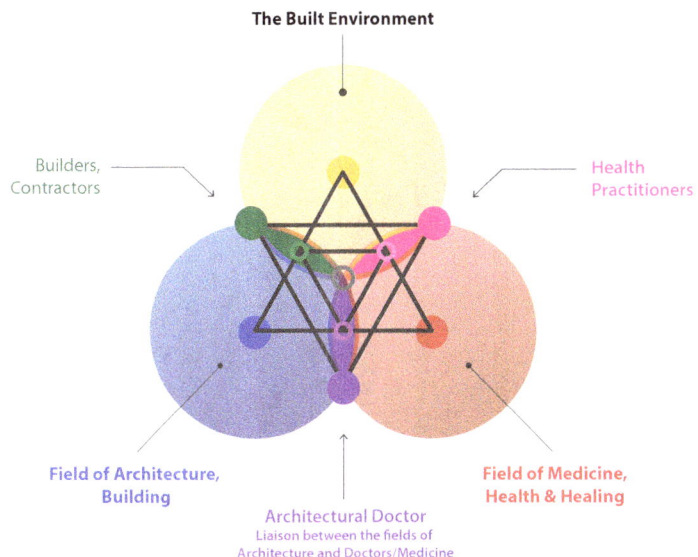

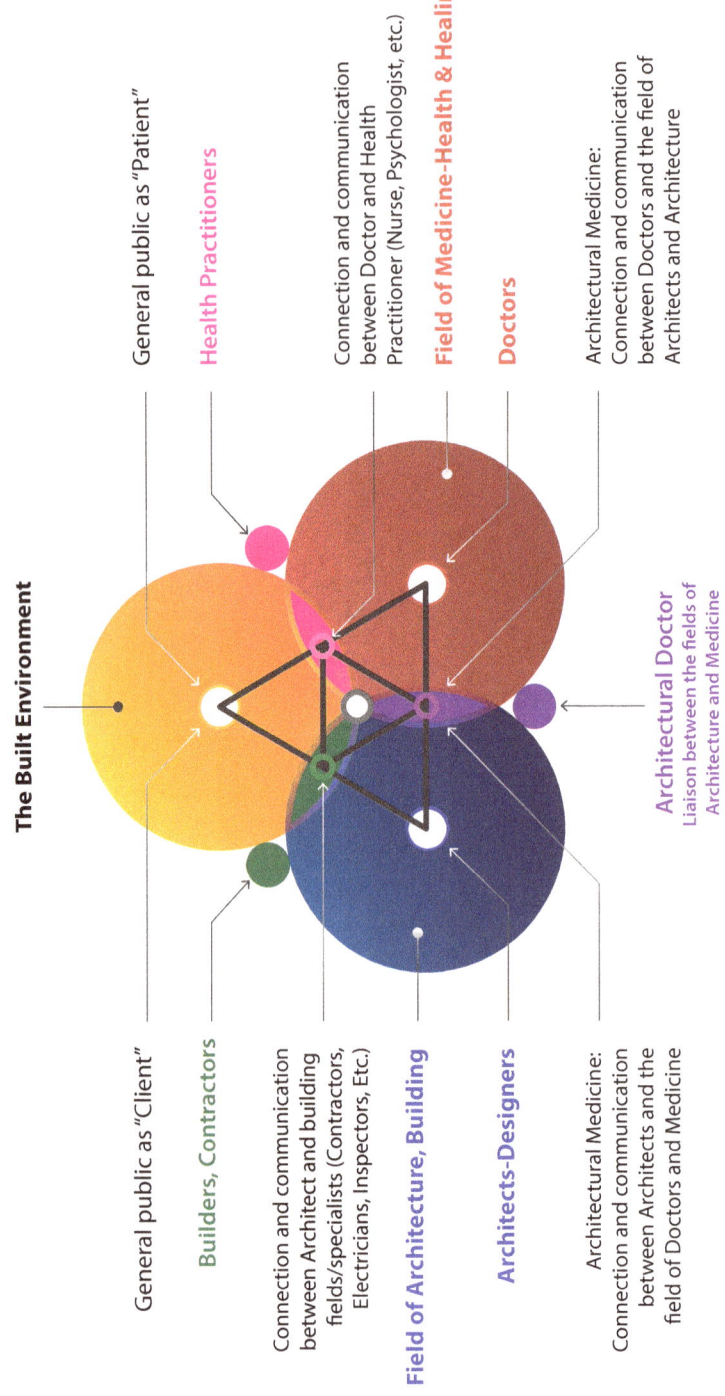

Chapter: 5   The Architectural Medicine System (AMS)

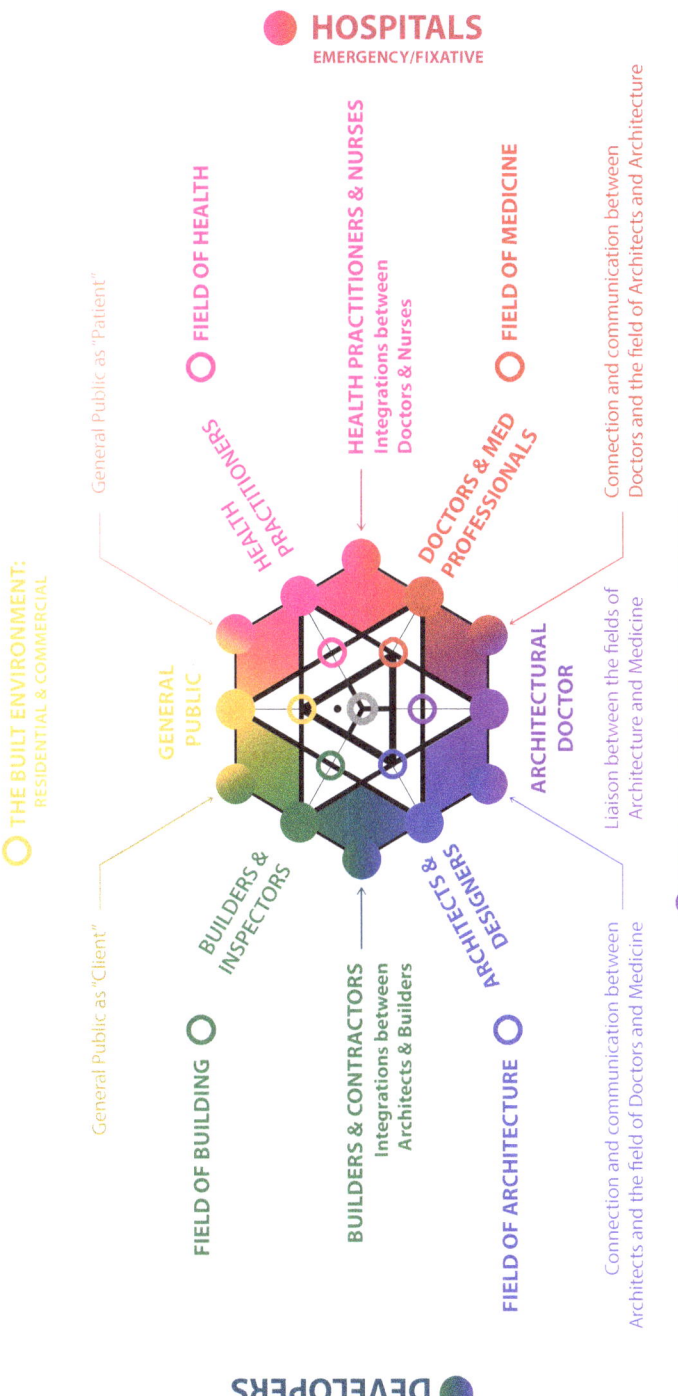

New Integrated Building Model for Health and Wellness

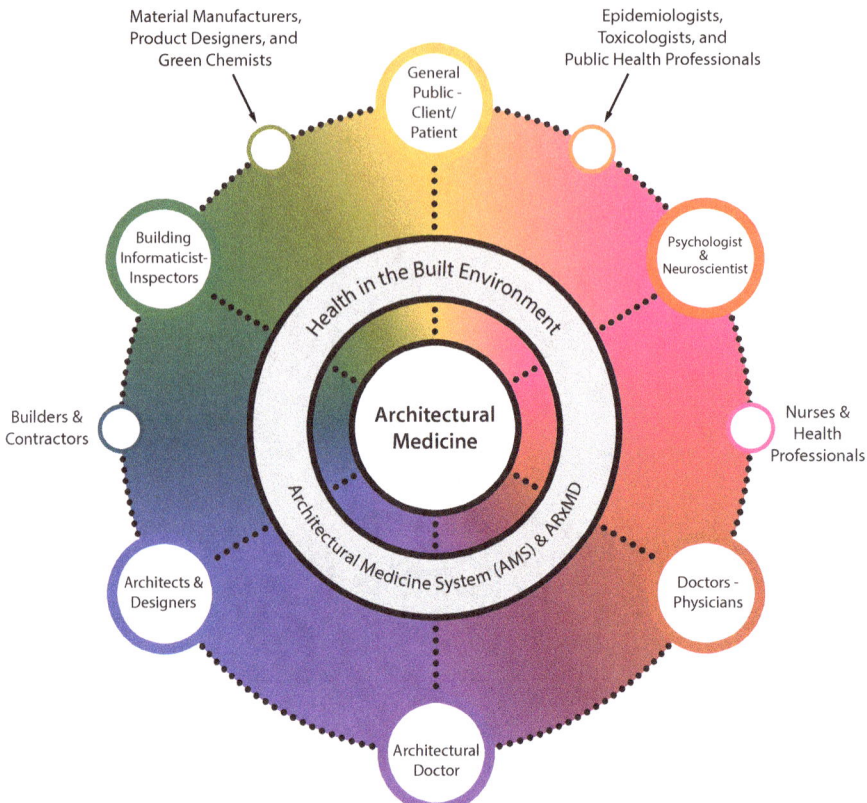

Often, there is a lack of awareness of the issues where certain materials and methods can cause health related problems, which is an essential part of the writing of this book.

While systems and procedures are required for these methods to be completed, it's also critical to bring awareness to these very complicated systems that we call buildings. Over the past fifty to a hundred years, buildings have gone from the typical simple structure to extremely complicated systems.

In my opinion, in the next several decades, buildings will be seen similarly to airplanes and vehicles as complex, integrated systems. This recalibration in viewing the built environment as complex systems requires a technological and functionally cohesive approach to designing, building, and maintaining these structures.

Towards the end of the book, I'll discuss some thoughts on the future of architecture, particularly concerning health and wellness. And one of these topics includes the idea that moving forward, buildings will likely be viewed and more aligned with advanced technological designs. They will be seen as analogous to an airplane or a sophisticated vehicular design and less so the old version of a building as an advanced shed.

The fact is these modern buildings as systems are multi-faceted and require many parts and pieces to fit and work together as a whole. This is often why many of these issues go unnoticed, as, over time, they've morphed from basic buildings into sophisticated technological structures. And many people do not understand the sophistication of the modern building until that is, an issue impacts the inhabitants of these structures.

Two takeaways can be gleaned from these comments moving forward. One is the recognition that buildings are complex systems that need to be evaluated on these terms and viewed in this manner by the professionals. Professionals involved in designing and building these structures need to work together, have some forward-thinking of the potential health issues, and work to resolve them before they become health hazards.

The second is to have more data collected, evaluated, and acknowledged for iterations of current practices. This can evolve into a knowledge base that each profession can utilize for their profession.

In this manner, large groups of people involved in building these structures can iterate before there are significant issues, instead of an afterthought or the need to fix something later in the building's life is recognized.

After all, buildings have a life as well, and if the building is healthy in terms of the structural integrity, then it is likely that this building's health will reflect on the occupants in the building.

Again, this is not to state that those involved are to blame for the lack of a current focus on building health, but instead a factor of the building's materials, methods, and systems changing so much over the past fifty years that it has been challenging to navigate.

In fact, many of these changes have occurred in the past thirty years in most of the world. Some of the world's most significant changes are areas where newer technologies in building materials have been implemented. These more contemporary building materials and methods have been utilized without much understanding of the impacts on human health in the short and the long term.

Many architects and doctors have never worked together or considered the overlap between their professions and the importance of working together. This is another reason why the focus on health and wellness in the built environment has been so elusive within these professions.

However, the time has come for the overlap between these professions to become more congruous. With goals of more significant overlap and the sharing of knowledge and best practices between each professional, the future can better support human thriving and well-being.

An active approach of working together between these professions, setting new protocols, processes, standards, and helpful systems to provide integrative solutions for better health in buildings, is ripe for change.

The advent of the novel coronavirus during the pandemic has also shown the importance and need for more focus on health in buildings — and is reason enough for this topic to flourish. Many building and health professionals, along with the general public, are struggling to navigate this pandemic even after several years since this first began. The need to work together to find solutions is more appropriate than ever and has not been as paramount as perhaps the 1918 flu pandemic.

Recipes for Better Health – The New Rx

If you are a medical professional, you're aware that the pharmacist's abbreviation of Rx is the shortened term for the word Recipe.[91] This becomes interesting when this symbol is used to define a recipe as a prescription or Rx for a healthier built environment.

The combination of professionals working together with increasing public awareness to support their health and wellness can produce a demand for professionals to provide solutions.

And these results require an integrated approach and process, from the example in the flow chart of the procedures to the information, education, and training necessary to fulfill these round trip, whole system solutions.

If these systems, as prescriptions or an Rx, can be put into place and utilized, then the collective collaboration could have a substantial positive impact on well-being for public health in the built environment. The synergistic effect this could have on the built environment, focusing on health and wellness, could support a better life for growing populations in current and future contexts.

The Architectural Medicine System can be realized in a practical format through the use of digital processes through the exchange and transfer of data between platforms and professionals.

These interoperability processes as an Rx or recipe and prescription can be defined as ARxMD. The use of this exchange of data and the systems required to perform these processes are discussed in the next chapter...

"My main task has been to show that there is a deep and important underlying structural correspondence between the pattern of a problem and the process of designing a physical form which answers that problem."

— Christopher Alexander

ARxMD – THE ARCHITECTURAL MEDICINE SOFTWARE SOLUTION (PART 1)

With this new system outlined, it may become apparent the current lack of systems existing between the medical and architecture fields. Recognizing the importance of such systems to provide better health in the built environment, the next step and question might be, "what can be done to help implement these systems?"

If you have followed along the trajectory of topics in this book, you might now be asking the question, "how would this Architectural Medicine System (AMS) function?"

And this is where the Architectural Medicine System (AMS) meets the actionable procedures of *ARxMD* — *the Architectural Medicine Software Solution*.

What Is the Architectural Medicine Software Solution – ARxMD?

ARxMD, pronounced "arcs-med," is a software solution that provides the nuts and bolts of implementing the Architectural Medicine System. It provides the methods that can be utilized between the many professionals involved, including the information provided to the patient and the general public.

This software is a solution that can record and exchange data for different professionals, and then transfer this information to ensure cohesive solutions can be completed.

Utilizing the ARxMD Software Solution for Interoperability Between the Architecture and Medical Fields

Interoperability is a term that provides an accurate overview of the ARxMD solution implementing the Architectural Medicine System. The overlap between the many professionals involved requires a group of specific procedures in order to function together. This can ensure that the processes are clear for each professional while also providing whole system solutions for the many interconnections involved.

To achieve this interoperability, there is a need for the exchange of data between different platforms. And this exchange is not just within each profession, yet the ability to transfer and share data between different professions.

In the field of medicine, this exchange of data has commonly been achieved using advanced procedures of code processing using standards specific to healthcare platforms. These have been created by the Health Level Seven International (HL7), a worldwide healthcare standards organization, mostly in the form of data exchange using XML and EDI communication interfaces. Health Level Seven International (HL7) is a "standards developing organization dedicated to providing a comprehensive framework and related standards for the exchange, integration, sharing, and retrieval of electronic health information that supports clinical practice and the management, delivery, and evaluation of health services."[92]

Over the past decade, the creation and use of a new standard defined as FHIR has become more prevalent, which enables the exchange of data using JSON and common API connections. This has the potential to allow the integration of information into a wider range of use. With this FHIR standard using RESTful API and JSON as the main source of data communications, this allows a larger scope of developers to provide software solutions that can "talk" between each platform using this new protocol.

The core of these new developments is based on REST APIs, which for those unfamiliar with this terminology, it is an "application programming interface (API or web API) that conforms to the constraints of REST architectural style and allows for interaction with RESTful web services."[93] Developed by computer scientist Roy Fielding, REST stands for representational state transfer[94] and is how modern computing can share data more easily between entirely different platforms, irrelevant of the platforms that the software is developed for.

These developments of FHIR, the Fast Healthcare Interoperability Resources (FHIR - pronounced "fire") is a "standard describing data formats and elements (known as "resources") and an application programming interface (API) for exchanging electronic health records (EHR)."[95]

HL7 FHIR can provide a larger scope of integrations and allow for a greater amount of software to share data, as JSON (JavaScript Object Notation) is a common API technology utilized in most modern day software. As a RESTful API, this also means that communications can exist beyond medical platforms and not only between the common hospital information system (HIS) and electronic medical record (EHR) platforms. It can provide a process to share data between software platforms outside of the common scope of medical software systems, including applications for professionals and patients to utilize for the best use of this information.

This critical development can allow for the Architectural Medicine System to provide interoperability between the medical and architecture professions, along with other software platforms that can exchange data using a RESTful API.

This method is how the ARxMD platform and solution can extend the exchange of data to other fields, such as the architecture, building, and inspection fields. It can provide round trip processes that span a larger group of professions that previously have not typically interacted together.

And this is because many architecture and construction platforms can also exchange data utilizing the RESTful API methodology. The result is the interoperability between new professionals, and new procedures, such as the Architectural Medicine System, can be properly implemented.

In previous chapters, I mentioned the many facets involved in creating the healthy built environment and the new professionals required to achieve this goal. This includes the Building Informaticist, the Healthy Building Inspector, and the Architectural Doctor. While the steps of the Architectural Medicine System were outlined in the previous chapter, the steps of this system were not clear.

In the rest of this chapter, I will provide details of the exchange of this data and the interoperability that can be achieved using these software solutions and the ARxMD software. This, along with the procedures of the Architectural Medicine System (AMS), forms the foundation to provide the actions for healthier built environment solutions.

The next step in this process is providing the necessary interconnections to allow all of these activities to function together. This includes the steps for each professional, along with the systems and software that can support these developments. And this is where the ARxMD software solution fits into the big picture of these integrations.

Blueprints for Health and Wellness in the Built Environment

As the subtitle of this book is "An Rx for Health & Wellness in the Built Environment," a question that might arise is to ask what exactly is meant by this? And what type of an Rx can be created for health and wellness relative to buildings?

Good questions lead to a better understanding of any topic, and this question is no exception.

An Rx is shorthand for Recipe and has often become known in the modern day as a prescription. This term recipe, in the older sense in English, "survives chiefly in the pharmacist's abbreviation Rx."

It is known from the 1580s as a "medical prescription, a formula for the composing of a remedy written by a physician, from French recipe, originally from Latin recipe as "take!" (this or that ingredient)." With a figurative meaning as, "a prescribed formula, from 1640s, is a word written by physicians at the head of prescriptions."[96]

Yet how can a building have a prescription or a form of medical processes related to this type of prescription?

In simple terms, a prescription viewed in its original form as a "Recipe" can be viewed as an instruction set to achieve a certain goal for good health, healing, and wellness.

In the world of architecture and building, an instruction set to achieve building goals are referred to as blueprints. A blueprint is any set of plans that defines an end goal or a system to achieve this goal. And in this manner, the Architectural Medicine System is the blueprint for these goals of health and wellness in the built environment.

The definition of a blueprint in verb format is "to create or provide a blueprint for (something); to design or plan out." The noun version is defined as "originally: a photographic print composed of white lines on a blue background, used chiefly in copying plans, machine drawings, etc.; (also) a blue-toned photograph. In later use also (more generally): any design or technical drawing. Something which acts as a plan, model, or template." [97,98]

So, a blueprint is originally called such because of the cyanotype chemical process of ammonium ferric citrate and potassium ferricyanide,[99] leading to the printing of plans having the famous Prussian blue color. The concept of a blueprint typically refers to a drawing that defines the schematic of a product or process. In the world of architecture, these blueprints provide visual plans of a structure showing different viewpoints of the design, such as the side views, front or rear elevations, and top view or plot plans of the entire site in which the building is situated. It also includes the construction drawings that define how the structure or the design should be built.

As the Architectural Medicine System provides a plan for providing steps to achieve better health and wellness as the goal, it is itself a blueprint. As with most blueprints, there are many variables and changes that occur, even up to the proverbial last person holding the hammer, as is referenced in the construction field as the last one providing the building processes and making the final changes.

Another way of stating this type of an Rx or recipe for health and wellness in buildings is as a "Blueprints for Health & Wellness in the Built Environment."

Plans for many design projects include a schematic utilized as both an outline of the design goals and to provide specific details on how to achieve these goals. It literally shows a big picture, macro view of what is being designed, and then provides the specific steps, in micro view, with detailed steps or construction drawings to achieve these goals.

This blueprint as a recipe or an Rx can help define the schematics and instructions for achieving these building health goals. In this manner, this is exactly what the Architectural Medicine System is striving to achieve.

Architectural Medicine is the process of providing an overview of the fields of architecture and medicine working together to provide solutions for better occupant health and wellness. The key part of this process is the working together between the two main fields.

It is this viewpoint in which ARxMD as an Rx, recipe, and blueprint for Health and wellness in the built environment is accomplished.

ARxMD can provide the bridge between the two fields, where both professions are working together to evaluate, measure, inform, and utilize certain procedures for better health for building occupants.

These evaluations and measurements are done in a myriad of ways, yet one key piece to the puzzle is the puzzle itself. If you do not provide systems and processes for both of these professions working independently and interdependently to evaluate, measure, and solve problems found, then the results are going to be very haphazard.

The requirement for such processes to be successful is education and training for both professions, as well as a system such as ARxMD to support these actions.

The Informed Patient Is a Patient Educated for Their Own Best Health

Before we get into the professional procedures of ARxMD, it's critical to remember that this work is being accomplished for the purposes of the building occupants and population health.

As such, it's extremely important to have professional systems in place. It's essential to be mindful that these are the homes and working environments of people whose spaces and places of work are often of critical importance in their lives for their health and for experiencing well-being.

An essential component of the ARxMD software is the patient's ability to receive and review these results. This allows them to be informed by the doctor, Architectural Doctor, and the other health professionals involved in this process. It can also ensure that the patient knows the issues that impact their health and can learn more about these topics for the empowerment of their own health.

After all, if the patient is not aware of the issues, they cannot contribute to their own good health. And when you scale this individual knowledge for the masses, it is either an empowering process for the public or a large-scale detriment to the overall health infrastructure of built environments.

The ARxMD software can exchange and sync this data to the patient's Electronic Health Record (EHR) or Comprehensive Health Record (CHR), as well as other applications created for this purpose. This information can be accessible for them to review in different formats. Ensuring the proper HIPAA compliance is followed using HL7, this information can be exchanged with the appropriate health systems and remain secure for their current and future review.

When the Architectural Medicine System is implemented properly, it involves all of the required professionals, as well as the proper education of the client as a building occupant. There will be more information about this accessibility relative to ARxMD in chapter 12, ARxMD – The Architectural Medicine Software Solution (Part 2).

The Doctor, Architect, Healthy Building Inspector, and the Architectural Doctor – New Systems and Solutions

The past twenty years have shown many changes and updates in the format of digital and electronic record keeping. The Electronic Health Record (EHR) and the CHR (Comprehensive Health Record) have brought the world of medical paperwork into the digital age.

In the US, the Centers for Disease Control and Prevention (CDC) enacted the Meaningful Use standards in 2009, defined by the "Health Information Technology for Economic and Clinical Health (HITECH) Act."[100] The CDC defines *meaningful use* as "the use of certified EHR technology in a meaningful manner (for example electronic prescribing); ensuring that the certified EHR technology connects in a manner that provides for the electronic exchange of health information to improve the quality of care."[101]

This helped support the transition from a paper-based medical system to an electronic or digital process. In this development, data sharing and data exchange between different medical systems, hospitals, and health professionals has been the end goal. While still a work in progress in the USA and worldwide, the electronic sharing of data has brought the possibility of integrated systems to another level. These new systems can allow for software to be developed to support many various healthcare factions. These systems range in scope from ordering and receiving test results to the sharing of examinations between health professionals without needing to be in the same network or even on the same software platforms.

This has continued to develop over the past decade in the USA with the advent of the 21st Century Cures Act (Cures Act), developed to "improve the flow and exchange of electronic health information." Advances in HL7, with these more recent developments of HL7 FHIR, combines the "best features of HL7's v2, HL7 v3, and CDA product lines while leveraging the latest web standards and applying a tight focus on implementability"[102] in providing the exchange of data.

And these procedures create opportunities for new systems to be added, integrated, and updated in formats that previously would have been extremely challenging, if not impossible.

An Evolution in the Architecture & Construction Fields

What's particularly interesting about the medical and health fields' history, in these updates to electronic records, is that a slow digital evolution in the architecture and construction fields has also been occurring over the past several decades. I mention that it's been a slow process, mainly due to the architecture and construction fields having complex systems as well, yet a lack of outside forces such as the healthcare requirements as the meaningful use act in the USA pressuring changes. These developments, instead, have occurred based on pioneers advocating changes and the capabilities of software developments as a choice. However, as the AEC fields have become more digitized and complex, it has required that architects, engineers, and construction professionals exchange data in more fluid formats.

The public knowledge of these developments in electronic health records (EHR) has allowed these updates to be more transparent and popularized. However, behind the scenes in the worlds of building and construction, this digital evolution has also been happening with the digitization of the architecture fields.

Chapter: 6   ARxMD – The Architectural Medicine Software Solution (Part 1)

From the developments of Computer-Aided Design (CAD) and the ability to create digital files from the 1960s onward, another data movement has been slowly developing. These advancements include Building Information Modeling, or BIM as it is known today. The roots of this information modeling began in the early 1990s as a group of leaders in the fields of building software created an organization to outline standards for the interoperability of data files. This group began to develop a standardized, digital description of the built environment called the Industry Foundation Classes or IFC.[103] [104]

Today these standards, which the buildingSMART International organization oversees, provide vendor-neutral standards that are usable "across a wide range of hardware devices, software platforms, and interfaces for many different use cases."[105]

The ability to exchange data can allow many building professionals to all work together, from architects, structural engineers, and the construction (AEC) professionals to mechanical, electrical, and plumbing (MEP) professionals. For example, an engineer can import designs from an architect, include their part of the building development into their software, and then export these updates back to the architect and construction management team. And this process can occur in real-time – or mostly real-time if the solutions are hosted in a cloud platform.

Essentially, the world of architecture has been slowly creating infrastructures to exchange this data electronically to enable construction professionals to work together. In a similar format to the electronic health record exchanges, these digital construction systems have also developed for better interoperability and functionality. With software having these integrations in place, the exchange of data between different electronic systems within the AEC fields can be properly supported. This opens the window of opportunity to provide integrations between these professionals, as well as other professions that can exchange data using the same technical capabilities.

This is where the *Architectural Medicine Software Solution – ARxMD* can enter the equation with greater possibilities in exchanging data between the architecture and medical fields.

Introduction to the Architectural Medicine Software Solution - ARxMD

These new integrations would ideally require a type of software to help the doctor request inspections when they discover potential health issues caused by the built environment. It can then allow inspectors to record appropriate testing and then send the data back to the doctor to review and analyze the results. Once issues are discovered, the subsequent information can be sent to the architect and building professional to provide solutions.

This process is something that I have been thinking about since 1999. After spending many years contemplating such a solution, the development began many years ago and now exists as the Architectural Medicine Software Solution – ARxMD.

This software allows each professional to log into their dashboard or specific platform, provide a process to evaluate with guides and protocols, and then evaluate their piece of the puzzle for best results.

An essential key to this whole process has not yet been adequately discussed, at least in the importance that it merits, and that is the proper communication and information provided to the "Patient."

Most of the time, the patient is left out of the equation in the process, and instead, the professionals focus on their work regardless of providing clarity to the patient. Yet, in my opinion, there is no greater focus and attention than to make sure the patient is supported and adequately informed throughout the entire process. Each professional should be helping the patient to better understand the steps that are taken for solutions.

After all, the whole purpose of this is to create healthier built environments for the occupants, not just to have a process of evaluations and improvements to do so without an end goal. The goal is to provide a solution for the patient and provide a healthier built environment to prevent disease and illness and offer solutions for wellness.

Architectural Medicine's whole purpose is to provide a bridge between these professionals to benefit the occupants and society at large. Otherwise, these are just systems in place for the professionals.

Another purpose of the Architectural Doctor is to help the patient navigate these steps and keep them informed and educated for their benefit. They can also help guide them through the procedures of inspections, evaluations, and potential building changes for solutions. This is also where developments in new technology can inform the patient, as more applications are becoming available for the patient to receive their healthcare data.

And because the Architectural Doctor is well versed in each profession, they have the knowledge required to help guide the patient through the process to become educated and informed on these issues and the solution process.

This is one of the critical differences between Architectural Medicine and the Architectural Doctor in reference to other fields discussing the topics of healthy building. After all, the goal is not to replace these various fields yet instead, to help integrate the knowledge and processes that are either available or potentially linked to creating a better understanding of health issues in a building. Architectural Medicine works to connect these fields using the Architectural Medicine System and ARxMD, from biophilia and epidemiology to environmental psychology and neuroscience in architecture.

These fields have valuable information that can help provide a better understanding of the built environment and provide integrations with the many pieces involved in the puzzle. The idea of integrating doctors with healthy building inspectors and building informaticists and then working with architects and builders to create solutions is where Architectural Medicine sees opportunities to provide these positive building solutions.

How ARxMD Came to Be and Why Is It Important?

This software concept is a big part of what first began my path toward Architectural Medicine. As I've mentioned earlier, this idea originated in 1999 when I first had the idea of what I called the electronic clipboard. It's a good thing this name has changed, as the electronic clipboard does not quite have the same word or brand recognition as the ubiquitous branding of the portable tablet – the iPad.

Yet essentially, an electronic clipboard or a mobile tablet as a device for professionals to use in the field and on-site is exactly what would have been ideal back then. In the late 90s, when I was working in the field with inspectors, I struggled with paper and clipboards to provide inspections, evaluations, reporting, and referencing for all of this new information I was learning.

As the goal of creating healthy built environments is extremely complex, having a mobile electronic device with the capability to record the testing and evaluations would have been very helpful. And as the modern tablets of today have powerful computing capabilities, there is a lot more that can be done than merely recording data for reporting.

I also recognized the importance of including doctors and health professionals when providing inspections for the building occupant's health. However, back in the 90s and early 2000s, there was no way to exchange data provided in building testing, and few healthcare professionals were aware of such building issues potentially causing health issues.

The Architectural Medicine Software Solution, ARxMD, provides several features that can provide a cohesive solution for each of the professionals involved. And, of course, this includes the focus on providing the best health and wellness for the patient as client and building occupant.

How Do We Get There? How Do We Create Healthier Built Environments?

While the systems and processes discussed in this book may seem to be either complex or daunting in scope, the alternative is to not work in some form of unison.

The past thirty-plus years of this process have shown me that a lack of integration as a team can end up being precarious at best. So, if there is to be a different outcome, there will need to be a different approach. And taking a proactive approach and taking the initiative for planned benefits seems to be a wise choice, at least in my book.

This process of reverse-engineering the desired goal, along with a forward-thinking design mindset, can help define and then create an action plan to achieve those goals. The lack of current systems to have these various professional fields working together is a roadblock to achieving any form of integrative solutions.

As mentioned earlier, with the advent of integrative medicine and a proposed approach of integrative architecture, combining these two developing fields opens the door for these professionals to work together in a synergistic format for exponentially beneficial results.

Next Steps and How Systems Can Be More Integrated to Support the Architectural Medicine Process

By defining six main groups, there can be processes put into place to help the evaluations of buildings and the development of procedures with an integrated systems approach:

- Patients
- Architects
- Doctors
- Inspectors/Building Informaticists
- Builders
- Architectural Doctor

The Architectural Doctor can be included as a unique component, as they can provide support in differing levels of involvement depending on the circumstances.

Some may find the listing of "Patients" in this list to be surprising. After all, they are not professionals, so why would they be listed and involved in the procedure process? As mentioned previously, the simple answer is that they are the focal point for all of this work. Leaving them out of the equation or eliminating them from any processes, protocols, and procedures is going against their better health goals. While they may not be involved in all decisions and may not be in the discussions for many of the protocols, they should be a part of the systems approach and be a critical part of creating healthier built environments.

How Does ARxMD Work and What Is Involved?

The following six steps outline the activities involved in the ARxMD workflow.

First, the software provides several vital functions that allow the Architectural Medicine System (AMS) to be implemented. From a big picture viewpoint, it allows different professionals to work together and provides a platform for each professional to work with, both independently and interdependently. It can give an overview of the processes and provide details for each step along the way.

The second part provides each professional a platform to utilize and achieve their facet of the work from a very granular perspective. For the doctor, the software allows them to request a building inspection when they see health issues with their patient – potentially related to their built environment. This can provide the physician with a system and procedures to better evaluate their patient's conditions.

The software can then provide a mechanism to create an inspection and then allow for the Healthy Building Inspector or Building Informaticist evaluation process. The testing and collecting of data to analyze the patient's built environment can then be recorded and sent back to the doctor. This data can be reviewed by the doctor and the Architectural Doctor, and when issues are found, it can lead to this information being shared with architects and building professionals to provide solutions. And with the support of the Architectural Doctor, it can lead to integrative, multi-disciplinary discussions with the doctor, architect, and builders to evaluate and provide solutions.

The third part is that the software provides an overview with guidelines for each professional's procedures. This can be extremely helpful when the doctor and architect's complex professions already have many protocols to follow.

Electronic Health Records, SNOMED, ICD, DSM, LOINC, HL7, IFC, BIM, and ARxMD

In the next sections, I'm going to get into the details of steps that require a plethora of acronyms utilized in both professions. For those unfamiliar with these acronyms, here's a quick listing of common healthcare and architecture nomenclature:

Architecture Acronyms:

AEC – Architecture, Engineering, and Construction

AIA – American Institute of Architects

BACnet – Building Automation and Control networks

BIM – Building Information Modeling

BMS – Building Management System (interchangeable with BAS Building Automation System)

CAD – Computer-Aided Design (also CAE & CAM – Computer-Aided Engineering /Manufacturing)

COBie – Construction Operations Building information exchange

FM – Facility Management

HVAC – Heating, Ventilation, and Air Conditioning

IAQ – Indoor Air Quality

IFC – Industry Foundation Classes

IOT – Internet of Things

MEP – Mechanical, Electrical, and Plumbing

OSHA – Occupational Safety and Health Administration

REC – Real Estate Core

VOC – Volatile Organic Compound

Medical Acronyms:

AMA – American Medical Association

CCD – Continuity of Care Document

CHR – Comprehensive Health Record

CPT – Current Procedural Terminology

DSM – Diagnostic and Statistical Manual of Mental Disorders

EHR – Electronic Health Record

HIE – Health Information Exchange

HIPAA – Health Insurance Portability and Accountability Act

HL7 – Health Level Seven

ICD – International Classification of Diseases

IHE – Integrating Health Enterprise

IOMT – Internet of Medical Things

LIS – Lab Information System

LOINC – Logical Observation Identifiers Names and Codes

SNOMED – Systematized Nomenclature of Medicine

SOAP – Subjective, Objective, Assessment, and Plan

With these basic terminologies outlined, the fourth part of this software system is the ability to provide proper communication, data, and procedures for each step of the way. These terms allow the sending and receiving of data to other healthcare systems using standards that are familiar within the medical community. By using the Electronic Health Record (EHR) and Comprehensive Health Record (CHR) in synchronization with Hospital Information Systems (HIS), the Architectural Medicine Software Solution can integrate with current medical systems and exchange data between fields.

This includes the use of standards such as SNOMED, ICD, DSM, and LOINC codes and expands the scope of these electronic records to incorporate this into more comprehensive information. The relatively new concept of the CHR as a comprehensive record can include the built environment and, for example, the social determinants of health as a tool for doctors to utilize for their patient's optimal health.

During the steps taken when the doctor requests an inspection of the patient's built environment, both the doctor and the inspector will need to follow standards that are codified in order for this data to be properly understood and utilized in a helpful format. While the built environment testing may be recorded directly on location, some tests may be sent to laboratories for analysis. In this manner, these testing processes will utilize the LOINC codes used in current medical lab testing. By using the ARxMD platform to record the on-site testing, this data can be implemented and exchanged with other systems using the common Health Level Seven (HL7) exchange standards.

It is of critical importance to ensure that this data and information is transferred in a secured format and to achieve this, the software will utilize the proper HL7 procedures. ARxMD uses the HL7 FHIR (Fast Healthcare Interoperability Resources), the most recent standards provided by the organization, to exchange data using these aforementioned common API practices. And while this topic may be new to many, the key is that it allows an exchange of data between many different platforms, and not just the common exchange between electronic medical record (EMR) software platforms. It allows for different systems to share and exchange data in a safe and secure format. The FHIR standard was "designed to enable information exchange to support the provision of healthcare in a wide variety of settings." [106] As of this writing, the most up to date version of HL7 is FHIR version 4.

While it's currently uncommon to exchange data between the architecture and medical platforms, this "wide variety of settings" provides EHR data to be exchanged and shared in new formats. There are many software processes currently used by architects that can be integrated for this use, such as BIM and the more recent developments such as the Brick Schema and the Real Estate Core (REC) ontologies. The recent merging of these two data ontologies, Brick Schema and REC, can provide more direct integration between the architecture and the medical fields in ways that previously would be impossible. With the advent of the advanced HL7 FHIR, this modern web-based API technology can provide interoperability with modern architecture and construction software systems.

This ability to share data using REST APIs can be seen as the fifth part of this system to provide round trip processes, and this exchange of data can be utilized for the best decision making for all involved. The Architectural Medicine Software Solution ARxMD is implementing these new procedures to provide supportive solutions for the architectural fields to connect with the medical fields with interoperability that has not been possible without these recent data schemas and ontologies. The cross-disciplinary procedures can provide the necessary integrations for each professional in working with each other across fields to achieve these goals of healthier built environments. This system can provide preliminary analysis for the doctor and final evaluations to utilize as a Comprehensive Health Record (CHR) from the pre-inspection to the post-inspection processes.

And the sixth and final step in this system — if consent from the patient is received — is the data anonymized and sent to a health data repository. This data can be analyzed and evaluated by the new building informaticist, along with public health professionals, epidemiologists, toxicologists, green chemists, building material manufacturers, and many others that can utilize this data to better understand built environments in relation to health. The results can then provide insights for medical and architecture professionals to offer valuable insights into overall population health. When analyzed, this data can also help determine standards for materials and methods to support healthier built environments for the future.

In chapter 12, ARxMD - the Architectural Medicine Software Solution part 2, I will go into more detail about the impact this interoperability can have on both local procedures for the individual, as well as the global impacts this can provide for public health and epidemiology, including the use of this data for Digital Twins.

And while all of this, in theory, might sound logical, let's dive into some of these details to see what this software looks like and how it functions.

The Architectural Medicine Software Solution – ARxMD in Use

First, let me state that this software is still a work in progress, and right now, it is in testing as a pilot program for a select group. The final writing of this book is in the fall of 2022, and the plan is to have the pilot program implemented from 2022 into 2023.

As the world is still suffering from the global pandemic of the novel coronavirus, this is both a tumultuous time to launch a new system yet also a timely opportunity to provide better health systems and metrics in the built environment.

There are six main segments of the software, and the graphic highlights the workflow process to help show each segment.. As you can see, each profession has its individual procedures, and in this manner, the software follows this structure. To discuss this in more detail, let's take a look at this swimlane diagram to 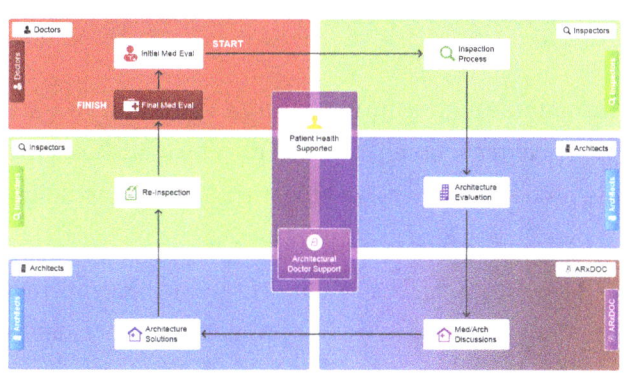 show how the flowchart shown earlier in chapter 5 can be implemented for each professional involved.

ARxMD – Swimlane Diagram of Processes

There are times when a swimlane diagram can provide more clarity as it segments each row as a "lane," and in this case, it can show each professional in their own row with each of their processes relative to the whole system.

As you can see in the following diagram, there are many steps that are occurring, and sometimes there are scenarios where multiple professions will review a process together, ensuring cohesive solutions are agreed upon.

THE ARCHITECTURAL MEDICINE SYSTEM (AMS) SWIMLANE DIAGRAM

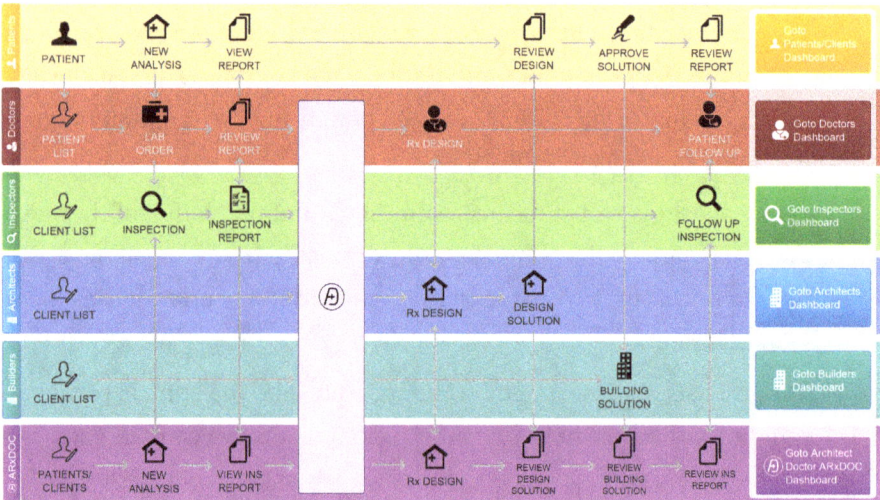

The graphic highlights the main groups involved and shows the importance of the center segment, in light purple, that shows the involvement of all of the professionals working together for cohesive solutions:

When this type of multi-professional analysis is provided, the complexity of these topics can be evaluated from each perspective, providing integrative solutions to ensure that more problems are not created. This is also where the Architectural Doctor can thrive as a liaison in the solution process. Providing questions to each of the professionals, it can make sure that the resolution will not exclude essential issues for the occupant's health.

While the swimlane shows a dynamic and sometimes non-linear process, it does have a structured format that can be viewed in the following steps:

- During the evaluation of the Patient, the Doctor requests a building inspection based on conditions that are possibly related to the Patient's built environment
- Inspector or Building Informaticist receives a request(s) to inspect the building and proceeds with the evaluation(s)

- Inspection data is recorded directly on-site or sent to the laboratory for test results
- Inspection data is reported and sent to the Electronic Medical Records (EMR) system for the Doctor and Architectural Doctor to review
- Doctor and Architectural Doctor work together and discuss issues related to health found in the built environment
- Patient is informed by Doctor or Architectural Doctor about the built environment issues
- Architects & Builders are included in the discussions when issues are found that need to be resolved
- Architect-Builder provides building solutions for the group to review
- Communication with Patient is provided by Doctor, Architectural Doctor, and Architect about the overall issues and solutions
- Solutions are approved for Builder to complete
- Builders implement solutions to properly fix the built environment issues
- Re-inspection of the built environment is completed and re-testing recorded
- Report on the re-inspection is provided to the Doctor and Architectural Doctor for evaluation
- Patient's health is reviewed after these healthy building re-inspections have been completed, and Patient's health is monitored over time
- * Data is anonymized and sent to a Clinical Data Repository (CDR) or Clinical Data Warehouse (CDW) for data analysis

* It is of critical importance to note that data is only collected as anonymous data and only after there is consent from the patient in full agreement. In the US, full HIPAA compliance is vital.[107]

The software provides a cohesive system for each professional to follow, implement, record, and exchange contextually appropriate data with the other professionals. In this format, each professional can provide their part of the process for completion.

In summary, the end goal is to provide an initial screening of issues that may be seen in the patient's health conditions relative to their built environment. Then inspections are completed to allow the doctor to analyze these issues.

The Architectural Doctor can support the overall process, especially when these different professionals have never worked together. And then, a building analysis can include the architect and builders to provide solutions. After solutions are approved and implemented, the eventual re-inspection provides the doctor with updated reports. These updates allow the doctor to evaluate their patient's long-term health.

The Clinical Data Repository (CDR) for data analysis can also provide insights and updates with new findings, which can then be included for each professional's education and training. The Architectural Doctor and the Building Informaticist can provide deeper insights into big data received to provide an iterative process. This can include an update in the multi-faceted evaluation processes and will lead to better solutions over time. As discussed previously, this form of a spiracycle process can iterate for beneficial developments over time. The opportunity of big data and data science to provide insights for better building health will be discussed in chapter 12.

In essence, the use of ARxMD allows the details of doctor analysis to be recorded and provides the methodology for the prescription as an Rx for building evaluation and inspections to be completed. The ArxMD solution provides the ability for the building evaluation to be recorded with specific steps and testing metrics to be recorded, and the reporting sent back to the doctor's electronic medical system to review.

The Architectural Doctor is available to support these reviews and to help the doctor include built environment issues impacting patient health. When issues are found in the patient's building, the proper data can be transferred to the building professionals using the ARxMD platform for them to review for solutions. In turn, these updates from the building professionals can be sent back to the doctor and Architectural Doctor to review for the next step and to provide clarifications to the patient.

Next Steps - How Each Professional Can Utilize the ARxMD Processes for Cohesive Solutions

In the paragraphs above, the details of how the ARxMD solution will function as a whole have been described and defined. Now that there is an overview of the software and how it functions using the Architectural Medicine System (AMS), the following chapters will dive into each professional's role and how this will function independently and interdependently.

To begin this discussion, in the next chapter, we will start with the role of the Healthy Building Inspector and Building Informaticist...

"The things to do are:
the things that need doing, that you see need to be done,
and that no one else seems to see need to be done."

— R. Buckminster Fuller

THE ROLE OF THE HEALTHY BUILDING INSPECTOR AND BUILDING INFORMATICIST

As I've mentioned throughout this book, an essential part of creating healthier built environments is to create systems. And along with systems is the need for those to support the procedures of these systems.

In this chapter, we're going to talk about the topic of the Healthy Building Inspector and the Building Informaticist who collectively can properly achieve these goals. I've chosen to start with the roles of the Healthy Building Inspector and the Building Informaticist for a few reasons, mostly due to these roles having the most direct connection with the steps in evaluating these built environments.

To start, it's important to note that the average building inspection in the USA and other sections of the world is completed to ensure the structural integrity of the building. These evaluations, in most cases, do not specifically inspect the building to discover issues related to occupant health.

I state "specifically," as there are inspections implemented where, if issues are found, they can be helpful to flag potential health issues. These include the discovery of lead paint, asbestos, and other problems identified, such as faulty HVAC systems, which can also impact health through air quality issues.

However, these are only a few topics that are evaluated, and there are many other issues that could be negatively impacting human health that are not tested. Too often, these go unrecognized. They are not part of the standard inspection, which means the building's inhabitants are also unaware of possible issues.

This is not to fault the current inspectors and building evaluation processes. After all, this is what the standards have been, and they are doing their work to fulfill the current standards. Yet the question arises, "can there be improvements focused on health?" Can these inspections be taken to another level to specifically look for built environment issues focused on health? And if yes, how would this be done, and what would they evaluate?

The awareness of Sick Building Syndrome (SBS) and Building Related Illness (BRI) that began in the 1980s and 90s formed a basic understanding of how health issues could impact occupants. However, the awareness of these topics has not been embraced in the professional world enough to provide active solutions. Therefore, creating a building inspection along with evaluations to address such issues has not seemed to be an essential priority in the building world.

The Healthy Building Inspector & the Building Informaticist

As discussed in the previous chapters, the systems required to achieve these goals have not existed, and due to the complex processes needed, the Architectural Medicine System and ARxMD platforms strive to provide such solutions.

To be clear, this does not mean that standards for health and safety in the building fields do not exist. On the one hand, there are the Industrial Hygiene professionals that utilize commercial building standards, such as OSHA – the Occupational Safety and Health Administration in the USA.

The American Industrial Hygiene Association (AIHA) defines Industrial hygienists as "scientists and engineers committed to protecting the health and safety of people in the workplace and the community. The industrial hygienist is part of a broader family of professionals often referred to collectively as the practice of occupational and environmental health and safety."[108]

While the AIHA is focused on these processes in the USA, the International Occupational Hygiene Association (IOHA) defines its mission as "enhancing the international network of occupational hygiene organisations that promote, develop and improve occupational hygiene worldwide, providing a safe and healthy working environment for all."[109]

This group was created to "ensure safe and healthful working conditions for working men and women by setting and enforcing standards and by providing training, outreach, education and assistance."[110] The main focus of this organization is industry and the workplace. As can be recognized in the above statements, there is undoubtedly a focus on building health and safety. Yet, in my experience, this is often specialized for commercial and industrial buildings.

On the other hand, there are others that offer inspections that view potential health issues in homes and built environments that are not necessarily industrial or commercial spaces. As independent environmental consultants, they have often been working on their own, providing information and solutions for clients. And this is extremely difficult to do, as it requires a large amount of knowledge and an even more considerable amount of education to provide to the client. This also requires working with other building professionals who have been trained to provide alternate solutions to meet more stringent standards. For many decades now, such individuals would work to help clients with building issues such as mold and volatile organic compounds (VOCs) before there was professional consensus that, indeed, these were health issues.

An example of this is the German organization IBN (Institut für Baubiologie + Nachhaltigkeit), which has set building standards focused on human and biological health. These standards are stricter to ensure that health is of the greatest importance in reviewing "physical, chemical, biological, indoor climate and other risks encountered in sleeping areas, living spaces, workplaces and properties."[111]

The industrial hygienist is a professional field with certifications on a national level in the US and worldwide. Environmental inspectors are often professionals that have gathered knowledge from many sources and work to fill gaps in the building inspection fields including human and biological health.

On the contrary, the environmental inspector is often an individual that offers an extension to the typical building inspection, with an added focus on health issues in residential construction.

For many individuals providing these services, this includes topics such as mold and moisture issues, pesticides in structures, and issues related to chemical exposures such as Radon, VOCs, and the many synthetic materials that can pollute indoor air quality. These issues can cause a wide range of health problems, from asthma and respiratory problems to endocrine and nervous system issues.

In my own experience, these environmental inspectors provide services to people who have not been able to find solutions from the medical community in typical formats. And as such, the lack of medical professionals having knowledge of building issues related to health problems is part of the origins of the Healthy Building Inspector and the Building Informaticist.

In my opinion, it would be great to have these Industrial Hygienists work directly with the medical and architectural communities to support the health evaluations for both residential and commercial locations. Obviously, their work is extremely valuable and important, yet it is my hope that more bridges between these professionals can support better health for occupants of all buildings.

Most of the general public has not been aware of the extent of building health issues, yet the coronavirus pandemic has brought the topic of health and wellness in the built environment into greater clarity. The historic pandemic of 1918 was the closest event that brought worldwide awareness to building health. Before the coronavirus pandemic, this topic had been out of sight and mind for most.

As the pandemic has been a harsh reality for most, this awareness can provide the potential for change in the built environment to support better health. As populations strive to get back to normality and spend time in buildings other than their homes, the recognition of ensuring that a building is safe from contaminants has never been higher on the list of priorities in the world than it is now.

The question is, how can we know if these environments, such as buildings for work, retail, shopping, and other locations, are safe from the coronavirus? And how can this be measured and resolved?

And what about toxins, contaminants, and other issues that can cause health problems? Are these being evaluated and included in some form of inspection process for best health?

The Healthy Building Inspector and Building Informaticist can help provide such evaluations, and in the following steps, I will go into more detail about how this works with the Architectural Medicine System.

These inspections include a wide range of issues, from the coronavirus to the many other topics that negatively impact physical, mental, and emotional health in the built environment.

Chapter: 7 The Role of the Healthy Building Inspector and Building Informaticist

The Healthy Building Inspection

A key element of this system is to have Healthy Building Inspectors and Building Informaticists trained to provide inspections focused on health. These new inspectors also need to be aware of the systems that doctors and health professionals expect in following the proper procedures and reporting in these health professions.

The first step is to require these three facets:

- Healthy Building Inspectors/ Building Informaticists
- Training for these new professional inspectors
- Protocols, processes, and reporting that will fit into the systems of the health professions

The next step in this process of the doctor recognizing an ailment potentially being related to a built environment issue is to have a need for systems in place to work with these new building inspectors. And as moving forward, these new building professionals will be trained and, hopefully in the future, certified.

In this way, the medical professional can order a building inspection with health specifications in testing and then receive a report and summary from the inspector about the issues found. This would be done in a similar manner that a doctor orders a blood test or an X-ray. They can request the reports of this testing, which can be sent from the inspectors to the laboratory professionals and then reported to the doctor. In this manner, the doctor has more information about their patient's built environment offering better insights into evaluating their health.

Yet right now, the profession of medicine is not typically connected to the building field in this manner. So, at this time, there is a need for both building inspectors that can evaluate structures based on health, and there is also a need for protocols to be put into place to support this integration between doctors and inspectors for round trip solutions.

As discussed in Chapter 5 with the Architectural Medicine flowchart, the evaluation process of the doctor and medical professional is required for the next steps to take place. With these steps, the doctor also needs to have the ability to order such building inspections.

While some inspectors and consultants do this type of work in the USA for residential buildings, only a few do this with a high level of integrated training focused on health. In places such as Europe, as in Germany, Switzerland, and a few other locations worldwide, they do offer such professional inspections, where there are some options in place for health-related building inspections. Many of these healthy building inspections are done in collaboration with the support of doctors who are more open to integrative approaches within these modalities. The training on health issues in buildings in certain places in Europe is not only more commonplace, yet more accepted and understood by certain doctors.

However, even with this greater awareness, there is still a need for doctors to have connections with each professional. And this includes the processes and knowledge of working with them to achieve the proper diagnosis to benefit their patients.

In this realm, providing these inspections for building health issues, the following is a list of requirements to achieve these collective goals as a second group of steps.

The second step is to provide these three facets for the Healthy Building Inspection:

- The processes, protocols, and technology to achieve these inspections – testing, equipment, laboratory results, standards, reporting, etc.
- The connection between professions – to work together for cohesive analysis
- The interest in creating healthier built environments – supply-demand

Chapter: 7   The Role of the Healthy Building Inspector and Building Informaticist

8 STEPS TO BETTER HEALTH IN THE BUILT ENVIRONMENT

1. The development of protocols for ailments potentially caused by built environment issues

2. The training of Doctors to utilize protocols during ailment analysis

3. The training of building inspectors and informaticists to evaluate topics related to health in buildings

4. Systems created to support this process, from the Doctor creating an Rx for a Building Inspection to the interconnected system of evaluation and reports sent back to the doctor for evaluation

5. The training of architects and builders to recognize health issues in the built environment

6. The development of protocols in the built environment that architects and builders are trained to evaluate and resolve

7. The training of doctors, architects, inspectors, and informaticists to work together to resolve health issues in the built environment

8. Software solutions created to support this process, from the Doctor creating an order for a Building Inspection and the inspection procedures to reporting for the doctors and subsequent prescription as building Rx for the architecture and building professionals to solve

As I complete the writing of this book, it is the year 2022, and the world continues to experience the global impacts of the novel coronavirus pandemic. Over the past several years, this has led to the stay at home initiatives, where people have stayed in one place in one building for several months at a time – and often all of the time. This situation has brought recognition to the impacts that the built environment has on one's health – physically, emotionally, and mentally.

Spending so much time inside a building for prolonged periods can often force people to realize the impacts of their built spaces. It can increase appreciation of how their built environment impacts their lives and possibly increase demand for better health designs moving forward. To bring things back to some level of normalcy, there must be health procedures and processes in the built environments of workplaces, retail stores, and many public and private buildings to ensure the health of the masses.

As people return to spending more time in large groups inside buildings, there must be processes required and implemented to ensure the populations' health. And this leads to the topics of how to achieve these goals, both as processes and protocols. These new professionals of the Healthy Building Inspector and Building Informaticist, combined with the Healthy Building Inspection, can provide better metrics through testing, evaluations, and relevant protocols to ensure that these buildings are safe. The healthy building inspection can include many physical and material issues in the structure that can cause health issues and problems, including impacts on the occupant's emotional and psychological well-being.

The Building Inspection and Evaluations Focused on Human Health

Below is a list of inspection topics that are focused on the advanced health and safety of the occupants:

- Air Quality
- Volatile Organic Compounds – VOCs
- Particulates

Chapter: 7   The Role of the Healthy Building Inspector and Building Informaticist

- Mold and Moisture
- Pesticides
- Allergens
- Lighting – Natural/Artificial
- Sound – Noise
- Material Toxicity
- Temperature/Humidity levels
- Thermal imaging/Thermal analysis
- Pressure testing – positive/negative pressure
- HVAC systems for health
- Water quality for health
- Extreme smells/noxious odors
- Radioactivity/Radon

Along with the physical issues, there may also be issues impacting the inhabitants' emotional and psychological wellness.

For the emotional and psychological impacts of the built environment, the healthy building inspector can work with psychologists and environmental psychologists, as well as neuroscientists and neuropsychologists.

Processes and Procedures for the Healthy Building Inspector

The healthy building inspector will have many variables to navigate, yet all of their procedures will follow a general pattern:

- Inspection setup process
- Systems and processes of working with the medical fields and medical professionals

- Inspection using standards and protocols
- Systems and processes of working with the architecture/building fields and architecture/building professionals

The associations and organizations for international standards and protocols can work with the medical, architecture, and other health and construction professionals with their professional organizations. This includes organizations such as the American Institute of Architects (AIA), the American Medical Association (AMA), the American Psychological Association (APA), and the many other groups and organizations involved in this large scope of topics.

These groups can span an expansive range from psychologists, environmental psychologists, and neuroscientists to public health professionals, toxicologists, and epidemiologists. These professional organizations can collaborate for integrative solutions for better health in the built environment.

Healthy Building Inspections and Integrative Systems Solutions

The physical components of the built environment that can be evaluated range in scope from some common issues of asbestos and lead in paints and products to the more complex topics such as VOCs, particulates, molds, bacteria, and pesticides.

And this is where we get into new territory for many health professionals. While there are many ways to review and order lab testing, such as blood tests, X-rays, and MRIs, how many medical and health professionals will order or request a building inspection focused on health-related topics?

And how many health professionals would be comfortable providing an Rx for a patient's building?

What's needed in this scenario is the addition of the Healthy Building Inspection, the Building Informaticist, and an evaluation process for the doctor and physician to include these potential issues in their patient's health analysis.

A key part of these new processes is to have systems in place for these professionals to work together and include these new procedures to implement, such as ARxMD.

The Healthy Building Inspection Process Using the ARxMD Software

This exchange of data and requests sent to the Healthy Building Inspector results in the next step, which is the actual inspection of the patient's built environment.

To show this in more detail, when you view the swimlane diagram and follow the processes of the inspector, the steps involved can vary depending upon the built environment issues. This can range from Indoor Air Quality (IAQ) problems and particulates to problems with materials, VOCs, and other pollutants.

The software shows the inspection details for guidance in gathering this data to support the inspection process. By providing specific instructions focused on building health issues, certain inspections can be performed related to these health ailments.

As mentioned previously in this book, most building inspections around the world focus on the structural integrity of the building and not on human health. Some structural inspections can overlap with health issues, such as building moisture issues and HVAC system problems. While these can sometimes flag potential health issues, the concern is often not focused on human health. Therefore, many building issues might be negatively impacting human health without the occupants being aware of such factors.

The Healthy Building Inspection focuses on these health problems and starts with a big picture view, literally, of the building plot plan. It then focuses on each facet of the building with a more detailed evaluation.

In the ARxMD software, there is also an interface for the Healthy Building Inspector as they begin their evaluations:

ARCHITECTURAL MEDICINE SOFTWARE SOLUTION – ARxMD
HEALTHY BUILDING INSPECTOR VIEWS

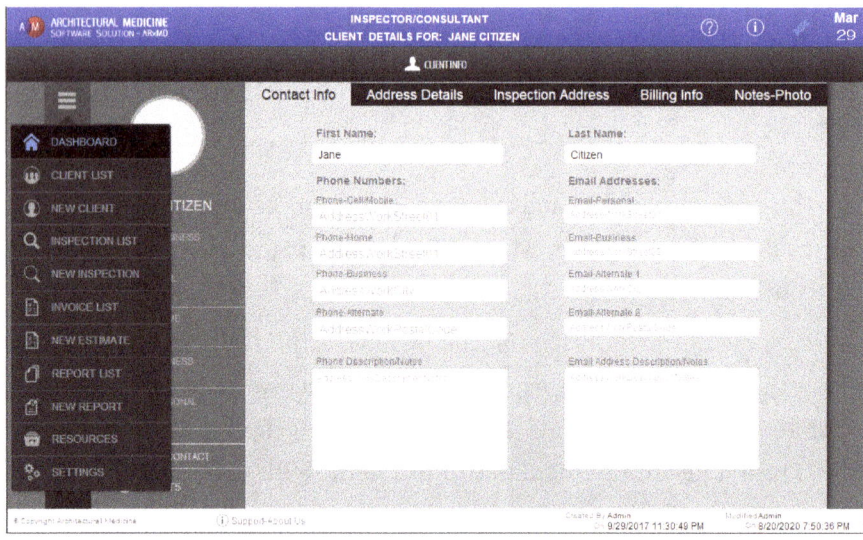

Once the patient's information has been sent to the inspector and an inspection date and time are set, the inspection process begins. Below is the interface for the start of the inspection process:

Inspection Process and Steps for Evaluating the Built Environment for Health

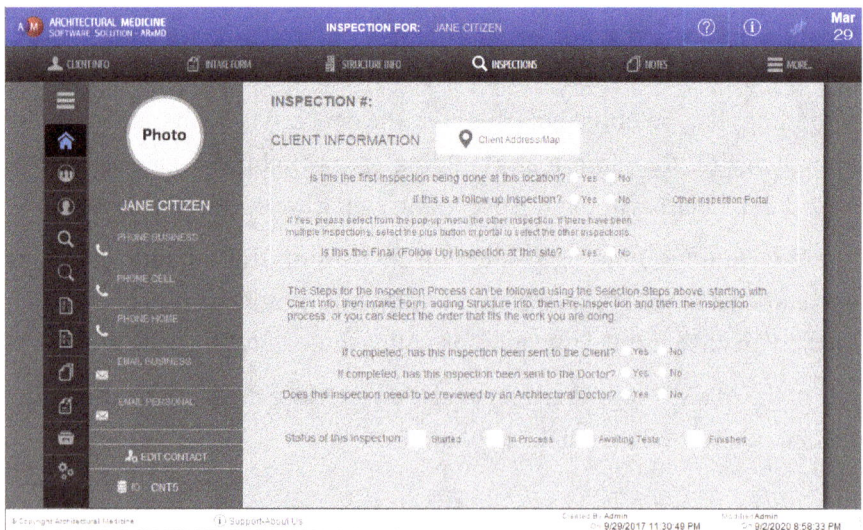

Chapter: 7   The Role of the Healthy Building Inspector and Building Informaticist

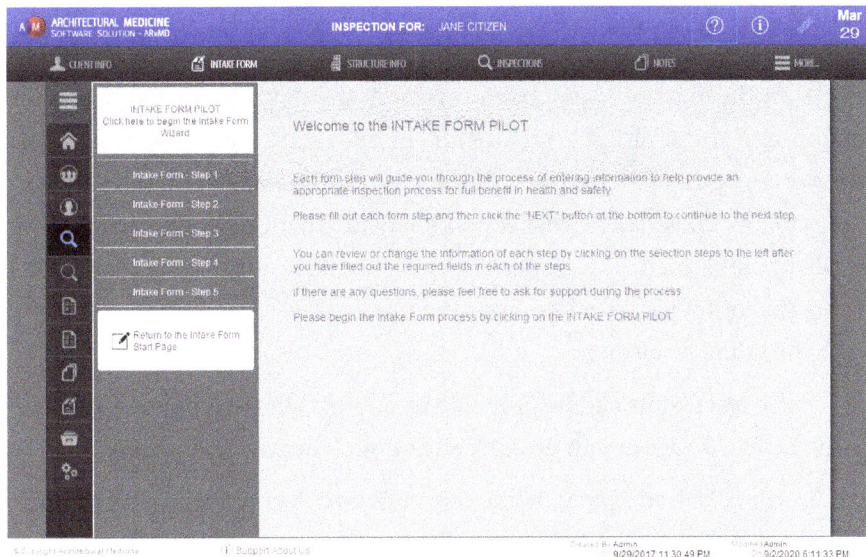

The software guides the inspector through the processes, from the pre-inspection and inspection to the room analysis and various testing modalities.

This reporting and raw data are recorded into the ARxMD software and, where appropriate, sent to labs for testing results. When tests are confirmed, they are sent to the ARxMD platform using the relevant LOINC codes using HL7 protocols.

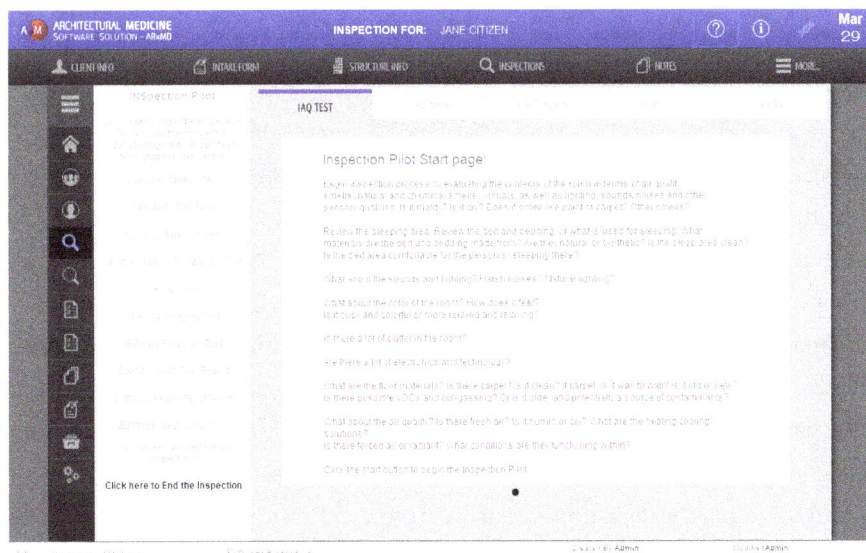

The Re-Inspection Process Using the ARxMD Software

After these issues have been resolved, the next step is to update the doctor and the Architectural Doctor to review the solutions. When they receive the updates to this work, they can notify the Healthy Building Inspector to follow up with a re-inspection to ensure that the work has been correctly implemented. The inspectors can provide re-testing of initial issues, using the initial test as a baseline. The updated results are then compared with the initial reporting.

These test results can be provided again through the laboratory systems using LOINC codes or can be entered as direct measurements on-site.

The data is then synced to the other ARxMD segments for other professionals to review, or the data can be exchanged to an EMR or HIS to ensure that the solutions were successful.

To achieve the goal of helping and supporting the patient's health, will require new training for the doctor and the architect with these new approaches, including the implementation of the role of the Healthy Building Inspector and Building Informaticist. This will require these new systems in place for the Doctor to request these inspections and request reporting that can provide lab test results from the built environment. It also means that there needs to be room for improvement for these new processes and systems to be implemented.

The Healthy Building Inspector is a key integrator in this process and acts as an important piece of the puzzle. They provide the doctor with the testing and laboratory results of their evaluations and deliver reports for the architect and building professionals to support the necessary information for a successful solution process. As an extension to this information, there are many other professionals, from epidemiologists, toxicologists, and public health professionals to those in the design and manufacturing of materials that can benefit from these inspection processes for future use. This includes emerging fields such as green chemistry for material and product developments. Each of these professionals can utilize this information in integrative formats to provide a collaborative process for cohesive solutions. They each add their knowledge and research to create best practices, yet only if there are sound systems in place as well as data to provide this information and expertise in multi-disciplinary formats.

And the data by itself will not be enough to enable a larger scale benefit for the masses. In order to utilize this data for achieving positive results, there must be others well versed in the analysis of this building data to provide deeper and more robust insights, especially those who are already familiar with healthcare and working with medical professionals.

Informatics – The Healthy Building Inspector and Building Informaticist

As discussed in the previous paragraphs, the professional organizations located in the USA, such as the American Institute of Architects (AIA) and the American Medical Association (AMA), are a part of a large global set of groups supporting their professions. The American Medical Informatics Association (AMIA) is another organization whose purpose is to support the field of informatics.

Informatics is defined as the "science of how to use data, information, and knowledge to improve human health and the delivery of health care services." [112]

> "Biomedical and health informatics applies principles of computer and information science to the advancement of life sciences research, health professions education, public health, and patient care. This multidisciplinary and integrative field focuses on health information technologies (HIT), and involves the computer, cognitive, and social sciences."[113]

The AMIA defines a list of informatics professions, such as the Clinical Informaticist and Public Health Informaticist, yet perhaps another facet of this process can be the addition of Building Informatics and the Building Informaticist.

After all, if evaluating buildings for health purposes can provide data for the health professionals to include for patient health assessments, then there is going to be a need for this data to be properly analyzed and utilized by doctors and other health professionals.

This use of informatics can provide "insights developed through data transformation, analytics, discovery and observations of clinical practices applied to a healthcare priority by a healthcare expert."[114] This use of data as informatics can provide a "key to ensuring healthcare data are translated into meaningful knowledge that helps healthcare professionals make appropriate decisions to assist people."[115]

With the increase in time spent inside buildings, the importance of data focused on health seems obvious. Yet as you review the expanse of informatics, there are limited facets that include the built environment. However, there is a great opportunity for the creation of a Building Informaticist to provide this analysis for healthcare professionals.

This is critical as the AMIA informatics organization stresses the importance of an expert in healthcare. As they state, "whether it is clinical care, public health, drug development or another domain that seeks to improve care decisions," a key to an informatics professional is in distinguishing "health informatics from data science and health information management."[116]

What I find particularly intriguing is the statement made by this organization with a focus on the stakeholders across the healthcare delivery system:

> "Informatics is the intersection between the work of stakeholders across the health and healthcare delivery system who maintain specific health expertise, committed to learning from each individual patient and seek to improve outcomes, increase safety and promote the high-quality services based on insights discovered in healthcare's data."[117]

This, in particular, showcases the potential for this type of professional to be a valuable asset in the Architectural Medicine processes bridging health and the built environment. The ability to discover data in buildings to provide insights into better healthcare is an excellent bridge to achieving these goals.

In terms of many professions becoming more integrated, in the past several decades, those with degrees in "computer science, statistics, epidemiology, nursing and population health recognized they can help countless people through informatics and embark on advanced education and training to have both the data science and medical expertise necessary."[118]

As the AMIA organization continues to define "credentials for professionalizing the field of informatics and the sub-specialties within it,"[119] perhaps they will soon include the subset of building health informatics into their catalog.

With the amount of data that continues to grow in exponential formats, it will require the management and proper evaluation of this data to provide helpful insights. People benefit from "informaticians' ability to collect, analyze and interpret data, which creates information and knowledge that is applied to healthcare decisions."[120]

This is a critical component of informatics, and extending these data sets to include building health data to overlap with healthcare data, can provide a tremendous amount of knowledge for public health.

The highlighted section below, from the American Medical Informatics Association, provides an overview of these informatics professions listing each of the specialties focused on healthcare topics.

If these issues in the built environment are to be properly evaluated and analyzed for the patient and public health, the inclusion of the Building Informaticist can provide this missing link.

These building evaluations can provide a wide range of data to analyze for data scientists to assess for public health insights.

And as most of these building evaluations are not currently being completed, there is the potential for extremely large data sets to be obtained and reviewed into the future.

THE FOLLOWING SEGMENT IS FROM THE AMERICAN MEDICAL INFORMATICS ASSOCIATION – AMIA

Understanding Why and How Informatics is Accelerating Healthcare's Transformation

Data science is the expertise of extracting knowledge or insights from the data in various forms. Data science is not limited to healthcare. To be able to extract and transform data into knowledge, one needs to apply computer science and mathematical techniques to a dataset or collection of data that is very large— often referred to as big data.

In healthcare *big data* comes from patient records, prescription records, genomic data, imaging, epidemiology studies, environmental data, clinical data or any other data set that in some way connects to care, treatments, patients or public health. Today, the amount of data are so massive that past methods used to collect, store and analyze it may no longer work—there are just too much data. Informatics is needed to assure that data are properly understood and analyzed and can be put to the best possible use(s). Informatics is what allows us to transform and make use of data.

Storing and collecting healthcare business data in accordance with regulations and laws, identifying errors and missing billing data and assigning codes to it is a necessary component of patient care that most accurately is considered *health information management* (HIM). This is a separate and distinct field from informatics. However, once this data, which is generated by the growing number of health information technology (HIT) applications, like electronic health records (EHRs), is collected it can be subjected to additional analysis by the informaticians who affect patient care.

During *data analytics*, researchers create models to analyze the data in different ways to identify patterns, evaluate findings, test hypotheses and further manipulate the data to achieve more precise analysis or results, if possible.

"AMIA® (American Medical Informatics Association®) is a community committed to the vision of a world where informatics transforms people's care. Over the last 35 years, the use of informatics has grown exponentially to improve health and to make better healthcare decisions. Today, informatics is the key to accelerating the current goals of healthcare reform."

SPECIALTIES WITHIN INFORMATICS:

Broadly, AMIA defines informatics as applying insights from data analytics to a healthcare priority by a healthcare expert. AMIA defines the specialties within informatics as:

Translational bioinformatics:
Applying informatics to optimize biomedical and genomic data into predicative, preventive and participatory health.

Clinical research informatics:
Applying informatics to discover and manage new knowledge related to health and disease, such as patient safety and clinical trials.

Clinical informatics:
Applying informatics to delivering healthcare services in care facilities, such as hospitals and community health centers.

Consumer health informatics:
Applying informatics from the perspective of multiple consumer or patient views, such as health literacy and consumer education.

Public health informatics:
Applying informatics to the areas of public and population health, such as surveillance, reporting and health promotion.

This information is from the AMIA PDF:

https://brand.amia.org/m/70d13c6fb0273972/original/AMIA-Media-Handout-pdf.pdf

https://whyinformatics.org/

Re-Thinking the Building Inspector as the Building Informaticist

In the above writings, the comments on informatics and the use of research are highlighted by the statement, "informaticians conduct research and apply findings to improve processes and propose solutions to technical, clinical, and organizational challenges hampering successful technology implementations."[121] When you view the Healthy Building Inspection in terms of a professional who is evaluating built environment issues focused on health and not just a structural inspection, then this viewpoint can be transformative. This process of informaticians who "conduct research and apply findings to improve processes and propose solutions" is very much in alignment with the goals of the Healthy Building Inspector.

Perhaps a better way to discuss these professionals is to define them as Healthy Building Informaticians or Building Informaticists. In this manner, they are providing research into the building, with a focus on building health issues and providing the data sets to evaluate the occupant's health. And their goals are to eventually provide data for professionals to create proper solutions to resolve building health issues.

After all, the Architectural Medicine System can be used as a process to evaluate building issues which can be measured and provide a template for each professional to work with, and this process of gathering data sets allows for the patient's health to be properly ascertained.

Another reason why a building informaticist is appropriate is based on the work being done over the past few decades by social workers and those in public health. They have been evaluating health topics relative to these determinants of health, and this includes the environment and buildings. Places and spaces where people live, work, and play, and the impacts of these places on human health, are becoming a more common topic and are a common definition of social determinants of health. While those in public health have been researching and reviewing this for decades, the missing piece, in my view, has been a complete round trip cycle of processes and the inclusion of the architecture and building fields into these equations.

Chapter: 7 The Role of the Healthy Building Inspector and Building Informaticist

Informatics, Data Science, and Health Information Management

Another vital component of these processes are data sets that can be collected as anonymous data and evaluated utilizing the methodologies of data scientists for this public health informatics.

As mentioned above, informatics is the overview or umbrella of the many facets of data evaluation processes, from big data and data science to data analytics and health information management (HIM), which includes health information technology (HIT) applications, such as electronic health records (EHRs).

And the reason why this is important is that the current scope of this data evaluation is merging with topics such as social determinants of health (SDoH), and as such, includes the built environment. The average person spends between 60 to 90 percent of their time indoors, and the amount of research and data collected in the built environment focused on health impacts is actually very small right now.

Providing more evaluations and data gathering in the built environment, it can provide a very large data set for both medical and public health professionals to determine best practices for better health in buildings.

Once the data is collected by the Healthy Building Inspector or informaticist, these larger data sets can be anonymized and shared by data scientists to provide more information for public health and medical professionals. These new data sets and resulting bioinformatics can then lead to better insights for the medical and health professionals to utilize for advanced understandings of how the built environment impacts human health and can, in turn, update their evaluation processes to include the environment in their analysis to diagnose their patient's health issues.

And this will then lead to the topics mentioned in previous chapters of the architecture professionals being involved in helping with built environment issues that are impacting occupant health. This cyclical process can then inform new updates in the architecture fields that are in alignment with the medical and health fields to provide better built environment solutions focused on health and wellness.

> "Biomedical informatics (BMI) is the interdisciplinary, scientific field that studies and pursues the effective uses of biomedical data, information, and knowledge for scientific inquiry, problem solving and decision making, motivated by efforts to improve human health." [122]

One of the first training programs in Biomedical Informatics was at Stanford university, with a degree program "initiated in October 1982 as Medical Information Sciences (MIS) and continues to emphasize interdisciplinary education between medicine, computer science, and statistics." [123]

This interdisciplinary education process is where informatics can provide new insights for developments in healthcare applied across several professions. While architecture and the AEC fields are not as active in these developments, there are architects and building professionals involved in Healthy Hospital Design, where some of these topics overlap. Extending these overlaps into average building construction, and not just hospital designs, can provide a wider reach to help impact the general public's health in broader terms.

The statement provided below, by Dr. William Hersh, a professor and chair of the Department of Medical Informatics & Clinical Epidemiology at Oregon Health & Science University, provides an interesting line of thought to ponder relative to these topics of health and data:

> "One of the biggest challenges for the field of informatics is the variability in the word(s) that precede informatics. The most comprehensive term to describe the field is biomedical and health informatics (BMHI). Sometimes just components of these broader terms are used, such as biomedical informatics or health informatics. But all of them refer to the field that is concerned with the optimal use of information, often aided by the use of technology, to improve individual health, health

care, public health, and biomedical research. Practitioners of informatics are usually called informaticians (sometimes informaticists) and view their focus more on information than technology."[124]

As I highlighted earlier, the expansion of these titles that precede informatics includes the following list of informatics professionals from the American Medical Informatics Association (AMIA):[125]

- Translational Bioinformatics
- Clinical research informatics
- Clinical informatics
- Consumer health informatics
- Public health informatics

At the core, the purpose of this proposed Building Informatics is to provide the "optimal use of information… to improve individual health, health care, public health, and biomedical research," as Dr. Hersh stated above so eloquently.

If this building data can be provided and analyzed in the same format as other bioinformatic professionals, then the future of building informatics for public health can become a valuable toolset. In the next section, I will elaborate on the use of bioinformatics and discuss how this can be connected to other emerging developments in both the building and medical fields.

Translational Bioinformatics, Building Informatics, and the connection to Digital Twins

Translational Bioinformatics, as defined by the AMIA, is the "development of storage, analytic, and interpretive methods to optimize the transformation of increasingly voluminous biomedical data, and genomic data, into proactive, predictive, preventive, and participatory health."[126] This includes research on the "development of novel techniques for the integration of biological and clinical data and the evolution of clinical informatics methodology to encompass biological observations."[127]

This viewpoint on the end goals of translational bioinformatics is prepared to provide "newly found knowledge from these integrative efforts that can be disseminated to a variety of stakeholders, including biomedical scientists, clinicians, and patients."

And this last statement, in particular, is where Architectural Medicine, the Architectural Doctor, and the interoperability between architecture and medicine can provide a great leap in building health and wellness. Utilizing the knowledge found from the big data of the healthy building inspections as building informatics and providing that knowledge for the architecture and medical professionals in a cohesive format, can be incredibly powerful.

By itself, this information can be valuable to provide insights for the doctor in delivering personalized medicine. This data, applied as informatics with genomic data, can be utilized to construct a medical digital twin for preventive and supportive health processes.

However, by adding the environmental and building health data into this equation, it can provide informatics for more cohesive health evaluations. In this manner, the digital twin representing a building can be overlapped with the medical digital twin for deeper insights into a patient's whole health analysis.

Not only can this provide new processes and procedures for both professionals, yet it can provide more information for the general public to better understand the relationship between buildings and their health and wellness.

These topics can also show the potential for more extensive overlaps between Biomedical Informatics and Digital Twins, which is also discussed in other chapters of this book. I provide more details on this topic and the digital twins of architecture and medicine in chapter 12, ARxMD – The Architectural Medicine Software Solution (Part 2), and in chapter 15.

Chapter: 7 The Role of the Healthy Building Inspector and Building Informaticist

A Summary - The Healthy Building Inspector and Building Informaticist

While these discussions on healthier built environments can provide solutions moving forward, many of these processes are complex and will require updates to previous procedures as well as new steps for many professionals in both the medical and building fields.

In this chapter, I outlined the steps and roles that the Healthy Building Inspector and Building Informaticist can take to provide inspections and analysis of the built environment for better health. Using the ARxMD software, processes were outlined to achieve the evaluations in a systematic format that includes the interoperability procedures required to function in the current medical and health systems. This also includes the integrations with the building and architecture professions to achieve the round trip steps for issues to be discovered and solutions to be created and implemented.

In order to ensure that these topics are viewed in a big picture format, and these overall goals maintain clarity, in the next chapter, I will discuss the foundation of these steps in a more simplified format. This way, while the complexity of these topics will emerge, an outline of these goals can be maintained and defined.

This will lead to a better understanding of how the doctor and architect function in this system and can provide an outline for these steps in a cohesive framework.

And this leads us into the next chapter — 8 steps to better health and wellness in the built environment...

"The reward for work well done is the opportunity to do more."

— Jonas Salk

8 STEPS TO BETTER HEALTH AND WELLNESS IN THE BUILT ENVIRONMENT

One of the main challenges in the modern day world is complexity, and as the world continues to become more complex, there is a need for a more simplistic overview. Otherwise, the complexities can overwhelm and can often deter people from understanding the big picture purpose of developments.

The topics of Architectural Medicine are inherently complex. They involve not only many different complex professions, yet the overlap and integrations require complex systems for beneficial outcomes.

Therefore, a simplification can help to comprehend the essence of the procedures, with the ability for this complexity to be navigated appropriately. In this manner, the depth of the procedures can have context and allow for these topics to be explored in an interconnected manner.

In chapter 5, the Architectural Medicine System was defined, showing the many pieces of the puzzle and how they can fit together for cohesive solutions. In chapter 2, I provided a brief overview of the goals of Architectural Medicine by discussing the "8 steps to better health and wellness in the built environment."

In this chapter, I will delve into these processes in more depth, utilizing the topics discussed in the previous chapters to form an overview of the work supported by the Architectural Doctor.

With the increasing number of people recognizing how the complex modern world, developed by humans, is negatively impacting human beings, there becomes questions as to what can be done about them. From indoor and outdoor air pollution to natural and human-created chemicals that are negatively impacting biological and human health, there are many variables to navigate. Topics of lead, asbestos, and newly formed synthetic chemicals impacting the endocrine system, there is an increasing number of toxins and contaminants in the exterior and built environments that are causing illness.

What can be done about these issues? Of course, many have already started, and their pioneering progress has brought awareness from the days of Florence Nightingale to Rachel Carson and, of course modern day pioneers who have kept the general public aware of these issues. While there are many who are pioneering the solutions, there are still big gaps in the processes and in the systems.

As mentioned previously, if issues in the built environment are negatively impacting health, then what is a doctor to do about this? And what's more, are doctors even aware of ailments that may be caused by issues in the built environment? And to make matters more complex, those involved in the built environment are rarely informed and educated about human health topics. And while the focus of these built environment professionals is to make sure the building maintains structural integrity to provide shelter, the processes that occur inside these structures may be affecting good human health.

There are many writings and commentaries on health in the built environment, yet for many years these concerns have often been left to individuals to approach and solve. With many new studies, research, and concerns about health in the built environment, how can these solutions that span many professions be more easily traversed to help support these goals?

A helpful step in this direction, in my opinion, is to recognize that inherent in the complex crossroads of multiple professions is the acknowledgment that there are problems. Providing clearly defined steps as an overview can begin new processes for solutions, especially when these main professions of architecture and medicine are often disconnected.

The Architectural Doctor is there to help be a liaison between these fields, and Architectural Medicine is provided to support and implement systems to support the education, training, and processes for protocols and solutions.

How can this clarity be achieved?

8 Steps to Better Health and Wellness in the Built Environment

If the doctor and healthcare professional recognizes these building health issues, the complex steps to provide solutions would need to be simplified for clarification.

As mentioned in the previous chapters, if the doctor or health professional does find issues in the patient's built environment, what steps can they take to analyze these issues creating or exacerbating illness. What would happen? Would a doctor be expected to go to a patient's home or work environment to check for issues? Not ideally. So, this is where the need for another group to be involved is required. As outlined in the previous chapter, this role could be that of a healthy building inspector, a healthy building consultant, or a building informaticist.

In the same way that a doctor would order bloodwork or an X-ray or MRI, the doctor could prescribe a built environment analysis to evaluate for health related issues in the built environment.

This would require that there be professionals trained in health related issues in the built environment. This could be a group already providing building inspections, where additional training is provided related to such health issues. Or this could be an entirely new group of professionals that are trained specifically on health related building issues.

Either way, there would need to be several things put into place for this to exist, most of which do not exist today. This list would include the training of doctors to include ailments that might be related to the built environment, as well as protocols created by medical professionals in which to follow. This would also require the Architectural Medicine System to be put into place for a doctor to order a building evaluation, much like a doctor would order a blood test or X-ray, as a building Rx and evaluation. And, of course, that would require building inspectors to evaluate topics of health. So, there are really four factors that would need to be created.

These first four topics are:

- The development of protocols for ailments potentially caused by built environment issues
- The training of Doctors to utilize protocols during ailment analysis
- The training of building inspectors and informaticists to evaluate topics related to health in buildings
- Systems created to support this process, from the Doctor creating an Rx for a Building Inspection to the interconnected system of evaluation and reports sent back to the doctor for evaluation

These, of course, would be added to the doctor's evaluation process in a similar manner that an MRI or X-ray would be used for proper analysis and diagnosis.

My direct experience of being involved in building inspections related to health, and my education from European professionals dealing with building health issues, led to this awareness of how complex this process really is. The lack of systems in place often prevents this whole systems health analysis and built environment solution from becoming a reality. In my work in this field to better support health in the built environment, I found that all of these facets, or lack of interconnections, led to way too much for any single professional to take on by themselves. And a subsequent lack of health and building professionals being involved in this topic has caused a lack of progress in building health to flourish.

My direct experience and education have led me on this path to become aware of these topics, to witness the lack of systems, and acknowledge the complexity required in this entire process.

These have been the seeds of Architectural Medicine and the Architectural Doctor, and as such, I've seen the direct results of not having integrated systems and the results. This lack of integration can leave many building health issues unresolved, and many occupants exposed to health issues that could be prevented. It also means there are many health professionals that are not aware of the origins of many of their patient's health issues, and the absence of public health insights into these metrics.

The Architectural Doctor is there to both help in the training and education of the medical professionals and the building inspection professionals, yet also as a liaison in providing protocols, processes, ailments, and the overall system implementation of these roundtrip services.

This is why the "systems" part of the equation is equally as important. Doctors are used to a process and specific protocols to order various testing procedures, so why not add an order for the built environment to be tested? This can then be followed up by a prescription as an Rx for a healthy building solution.

And then the question of what happens if and when issues are found in the built environment? While there are very few doctors who might work with a building inspector on health related issues, there is the question of how doctors would work with architects and builders to find and resolve built environment issues.

While there is the emerging field of doctors and architects working together in healthy hospital design, can this scope of work include the entire built environment of all places and cities and not just hospitals? Again, this is where the Architectural Doctor plays an important and helpful role in supporting these liaisons for healthy building solutions.

If a system is created for a doctor to order a healthy building inspection, then can a system be created for a doctor to write a prescription for a healthy built environment?

In architect Paula Baker-Laporte's book *Prescriptions for a Healthy House*, she joins the medical doctor Erica Elliott and the builder John Banta in penning a book that deals with topics related to health and the built environment, and, as the title suggests, solutions to such issues.

I first met Paula Baker at her first ever healthy building presentation in the 1996 conference "Building For Health," with teachers who have also been pioneers in the field, including Cedar Rose Guelberth and Carol Venolia. Several months before meeting Paula Baker-Laporte, I met builder Robert Laporte, the founder of the Econest Building Company and the Natural House Building Centre. After the two met, they joined forces to write the book *EcoNest,* a book that I recommend for those seeking more natural building solutions for healthy building.

While their book provides solutions to many building health issues, there is a need for these health and building professionals to evaluate buildings and for systems to provide interoperability for this to occur. And if these topics were then formed into protocols that doctors were familiar with as possible built environment ailments, and allowed a process to order a building inspection for health, then the first half of the equation would be met. And adding in an Rx for a healthier built environment would then complete the cycle as a round trip process for the patient and all professionals involved.

Yet the procedures required to achieve these goals, once again, do not exist. So again, this is where the goals of Architectural Medicine and the role of the Architectural Doctor can support these systems. If the Architectural Doctor is there to support the doctor in analysis, which can help bridge the doctor with healthy building inspectors, they can act as a liaison to support the connections between the doctors, inspectors, and the architects and builders. This process, from analysis and evaluations to solutions, can be formed and implemented as this full system solution – the Architectural Medicine System.

The four topics above dealt with the steps that would be taken in the analysis and evaluation for the doctor and the building inspector. As such, there are four more topics to be added to this list:

The second four topics are:

- The training of architects and builders to recognize health issues in the built environment
- The development of protocols in the built environment that architects and builders are trained to evaluate and resolve
- The training of doctors, architects, inspectors, and informaticists to work together to resolve health issues in the built environment
- Software solutions created to support this process, from the Doctor creating an order for a Building Inspection and the inspection procedures to reporting for the doctors and subsequent prescription as building Rx for the architecture and building professionals to solve

When you have the full cycle of processes defined and provide procedures that each group can follow, the result can be a cohesive solution process from start to finish.

As mentioned earlier in the book, I've used the term spiracycle to define these round trip solution methods. As the process is a circle, the end result will either help or hinder a positive result. In this format, a cycle will either spiral up as a benefit, or down as a detriment in a spiral format.

The Architectural Medicine System (AMS) and the ARxMD software function to provide the structure and procedures to utilize this whole system solution, with the focus on the positive spiracycle for better health and wellness in the built environment.

These procedures can also support topics related to social determinants of health, as well as the large increase in potential toxins in the modern day world. As the medical profession and doctors become more well versed on environmental issues, there will be a greater need for their procedures to include these building issues for patient health and utilize systems for solutions.

With the addition of the healthy building inspections, processes can be implemented with scientific evaluations and testing, providing more building data to work with.

Each professional can provide their piece of the puzzle to an extremely complex jigsaw puzzle, with the focus on the end result benefitting the patient and the general public at large.

Every step along the way can lead to positive benefits, which can form a database of solutions for each professional to continue to learn from. This can form a synergistic benefit that can become exponentially valuable for both the individual patient, as well as the collective of humanity.

By sharing these results and then adding to the education of each professional as integrative solutions, each professional can work with each other for collaborative, beneficial results. Over time, these topics can expand to many other professionals that are indirectly involved with the fields of health and the built environment. This synergy adds to the spiracycle of benefits when providing new materials and methods that form the many facets of health and wellness in society.

The additional developments of Integrative Medicine for medical professionals to include determinants of health and the built environment, and the developments of Integrative Architecture for building and construction

8 STEPS TO BETTER HEALTH IN THE BUILT ENVIRONMENT

8 STEPS	SCALE: 1:1	CLIENT: GLOBAL CITIZENS	DRAWING 1 OF 2
	PROJECT: THE ARCHITECTURAL DOCTOR		
HEALTH IN THE BUILT ENVIRONMENT			
DATE CREATED: 4/22/2014			
DATE REVISED: 12/27/2021			
DEVELOPED BY: TIMOTHY D. ROSSI			

① The development of protocols for ailments potentially caused by built environment issues

② The training of Doctors to utilize protocols during ailment analysis

③ The training of building inspectors and informaticists to evaluate topics related to health in buildings

④ Systems created to support this process, from the Doctor creating an Rx for a Building Inspection to the interconnected system of evaluation and reports sent back to the doctor for evaluation

8 STEPS TO BETTER HEALTH IN THE BUILT ENVIRONMENT

8 STEPS	SCALE: 1:1	CLIENT: GLOBAL CITIZENS
	PROJECT: THE ARCHITECTURAL DOCTOR	
HEALTH IN THE BUILT ENVIRONMENT	**DRAWING**	
DATE CREATED: 4/22/2014	2	
DATE REVISED: 12/27/2021	OF	
DEVELOPED BY: TIMOTHY D. ROSSI	2	

⑤ The training of architects and builders to recognize health issues in the built environment

⑥ The development of protocols in the built environment that architects and builders are trained to evaluate and resolve

⑦ The training of doctors, architects, inspectors, and informaticists to work together to resolve health issues in the built environment

⑧ Software solutions created to support this process, from the Doctor creating an order for a Building Inspection and the inspection procedures to reporting for the doctors and subsequent prescription as building Rx for the architecture and building professionals to solve professionals, can provide an overlap for the Architectural Medicine System (AMS) to be successful.

In summary, these are the 8 factors and steps that would need to be created, which many today do not exist.

These first four topics are:

- The development of protocols for ailments potentially caused by built environment issues
- The training of Doctors to utilize protocols during ailment analysis
- The training of building inspectors and informaticists to evaluate topics related to health in buildings
- Systems created to support this process, from the Doctor creating an Rx for a Building Inspection to the interconnected system of evaluation and reports sent back to the doctor for evaluation

The second four topics are:

- The training of architects and builders to recognize health issues in the built environment
- The development of protocols in the built environment that architects and builders are trained to evaluate and resolve
- The training of doctors, architects, inspectors, and informaticists to work together to resolve health issues in the built environment
- Software solutions created to support this process, from the Doctor creating an order for a Building Inspection and the inspection procedures to reporting for the doctors and subsequent prescription as building Rx for the architecture and building professionals to solve

What is created are the 8 steps to a healthy built environment in this health evaluation and solution system. This is why ARxMD — the Architectural Medicine Software Solution, was created, which provides connections between the medical, architecture, and inspection fields, including other health and building professionals that may be involved.

A key to this process is also the care and proper communication with the patient. The Architectural Doctor is there to support the integration between the doctor, the inspector, architect, and builders, yet also to be supportive for patient care. After all, it is the patient's health that is at focus. While this process provides orders for inspections and an Rx for a healthy built environment solution, there is a critical requirement for the patient to not only be informed in this process, yet also educated and properly communicated with all of these processes.

It should not be forgotten that people's homes and buildings that they live in are very sacred places and provide space for human health and well-being. It's not just about the physical structure. It's about how comfortable the occupant "as a patient" feels in this entire process.

It's akin to the bedside manner of a doctor talking to another doctor or health professional about ailments or health topics right in front of their patient. Professionals should be concerned about this in a caring manner, and when a built environment issue needs to be evaluated and then fixed, it's no minor issue. Ignoring the emotional and psychological impacts these changes may have on the patient should not be taken lightly. If the patient is already suffering from an ailment and feels uneasy and at dis-ease with these issues, their built environment and home will be an essential place for their healing and mental and emotional well-being.

So there needs to be proper communication and support from someone in this round-trip process between the doctor, inspector, architect, and builder, which can also be a role of the Architectural Doctor. To help ease the pain of the process and to support and integrate the approach for a smooth and successful solution.

I believe the topic of health in the built environment has been slow going due to this lack of systems and general protocols between doctors and architects. It also should be noted that there's been an increase in healthy hospital design as a focus because if there are designs and processes in hospitals that can support better human health and healing, then there must be a wealth of knowledge that can be translated for general buildings.

Analemma, the Figure Eight, DevOps, and the Infinity Symbol

As a society, we can choose to either repeat cycles without changes, or we can utilize these cycles to learn, adjust, and make updates to systems and processes that are beneficial.

However, to simply expect this to happen without any systems in place or any planning for this to occur is a bit absurd. And as I've mentioned in this book many times previously, the fact that many of these processes with a focus on health in the built environment do not currently exist, it would be a bit far-fetched to believe that positive changes can occur without the proper effort.

This is not to say that changes have not occurred and there have not been beneficial changes and updates in the realm of health in buildings, yet to state that there is a comprehensive format that is integrative and inclusive is not exactly accurate.

These simplified processes, as eightfold steps, can set a baseline and blueprint for developments to provide more complex procedures to be examined, evaluated, and included in the professional processes for the architect, doctor, and many other professionals involved. This synergistic overlap that can occur between the different professions is, in my honest opinion, one of the great benefits that integrative processes can yield.

The software world has utilized this similar process of iteration to develop, build, and offer software solutions in a process known as DevOps. The term is a portmanteau of "a compound of development (Dev) and operations (Ops), DevOps is the union of people, process, and technology to continually provide value to customers."[128] A common symbol that is used to define these processes is the figure 8 as an infinity symbol:

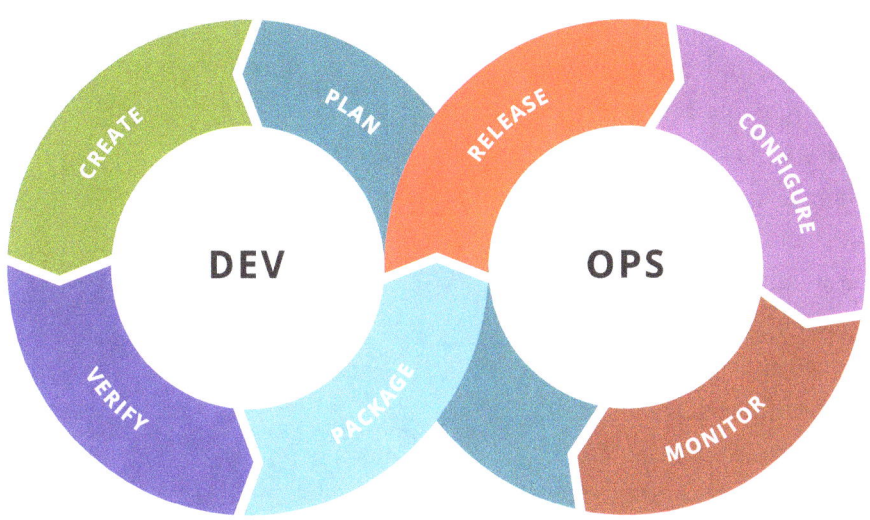

"Devops-toolchain" illustration showing stages in a DevOps toolchain by "Kharnagy"[131] – CC-BY-SA-4.0[306]

The process is often discussed in the software world as continuous integration (CI) and continuous delivery (CD). It is known as CI/CD to provide a "faster and more precise way of combining the work of different people into one cohesive product."[129]

In these development and operations processes, the general concept is to provide the continuous integration (CI) and continuous delivery (CD) to a DevOps process that can provide updates to software code in increments, which can allow for an agile development process. As defined by IBM, by utilizing this system, the "methodology is iterative, rather than linear, which allows DevOps teams to write code, integrate it, run tests, deliver releases and deploy changes to the software collaboratively and in real-time."[130]

A key component of this definition is an "iterative, rather than linear" process, hence the shape of the figure 8, which also denotes cyclical advancements. These updates allow a format that can utilize learned knowledge and provide new knowledge to be applied with all fields involved. While DevOps and CI/CD is a software world terminology, they can also be applied to developments in other fields. In fact, as the world of software continues to become more integrated into each profession in the real world of human processes, these integrations require systems to allow for such iterations.

Applied in this way for Architectural Medicine, the Architectural Doctor, and ARxMD, the big data science results as informatics can then be utilized as a constantly updated iteration to provide better solutions across many fields while encapsulated in a cohesive format. The

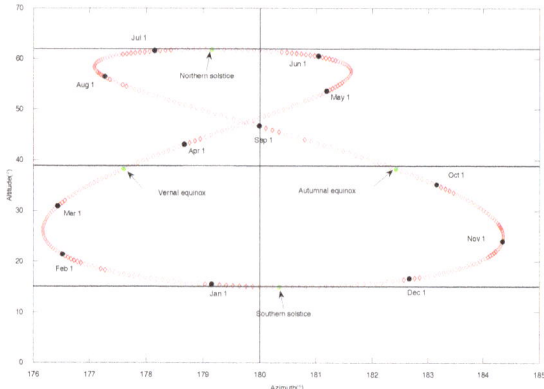

"Analemma Earth" by "PAR - JPL Horizons"[307] – Public Domain

iterations of 8 steps to better health and wellness in the built environment can be followed as a blueprint to achieve goals of better health in buildings while also providing a foundation for a system to be implemented between each profession.

As each of these 8 steps of Architectural Medicine and the Architectural Doctor can include extensive procedural updates for each professional, there will be requirements for each facet of these steps to be defined in more depth. Yet as mentioned earlier in this chapter, if there clear goals as steps are not communicated, there can often be confusion as to the goals that are striving to be achieved.

As another reminder of recurring movements, the analemma can also be utilized as an image denoting

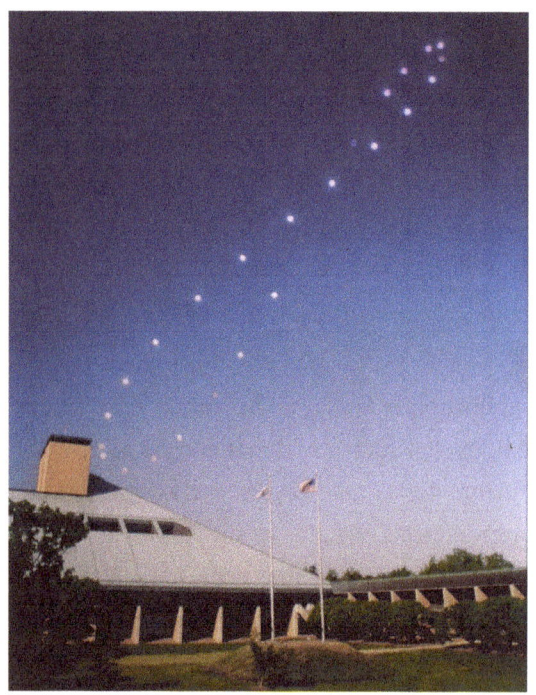

"Analemma fishburn" by "Jfishburn at English Wikipedia"[308] – CC BY-SA 3.0

these cycles. Due to the Earth's axis angle and the rotation around the sun, when you plot this path over time as a graph, it forms a figure 8, which is also the infinity symbol. This can suggest a process of repetition and can also convey an iterative process.

Whether it be an infinity symbol or the skyward movements of an analemma, these representations of a cyclical, iterative 8 step process can be reminders of the importance of such systems. The reduction of complex steps is obviously not to infer the simplicity of these procedures, yet it can be a reminder when complex systems may become extremely challenging to achieve. The changes applied in these steps can either spiral downward in a negative format or provide an upward spiracycle for overall benefits in building and public health.

In the following chapters, the individual steps for each professional will be discussed in more detail relevant to these 8 steps along with the Architectural Medicine System and ARxMD. In chapter 7, I discussed the role of the healthy building inspector and the building informaticist, and in the following three chapters, I will delve into the individual processes of the doctor, architect, and the Architectural Doctor relative to this whole system approach.

As many of these processes may begin with the doctor, in the next chapter, I will start this conversation with the roles and procedures of the doctor and the health professionals...

"Cure sometimes, treat often, comfort always."

— **Hippocrates**

THE PROCESSES OF THE DOCTOR AND HEALTH PROFESSIONALS

I would like to begin this chapter by asking you a question. If you are a doctor, have you ever considered, inquired about, or included the built environment when assessing your patient's health? As a patient, has your doctor ever inquired about or included your built environment when assessing your health?

Why or why not?

My guess is the answer to both of these questions, relative to your position as either patient or doctor, is "no." Or at least, I'd be fairly confident that the answer is no for over 95 percent of those being asked this question, if not a higher percentage.

While I may have some confidence in this answer, it is not to infer this as a positive affirmation. I've spent enough time around the focus of this question to feel confident in my guess, yet I am not happy with the common response.

Of course, this answer is mainly relevant in modern medicine, and for those whose medical modalities expand outside of common medical practices around the world, your answer might be different. To be extremely clear, this is not a negative connotation to modern doctors or the modern health processes of today.

I have benefited from modern medicine and know that doctors and health professionals today have a system that is utilized, and this system works.

My question and suggestion is this — can it be better?

My reply is yes, but I certainly understand enough about systems to know that changes are complex and the topics outside of the scope in which doctors and health professionals perform their work are not easily navigated.

Let me actually take a moment to recognize the value of our healthcare professionals and doctors.

They are often working in high stress positions, looking after your health and a large number of patients, and have endured years and years of extremely challenging and difficult content and situations. Many modern doctors struggle with fatigue and worker burnout, which is a terrible reality. With all of the work they've had to put into their careers, this is a sad reality.

I think doctors deserve better conditions to work within, especially better built environments in which to work.

With many updates and benefits in healthy hospital designs, there is still much work to be done for doctors in their working spaces as places for them to thrive. I believe that those who provide so much support to so many people deserve environments that offer their optimum thriving capabilities.

With all due respect, as I go back to this question, I do so with respect to the workloads of doctors and their years of study and experience.

And my question still remains as such:

> "Does the modern day doctor and health professional utilize the patient's built environment when evaluating patient health?"

While most of the time, the answer is no, what I think is important to write is that I also know why. Or at least, I can state that I have observed enough in life to answer with some clarity. The reason why is often based on a lack of systems, and as such, I'm not inferring this is not possible, nor am I inferring that doctors do not care about this.

The real answer, again, stems from the fact that the medical professionals require systems and, of course, the proper education and training in order to utilize these systems. The addition of including the built environment in evaluating their patients' health would require both education on this topic and appropriate systems in place to support these processes.

The doctor cannot merely inquire to the patient and ask, ponder, or postulate that the built environment may be impacting their patient's health. And even if they did have an inkling of this knowledge, what would the doctor do about it? Would they write the patient an Rx for a healthier building?

Actually, yes. But right now, at this time, this would not really be feasible.

The Addition of the Healthy Building Inspection in Medical Processes

In previous chapters, I discussed the addition of not only the Architectural Doctor but also the healthy building inspection. As all systems need the proper components to make the entire system function, there are parts to this big jigsaw puzzle that are required.

I believe these systems should exist, hence the creation of this book, as it is a wish of mine that populations can achieve better health and wellness, especially in the built environment. With professional inspectors in place and the proper training for the doctor and this new inspector, the doctor could include the patients built environments into the equation of health evaluations.

And being that most people are spending from 60 to 90 percent of their time, and sometimes 100 percent of their time, indoors, this lack of inclusion to evaluate these spaces can be a huge missing piece of the patient's health puzzle. If doctors are truly evaluating their patient's short and long-term health, the factor of their building health should also be included in this assessment.

And so, with this stated, I can begin to discuss the process and first steps in these evaluations.

The Doctor's Process - Including the Built Environment in Evaluations

This first step of the process is to ensure that doctors and health professionals are educated and trained on the range of health issues that might be caused or exacerbated by building issues.

During the medical evaluation process, often known as SOAP notes, when there are ailments that fit the SOAP note medical evaluation procedures, the next step would be for the doctor to write a prescription to have this building evaluated by a healthy building inspector. The Subjective, Objective, Assessment and Plan (SOAP) note process can include the built environment in the doctor's "objective" considerations. For instance, this segment of the physicians' review "documents the objective data from the patient encounter," including "vital signs, physical exam findings, laboratory data, imaging results, other diagnostic data, and the recognition and review of the documentation of other clinicians."[131]

This sounds like a prime opportunity to include the proper building inspections to fit in with these health procedures.

This inspection process will follow the regular procedures and steps that a current doctor takes by including an intake in the process and then submitting this request in the same way an Observation/Result (OBX) is requested in the electronic health record platform.

The main difference is that instead of a laboratory technician, nurse, or other health practitioner being presented with this request, it is sent to the healthy building inspector or building informaticist to provide the appropriate building information and the results.

The building request would be based on the premise of the patient's ailments, and each request can be very specific for each inspection, or a wide ranging request to inspect the patient's building spaces can be created.

In this manner, it is similar to a doctor requesting a blood test for a general evaluation to be performed, as opposed to an X-ray completed at an exact location of the body. The request for an inspection can be very specific or wide ranging to provide a more in depth analysis of the structure.

And this is where the modern electronic record systems can be of benefit. In this manner, utilizing the OBX as a request for a laboratory test, the healthy building inspector can receive the request from the doctor with only the necessary PID (Personal Identifiable Data) and OBX requests in order to do their work.

Once they have provided the evaluation and inspections, their results can either be sent to a lab to provide detailed results, or the data can be recorded on site. The resulting reports can then be sent back to the EHR. And when this is achieved, either by the inspector or the lab technicians, the HL7 processes will automatically send these results and reports back to the doctor to flag for their review.

All of these activities are possible due to the Health Level Seven (HL7) communications protocols, whether the system is based on the HL7 v2 or FHIR messaging approach. It is this system of communications that can allow data to be processed and sent to the inspector, ensuring that only the necessary PID and OBX requests are sent while maintaining the privacy of the patient based on HIPAA regulations.

The Doctor's New Education and Training on Health in the Built Environment

Due to new education and training for doctors to recognize and evaluate potential health issues related to the built environment, there can be a better understanding of the results sent back to the doctor to include in their patient's health analysis.

This extra level of knowledge and insights into their patient's health can be particularly helpful when it comes to issues related to the respiratory system and endocrine system, as well as a large range of topics that could be seen in long-term health issues.

The core of these comments is based on the fact that with most people living in the same places for prolonged periods of time, they can be negatively impacted by scenarios in their building that they may never be able to overcome with the common medical practices and pharmacological solutions.

This can mean that the patient can make changes in their diets, changes, and increases in medications, and perhaps the addition of other modalities for their medical health support, yet all along could be fighting against an issue in the built environment causing or intensifying the initial health issue.

Over time, many of these built environment issues can worsen health conditions, such as being around indoor air quality that is toxic in some formats and being around materials that emit toxins. These problems can be wide ranging, from impacting the respiratory system to negatively impacting the endocrine and hormonal systems. They can impact the skin and can cause issues such as asthma with an increase in particulates in the air. Harmful bacteria and contaminants existing in their building spaces can also create health issues.

All of these symptoms can be treated with different modalities to provide some comfort, yet if the root cause is something existing in the building spaces where the patient lives and spends a large amount of time within, then no amount of modern day solutions will be successful for best health. The lack of discovering and addressing the root cause may never allow them to heal properly.

And you may not think that a building has many possible detriments to health. However, in today's modern building processes, especially if built within the past 30 to 50 years in most parts of the developed world, you may be surrounded by toxins that you never knew about.

For those in the know, these toxins have been known for a while, including substances such as lead in paint and in pipes impacting drinking water, as well as asbestos for insulation – if it exists in a friable state. There are also other contaminants that may exist in modern buildings, such as particulates in the air from heating and ventilation systems and toxins from newer materials outgassing in structures that are built more airtight. The decrease in fresh air circulation and the possibility of high VOC (volatile organic compounds) levels can cause issues. There can also be the prevalence of toxic gases such as carbon monoxide, carbon dioxide, and nitrogen oxides, especially during the use of gas stoves and natural gas leaks. Even if these levels are low and might be acceptable for many, they could be causing health issues for those whose immune systems are more sensitive.

And this includes the health of children and the elderly, as these generations have greater sensitivity to contaminants, and children's systems cannot be viewed as little adults. Their systems have greater sensitivity to many contaminants, and even if the adults are ok with certain levels, the children and elderly may not.

As an example, according to the latest statistics from the WHO, around "2.4 billion people worldwide (around a third of the global population) cook using open fires or inefficient stoves fueled by kerosene, biomass (wood, animal dung and crop waste) and coal, which generates harmful household air pollution."[132] And household air pollution was responsible for an "estimated 3.2 million deaths per year in 2020, including over 237, 000 deaths of children under the age of 5."[133]

While these statistics may focus on the lower income locations in the world, household air pollution and exposure can lead to "noncommunicable diseases including stroke, ischaemic heart disease, chronic obstructive pulmonary disease (COPD) and lung cancer"[134] regardless of location if the indoor air quality lacks appropriate fresh air exchanges.

What's worse is that women and children often bear the "greatest health burden from the use of polluting fuels and technologies in homes,"[135] based on the reality that women and children are often responsible for cooking activities.

In the United States, millions of homes and apartments utilize gas appliances for heating and cooking. However, the use of gas cooking appliances in buildings "is not only a threat to climate action but also to human health, as these appliances are sources of indoor air pollution. Gas stoves, particularly when unvented, can be a primary source of indoor air pollution... a robust body of scientific research shows the pollutants released by gas stoves can have negative health effects, often exacerbating respiratory conditions like asthma."[136]

Who Is Responsible for Reviewing Building Health Issues?

As you read about these health issues caused by a variety of building scenarios, you might be asking who is responsible for considering these potential health problems in buildings. Is this the responsibility of the doctors and medical professionals? Is this the responsibility of the architecture and construction fields?

The unfortunate answer right now is there are few organizations that are monitoring these topics, as there's been a gap between the topic of health and the built environment. A recent report from RMI stated, "despite this growing body of evidence, indoor air pollution remains largely unregulated."[137]

However, this organization RMI has published a report which gathers data from research over two decades and offers "recommendations for policymakers, researchers, health care professionals, and the public to work to swiftly mitigate the health risks associated with gas stoves." As the report summarizes, "air pollution is preventable, and we hope this report can spur the necessary action to protect public health." The publication provides research from a collaborative of concerned groups consisting of; Physicians for Social Responsibility, Mothers Out Front, Sierra Club, and RMI (Rocky Mountain Institute).

When reviewing these wide ranges of building topics, you can also add into the equation modern building materials. Some new building methods create an easier way for mold to populate in building cavities, causing toxic mold spores and mycotoxins to emanate into the air. This can cause a wide range of health issues that are often not easy to ascertain.

On top of this, other materials in the news, such as BPA can also cause health concerns in buildings. The negative impacts of BPA over the past few years in water bottles are not just limited to drinking devices. BPA stands for "bisphenol A, an industrial chemical that has been used to make certain plastics and resins since the 1950s. BPA is found in polycarbonate plastics and epoxy resins."[138]

This chemical is also used in many modern building materials, and the fact that most current structures are designed to be airtight with a reduction of fresh outside air for energy efficiency purposes, can also mean that any toxins from materials such as BPA are left to linger inside.

According to the Mayo Clinic, "exposure to BPA is a concern because of the possible health effects on the brain and prostate gland of fetuses, infants and children. It can also affect children's behavior. Additional research suggests a possible link between BPA and increased blood pressure, type 2 diabetes and cardiovascular disease."[139]

These topics have a greater detriment to those who are immune compromised. They can also create increased vulnerability to children and pets due to being closer to ground level, where these toxins can collect in larger amounts.

Health and Sickness in Buildings – An Unorthodox Example of Problems and Solutions

As a side note and example of these types of health problems, I was once involved in a healthy building inspection with a mentor, who was hired to provide an inspection for a famous animal. This famous pet was reported as having health issues that were an anomaly to the veterinarians and professionals striving to help with their health. They were at a loss as to the animal's illness, and we were called in to provide a full building evaluation to explore a possible cause of these health concerns. While the entire inspection process went forward without any issues found, as we were completing the inspection process, we noticed something different about this structure that caused us to pause.

Most buildings in this location were slab on grade, and therefore inspecting a basement or crawl space was not an option. However, we noticed one of the rooms of this rather large house seemed to be elevated, and after a quick review of the structure, we noticed there was a crawl space under one of the rooms. After we suited up in our inspection outfits from head to toe, we were prepared to venture into the crawl space to discover any issues. After only a few moments, my mentor knew right away what the problem might be, so we spent a short time recording the problem, taking photos, and then preparing to talk with the clients.

It turns out the entire crawl space was filled with mold and fungi, with extremely high levels of mycotoxins. Later, after our conversations with the clients, we found out there had been a pipe burst in the building some time ago. But after this had been resolved, no one thought to check to see if there were any leaks or issues in this crawl space. It turned out the client knew about this pipe burst but never checked this space as the burst had happened in another part of this large house. Little did they know, the result was excess water damage that resulted in a massive amount of toxins created from mold spores and mycotoxins from mold and fungi.

While the owners of the house were not impacted by these mold spores and mycotoxins, their pet, living much lower to the ground and often spending most of their time living and sleeping in this room all day and night, was negatively impacted with severe health issues.

The good news is that the remediation process was completed, with the abatement successful in removing the mold and fungi, and all of the contaminants. The use of abatement protocols to prevent any leakage of these contaminants from entering other building spaces in the rest of the house provided safe air quality for the other rooms and all inhabitants.

Soon after, the animal's health was better, and a success story was the result.

The only thing that would have made this inspection and abatement process better is if the actual story of this famous pet's sickness had been popularized, providing education to the masses. Unfortunately, we all had to keep this information private, and to this day, I cannot disclose specific details about the animal from the inspection.

That was over 20 years ago, so quite a while in terms of my experience with buildings impacting health issues. This story was about a pet, yet my experiences in these evaluations have led to many other results to help human health. There are stories that my fellow colleagues could provide that span a time period of over 30 years, although many are not disclosed due to the privacy of those inhabitants. Perhaps over time, they may share their stories with the public. A big part of the challenges in the work that these environmental consultants and inspectors have navigated is a lack of systems between the medical and building professionals. And this means a lack of client and patient information that can be provided for many who are suffering.

This, to me, is a sad reality, in which many people could be offered better health solutions, yet also another reason why I'm writing this book and have created Architectural Medicine. The inclusion of the Architectural Medicine System and the work of the Architectural Doctor are inherent in these stories and have inspired the seeds of these ideas in providing better health evaluations and building solutions for the future.

If updated building protocols and processes are included in the modern medical system, they can provide solutions for those whose health may be negatively impacted by their buildings. The places where we live and work have the potential to create sickness or health — the resulting decision will be determined by us as a society to provide appropriate systems and solutions, or not.

Chapter: 9 The Processes of the Doctor and Health Professionals

Software Application Views – Inspector, Doctor, Architect, and the Architectural Doctor

Now that we've discussed the theoretical aspects of this process, it's time to review the details of how this functions in real-world scenarios.

The first process is to review the Architectural Medicine System graphic of the six segments as a reminder of the round trip steps that will be taken.

The first image of the six main segments of the software shows an overview of the ARxMD software cycle, starting at the top left, where the patient visits 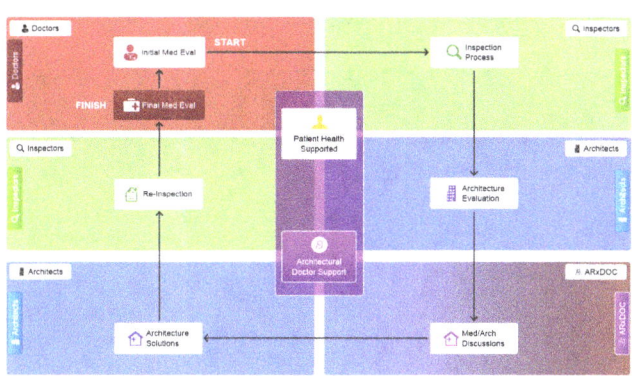 the doctor and then continues clockwise to the inspector. It continues to the architect and then the doctor, architect, Architectural Doctor, and the inspector's collaborative process if their feedback can be of value. It continues with the architect and builder providing the solutions for issues found and then a re-inspection to confirm changes have been resolved. These reports then return to the doctor and the Architectural Doctor, if required, to evaluate the patient's health for both short and long-term analysis.

The interface of the doctor's segment of the Architectural Medicine Software Solution – ARxMD consists of the main screen in a common CRM or EMR format when going to their portal page or dashboard.

The ARxMD screen is likely familiar in that it consists of the common Customer Relationship Management (CRM) fields. It is likely what health professionals view when they log into their Electronic Medical Record (EMR) system or their Health Information System (HIS).

It's important to note that doctors and health professionals may not be accessing the ARxMD software and instead might be utilizing their own

EMR or HIS system. As mentioned earlier, due to the advancement of the HL7 FHIR mapping process, the necessary information can be exchanged between systems.

In this doctor's ARxMD portal, the doctor has the ability to record the ailments of their patient, which might be caused by the patient's built environment. They can then request an inspection using the proper coding. This process is similar to a doctor requesting an MRI or X-ray, yet the request is sent to a different group of professionals.

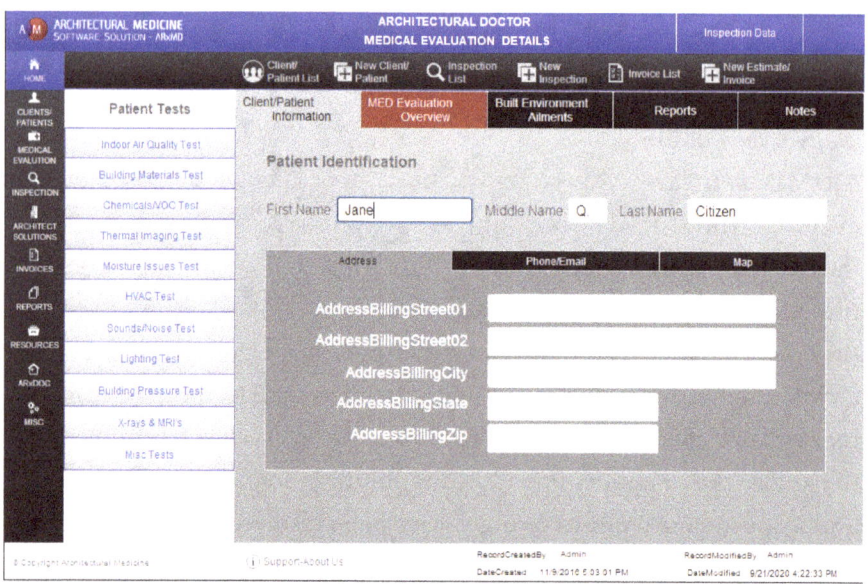

ARxMD portal for doctors and healthcare professionals

A building analysis or observation request can use a common medical process, using the SNOMED and ICD codes for the appropriate conditions. The relevant LOINC codes would be recorded from the lab testing completed by the inspector. However, there will also be a need for additional SNOMED, ICD, DSM, and LOINC codes that will be in alignment with these building issues and laboratory results.

At the time of this writing, there are some SNOMED, ICD, and LOINC codes that describe and define assorted built environment issues based on the topics such as social determinants of health. So, where there is an overlap between codes, they can be utilized appropriately.

Where there are new codes to be developed, we will discuss the topic of the ARxMD standards and protocols in a later chapter.

When a patient's condition may require further building inspection, the doctor can now request this to be completed by the inspector. Once the request is routed to the inspector, the software sends a message using the secure HL7 protocols, and the inspector receives this request.

The benefit of using HL7 is that only specific information that has been appropriately mapped is sent to the inspector, which can alleviate any HIPAA compliance concerns. In this way, only the Patient Identification (PID) information, such as name, address, and the requested inspections, are sent to the inspector for them to complete the building evaluations.

The advanced mapping features of HL7 FHIR allow the exchange of complex data between systems in a bi-directional format. Therefore, once the inspection is completed, the results can be sent back to the EHR or HIS for the doctor to review the results.

The Evaluation of Inspection Results by the Doctor & Architectural Doctor

Once the inspection results are completed, the data and reports are then sent back to the doctor and Architectural Doctor for review.

In time, with additional education and training in the medical fields, this review process can be supported with advanced help from the Architectural Doctor.

As this field begins to embrace additional data, the Architectural Doctor can work with a Building Informaticist to support the doctor in these procedures. This can be especially helpful if the MD is a general practitioner and would benefit from this additional specialized support.

As time goes on, the Architectural Doctor may also become a specialized practitioner. Just as the doctor can be listed as a family medical professional or an internal medicine professional, the Architectural Doctor may become recognized as an external medicine professional.

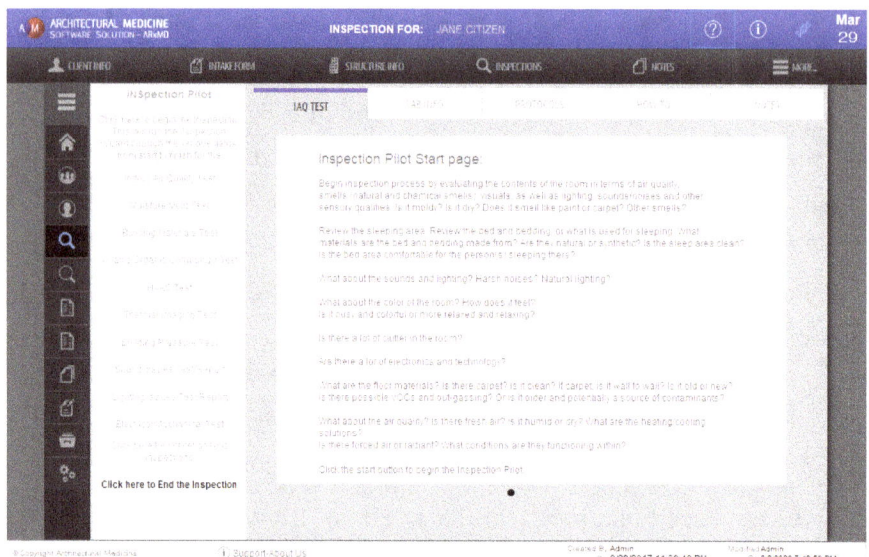

ARxMD layout for building inspection data entry and inspection procedures

In tandem, these professionals can support internal and external medicine to achieve the goals of Architectural Medicine to provide optimal health and wellness in the built environment.

Initially, the Architectural Doctor can evaluate the inspection reports and guide medical professionals to achieve their work. The Architectural Doctor can also support the doctor and the patient by assisting in the next steps if and when issues are found.

The Collaboration Process Between Doctor, Architect, Inspector, and Architectural Doctor

When there are issues found that are impacting the patient's health in their structure, the next step is to involve the building professionals. Therefore, there is an ARxMD software segment for these architects and building professionals to access these inspection reports.

It is crucial to ensure that all of these professionals can work together in a collaborative process during these findings, and ARxMD can ensure that the communication of the issues are provided in a systematic process. This includes the building solution itself, as well as the subsequent steps to implement the necessary procedures.

These next steps will depend upon the review of the building professionals based on the building solutions required for the problems.

In the next chapter, I will discuss the ARxMD steps and software interface of the architect and builder's view in their portal. This will provide the appropriate building piece of the puzzle for review and analysis.

As stated in previous sections, the currently limited connections between architectural and medical can be bridged with the ARxMD software, especially with these topics related to medical workflows. And as software systems advance, the ARxMD portal that the architects and builders view right now can extend by connecting to their software with the appropriate API and technology integrations. The ARxMD platform can extend its interconnectivity to provide this interoperability.

An Overview of Building Related Health Issues for the Health Professionals

With the processes of examining the built environment for health issues, there is a need for education and training, along with new procedures to ensure the doctor can have systems in place to achieve these goals. In the same manner, as the doctor utilizes other lab testing, such as X-rays and MRIs, the evaluations of the built environment can add to the whole picture of patient health.

Due to the average person spending from 60 to 90 percent of their lives inside of buildings, it seems strange not to include these building reviews in clinical evaluations.

To not utilize these building insights for patient health is to ignore a large range of issues that could be creating health problems. The range of these health issues can be from respiratory and endocrine problems to issues related to the nervous system and circulatory concerns.

In the modern world of medicine, the doctor initiates and records all of these processes for their patient using an electronic format, such as an electronic health record, which can be recorded in a HIS or Hospital information system.

In this process, there is a need for an interface that allows the doctor and health professional to record the evaluations, diagnoses, and requests for tests that are outsourced to other medical professionals.

This interface today is a digital platform, which provides a process for the doctor to record all of this information, to eventually become the patient's EHR.

Expanding some of these capabilities, which can include the patient's environment, can extend the EHR to become a comprehensive health record or a CHR, as it is sometimes called today.

And including these topics of the patient's environment in their health analysis requires more education, training, and of course, systems to enable these steps. It also requires the interface and digital steps to include the ability to record and request these as other options.

The Architectural Medicine System and the ARxMD software platform can support these new processes, as well as help define these new systems for the doctor to implement in their workflows.

Obviously, if you are a doctor and reading this, you already know all of this, yet as this book has a wide range of professions that may be reviewing these processes, it requires that we discuss what these are and how these systems in the medical profession function.

What You Should Know About the Architecture Professions and What They Might Be Asking of You

One of the differences of Architectural Medicine and these systems is the involvement of both the doctor and architect working together. Up to this point in history, this integration between professionals has been limited, except for the few doctors and architects that may work together in the hospital designs.

As these interactions will be new for most healthcare professionals, there will be a need to understand some basic principles of how these professionals function. As the healthcare professions are already incredibly complex, adding more complexity to their daily processes will require two main components. One is the education and training that is established in their curriculums, and the second is the provide procedures that enable them to provide these services in an efficient and systematic manner.

As mentioned throughout this book, the built environment can impact many facets of health, from the physical to the emotional and psychological, and each professional needs to have an awareness of these factors. In terms of physical health, the range of these issues can be from respiratory and endocrine problems to issues related to the nervous system and circulatory concerns.

These topics will need to be part of the medical training methods, and in the United States, this should be where the AMA and the AIA will need to work together as professional organizations to set these training guidelines to update the education of these professionals.

When the medical analysis includes the built environment topics and can be flagged for the doctor during their SOAP note evaluations, this can trigger a process for a building inspection and initiate the steps using the ARxMD software system to begin the evaluation process.

How to Work With the Architecture, Building, and Construction Fields

The medical professional is used to requesting testing provided by other professionals, such as requesting a nurse to provide blood tests and those in radiology to perform medical imaging procedures, such as X-rays, computed tomography (CT), magnetic resonance imaging (MRI), positron emission tomography (PET) and ultrasound.[140] Working with a Healthy Building Inspector and the Building Informaticist would be akin to them working with a radiologist, where a process is in place, and they are both familiar with the procedures working together.

Once their education and training include the topics of the built environment and the Architectural Medicine System can be utilized in their evaluations, then the steps taken will become more familiar over time.

Best Practices in Creating Healthy Building Solutions

These practices will also require that the medical doctor has an understanding of what to expect from the building professionals, and this includes the procedures, yet also the communication and proper nomenclature.

This is an important part of how the Architectural Doctor can support these connections, especially in the beginning when this is new for these professions o work with each other.

The most important part of these connections is to ensure that each profession is informed of the big picture process, as it will provide context for their work. The doctor does not need to know the details of the inspections and building steps and solutions, yet they will benefit from having a big picture view of such matters so that they may provide their part of the equation in a cohesive manner.

I will go into more detail about this training process in chapter 11, as I outline the role of the Architectural Doctor.

Interoperability Between the Fields of Architecture and Medicine

With the combination of the essential 8 steps outlined in chapter 8, the Architectural Medicine System defined in chapter 5, and the ARxMD software explained in chapter 6, the next question is how these procedures can be implemented into the modern day systems for architects and doctors.

The good news in terms of processes, as discussed in chapter 6, is that the current digitization and sharing of data electronically can provide a platform for all of these steps to be implemented.

Due to the modernization of both the building and health field utilizing computing processes to share data, each using taxonomies that set a baseline for communications both within and between professions, the extension of this data exchange can bridge each of these new professionals working in unison.

The status of modern medical systems includes interoperability, which can allow the transfer of data, including requests for medical procedures. If the building inspection were added to this request, which is included in the observation category in medical systems, then steps can be taken for the doctor to request these inspections by the Healthy Building Inspector and the Building Informaticist.

As well, the building and construction professionals utilize the ARxMD software that can include new requests and the sharing of data across the architecture, engineering, and construction professions (AEC). This interoperability, achieved using the Health Level 7 (HL7) FHIR processes, provides the ability to transfer data between not just medical software but any software systems that utilize a REST API.

This means that data can be shared between medical software, inspection software, architecture software, and any other professionals involved in this cyclical process. This opens up opportunities for these professions to work together and achieve these round trip systems to be implemented.

Looking Ahead - Viewing the Big Picture

Of course, this is only one piece of this complex puzzle. If issues are found by the Healthy Building Inspector and Building Informaticist in the inspection process, there still needs to be a solution provided, and who's going to do that? What would the doctor do, request a healthy building prescription or an Rx?

Actually, yes, that's precisely what they would do.

And in the next chapter, we'll discuss the next steps in this evaluation process, adding the architect, building, and construction fields into the equation...

"The architect should also have a knowledge of the study of medicine on account of the questions of climates, air, the healthiness and unhealthiness of sites...for without these considerations the healthiness of a dwelling cannot be assured."

– Vitruvius

THE PROCESSES OF THE ARCHITECT AND BUILDING PROFESSIONALS

In the previous chapter, we discussed the new role of the doctor in evaluating their patient's built environments for potential health implications for their patients. In discussing these procedures, I began the chapter with a question to those from both the perspective of a doctor or a patient as the general public. In this chapter, I'm going to start by asking a similar question:

> "As an architect, have you ever asked how the built environment that you're designing is impacting your client's health?
>
> If you are not an architect, have you ever had an architect ask you how your health has been impacted in a building that they have designed or built for you?"

In reality, the answer to these questions in this chapter may receive more replies of "sometimes" than the previous chapter's replies. There may even be some that would answer "yes." However, these replies are often based on rudimentary issues related to health as that of basic indoor air quality issues, such as carbon dioxide or carbon monoxide topics, or fresh air intake and issues related to radon in certain locations of the world.

In climates that are hot and more tropical, the questions of mold and mycotoxins may be more dominant, and in today's building world, we can even have discussions about lead paint, asbestos, and other contaminants that might exist in current and previous buildings that are being retrofitted.

These are all important developments, as many of these building issues were not even on the radar for building professionals some 30 to 50 years ago. The most recent topics, being mold and mycotoxin issues, has been a relatively new contaminant and health issue in the building world.

The Processes of the Architect and Design Professionals Creating the Healthy Built Environment

Relating to chapter 7 on the healthy building inspector and building informaticist, most building inspections today have nothing to do with health unless they fall under the category of HVAC systems or water damage, which can impact health. But the focus of these inspections is most often centered on the structural integrity of the building and its various systems.

While mold is a flag for many building inspections, it's typically a flag to show that there are functional problems with water infiltration, which can have negative impacts on the structural integrity of the building. The same is true for faulty HVAC systems, in that these issues can cause building problems, not necessarily a high priority related to occupant health issues. These health issues are often a by-product of other building issues, the focus of which is building integrity, not the health of the occupants.

There are a few contaminants in buildings that are currently focused on human health, such as lead in paints and pipes along with asbestos, which is analyzed according to occupant health. While it is good to see that there has been an increase in these inspection developments focused on health, there is still a lot to be achieved to ensure optimal health and safety in buildings for health and wellness.

And this small scope of focus on health is due to two main factors. One, the field of architecture and construction has not explicitly focused on these health issues in a professional format. Architects and contractors are not trained to know about human health, and many do not consider this topic relative to their work. The second is that many building materials are not vetted for building health issues.

To make matters more challenging, many of these health issues are caused after the building has already been built and is not always a direct result of a toxic building material. A case in point is mold and fungi. Many homes are built using airtight building procedures, and in many climates, this can promote mold growth in its design essence. What makes it worse is that many building materials can act as food for this mold, such as the paper existing in the commonly used sheetrock in North American building processes.

And so, when you have this combination of airtight buildings and materials in the building wall cavity where mold can feed upon, you can have mold issues that can persist over time without the knowledge of the inhabitants. And being that the spores of mold and the mycotoxins fungi are the causes of health issues for the occupant, these air quality issues often impact health without the knowledge of the inhabitants.

In North America, this is a significant problem, especially in warmer climates with higher humidity. However, in other parts of the world, where this building process of using light frame construction is not utilized, it is not as much of an issue. So, what you then have are certain materials and methodologies of buildings that can cause issues in certain parts of the world, and in others, these are non-issues.

This diversity in building processes is great to have, yet also challenging to navigate.

In reference to the previous chapter, where the medical professionals are not trained to recognize that potential respiratory issues could be caused by the aforementioned air quality building topic, it can lead to a lack of knowledge for the architect and building professionals to provide proper solutions.

The inclusion of a building inspection and the doctor's evaluation finding issues related to the patient's health at this time, are rare. Few, if any, doctors can reach out to an architect or building professional to request a remedy to resolve the built environment problem.

And in this chapter, an important facet we will discuss is this very issue of integrated solutions and interconnected approaches for the architect to support occupant health.

What You Should Know About the Medical Professions and What They Might Be Asking of You

To start, it should be noted that the current day architect may not have the bandwidth to provide the support that the ideals of Architectural Medicine aspire towards. Not as a lack of ability but as a lack of training and education.

Just as the medical profession should embrace this training as part of their systems, it's crucial to recognize that this form of education should begin in the architect's formative years as architecture students. In this manner, human health and biology education can be included in the cohesive teaching matriculations for undergraduate and graduate studies.

This way, the knowledge can be appropriately communicated to the student in terms relative to their profession, and this can make a huge difference, especially when working with the health and medical fields. Having the knowledge of these basic health topics, as well as the context for their roles, will be important to ensure communication is clear.

For instance, if there are health issues in the built environment caused by mycotoxins or other toxic materials, the architect educated on these topics will have enough context to understand the core issues and then be prepared to create design solutions appropriately. This will be particularly helpful when discussing topics with the doctor and the Architectural Doctor.

Patient as Educator and the Absence of Building Health Knowledge

In today's world, the person who is striving to have this solution created is often the client as the patient, and to have to educate the architect, designer, and contractor at the same time as they learn about their health issues is too often a massive lift for them to achieve. This is especially important if they are already sick and not able to have the energy to navigate these building problems.

It's unfair for the client to have to provide the education and the knowledge for these solutions, and instead, it would be more logical for these professionals to already have context to review the issues and provide solutions.

And the proper way for this to unfold is for the building professionals to know the main issues and to have the proper context to provide solutions.

In my formative years during college and after my education working in the construction fields, I learned a tremendous amount of information that was either not in the textbooks or impossible to convey in the classroom. Fortunately for me, I was a healthy young worker, and while I was exposed to many building materials at that age, I had no idea that many of them were and could be toxic.

In my later education, which fortunately I was able to receive in terms of building health, were at the time considered an alternative to modern building courses. Health was not the main focus in construction, which was something I learned working in the construction field. In fact, most builders are merely receiving instructions from the architects and designers who are providing the building requirements. And to make matters worse, the client would often work with designers who had no knowledge of specific toxic substances, as neither group involved in the design process was educated on these topics.

Architects and building professionals weren't and still often aren't educated on these matters, and so they have no information to provide for their clients. As is often the case, the construction managers and workers are providing the building solutions and are merely given the material specifications to complete the job.

In the mid to late 90s, I had the good fortune to work with healthy building pioneers, such as Cedar Rose Guelberth, and was educated by Paula Baker-Laporte, Mary Cordaro, and Carol Venolia about these building health issues and how to address them. Paula's book *Prescription for a healthy home*, as of this writing in its 4th edition, is a must-have for those involved in healthy construction.

I then worked with the building inspector Richard Scarborough and was taught by another building consultant Will Spates as to building procedures to provide healthier solutions.

However, one of the most important aspects of these experiences that I learned was the process itself. Working with either clients who wanted to have healthier built environments or working with those who were sick and were seeking solutions for their own health, provided insights into the processes that, in many ways, led to the creation of Architectural Medicine and the Architectural Doctor.

These insights were based on the fact that every time a new project was begun, all people involved, from designers, architects, contractors, and even medical professionals, had to be educated about the issues and the design solutions.

This was a heavy load to lift for every client, as each time a new project was entered, an entirely new group of professionals was involved and had to be educated, along with the client's education. There are not enough hours in the day to achieve this, and as such, these projects would often become giant problems caused by a lack of information for each professional involved, along with an absence of communication between each professional.

This is not a criticism of any of these professionals. In fact, the reality of these few professionals being open enough even to consider such "alternatives" to building issues shows the resiliency and interest of those who strive to help their clients.

Another major issue was that, too often, these topics would be brought into the design-build discussion after the majority of the design had been completed. As such, these design revisions were often seen as a hindrance to the project to be navigated for the other professionals. It meant that design solutions were often altered, instead of the implementation of these design solutions from the beginning. Being that some of these solutions required different materials and methods, unknown to many in the design and construction field, meant an unease of these professionals striving to achieve the design goals.

And as any construction project is already a stressful process, this added more complexity to an already stressful scenario.

The psychological ramifications on both the building professionals involved and the client as the customer were evident in most of the projects I worked on. And unfortunately, it was a major detriment to the end result.

As I write about in the introduction and provide some more details on the about the author page, these experiences provided a tremendous learning opportunity, yet at a high price with on the job training and dealing with complicated real-world building projects. The takeaway was clear to me — if there are to be whole system solutions, there must be education and training for each professional and a baseline knowledge of each of these professionals working together.

Hence the tagline for Architectural Medicine is "Building the Bridge to Wellness." The building portion includes the bridges between professions, and the content required for these healthier building goals to be realized.

The Architectural Doctor has to be knowledgeable about these topics and be able to discuss these issues with different professionals, from the doctor to the architect and beyond.

The architect must have context for their role and the role of the doctor and the Architectural Doctor if the Architectural Medicine System is to be utilized in a successful format.

The good news is that if these steps are taken, the designs don't have to be formulaic, and the architect can navigate these design processes in a creative format. This can be achieved with solid engineering required and the goal of proper biological and human health considerations included in the core of the design. These important topics should not be an added segment that is included after the design process; otherwise, the goal of healthier buildings will be a challenge to be achieved.

How to Work With the Medical and Health Fields

This process also includes the need to know how to work with health professionals and their perspectives on these topics. As written in a previous paragraph, it's not expected for the building professional to know the details of these health problems. Yet, it is expected for them to have a brief overview of these topics and how to handle both communications with other professions as well as to provide solutions for them and their patients.

In this way, the current format of the patient being the hub of all this knowledge is now moved from the patient to the direct communication between these professionals. As such, this statement may become more obvious as to the value of the Architectural Doctor and the importance of this new professional. The architect and doctor will have some context, but in terms of the details, there may be many gaps.

In some cases, the architect may need to discuss the solutions with the patient as the client, and this will require a baseline of knowledge relative to both health and the building processes.

What this also means is that a close working relationship between an architect and a medical professional can be critical. The Architectural Medicine System provides a blueprint for these processes and can function as a starting point to dive into more in depth solutions based on this framework.

Integrative Systems Working With the Building and Health Professionals

Another essential professional connection for the architect will be with the healthy building inspector. When the inspector finds issues that need to be resolved, the architect and builder will need to know the inspector's reporting results and be able to evaluate the problems encountered. If taught in architecture and building programs, at least with some basic context, the ability for the architect to work with the inspector and the doctor will not be so foreign.

Some architecture education programs will include building and materials and methods courses that provide an overview of how things are built. Having this knowledge will give these architects a core base and familiarity with building problems that can create health issues. And an important part of this equation is that when they draw up plans to fix these issues, it's imperative that in the process of solving one problem, they do not create others.

For instance, asbestos, lead, and mold remediation all require a similar process, where the removal of the materials must be sequestered from the other parts of the building. In this manner, the removal of the issues will not contaminate the different parts of the building or spread to other rooms during remediation.

Otherwise, the solution to one issue could be creating more significant and more expansive issues that, over time, can be deadly for the occupants. These topics should not be taken lightly and require professional knowledge for the architect, even if they don't have the depth of knowledge that the remediation experts will have.

They need to know that these issues require such steps, and can design solutions that meet the current requirements that are causing occupant health issues but do not cause more problems in the solutions process.

An Rx for Building Solutions – From the Fields of Medicine to the Fields of Architecture

And an Rx or prescription for a building solution is precisely what should be ordered. This resolution can be similarly requested from the medical professional in requesting a healthy building inspection, but the problem is that most architecture software solutions are not designed to accept these requests.

As such, the ARxMD system is available in the same manner as the Healthy Building Inspection, yet it can also be formatted to function with architecture and AEC software. This is because most modern AEC software is prepared to handle API integrations and the use of IFC standards, or what's known to many as BIM. Building Information Modeling, or BIM, is a process of defining design elements in software that creates building information that can also be shared across different AEC platforms. In essence, it can be shared across any digital platform as long as they share the same language.

So what ARxMD can provide is not only a software solution, but it can also support software communication between platforms. The way it handles this is through proper mapping utilizing interoperability processes, such as HL7 communications.

What this means is that HL7 can provide interoperability formats, not only for different medical platforms, but using HL7 FHIR, it can communicate with a common language format called JSON. Typically, HL7 uses XML as its base language, and in this process, it can be configured and mapped to talk to other medical platforms. Yet these new connections using the modern API and JSON means that by utilizing the newer APIs in AEC software, these new HL7 FHIR communications can exchange data that is not just between other medical systems, it can be poised to talk to these AEC platforms as well.

While this is not common practice today, there is the capability for this to function in this format. And with the world of software becoming more agnostic, such as SMART on FHIR applications, the scope and reach are going beyond the typical interconnections and expanding to a broader range of platforms. We are now seeing this with smart devices and sensors such as the Apple Watch and the FitBit, as well as many other software applications sharing data in previously impossible ways.

And to describe how these systems would function in sharing data between an EHR and the AEC fields, let's take the example used previously where a mold issue was creating toxins as an IAQ issue. What's required in this process is a request sent from the medical platform as an EHR or HIS, and then this request or OBX for a resolution would be sent to the architect or building professionals.

This messaging would only include the PID and the OBX, yet no other information based on HIPAA standards. In this format, only the required information would be provided for the AEC teams to provide appropriate solutions. Building professionals can attend to and address the building issues, yet can do so without revealing patient information, which should remain private.

In this way, the inspectors and building professionals can propose solutions and then report this back to the doctor using the HL7 FHIR methodologies providing details for both the doctor, the Architectural Doctor, and the client as a patient with pertinent information to decide a resolution.

Once the approval has been given for these updates to be fixed, the completion of this process is communicated to the doctor, the Architectural Doctor, and the patient as the client. In this format, the value added by the Architectural Doctor can be critical. In the same ways that the Architectural Doctor helped provide any feedback about the building issues to the doctor, the Architectural Doctor can also discuss the resolutions with the building professionals and then offer more clarity to the doctor and patient.

The Architectural Doctor can also update the doctor on processes and then update the patient on the next steps and how to proceed. This can provide a bridge between each group, who at first may be confused as to the next steps and what to expect, and provide guidance in appropriate actions for each group involved. The Architectural Doctor can also discuss any issues that the architect and builder may need to confirm to ensure that solutions are done in a proper format to prevent other problems from occurring.

This round trip process will then be reflected in the building solution reports, which are then sent back to the EHR and the HIS to ensure that the doctor and Architectural Doctor receive updates. The Architectural Doctor can provide feedback for the doctor and help assist the patient in answering questions or issues that can arise. Once the work is completed, the final step includes the report being sent to the Healthy Building Inspector to provide a final inspection of the provided solutions. This round trip system allows each professional to deliver their tasks and for the Architectural Doctor to be a liaison in the entire processes where needed, supporting each group as necessary.

They can also be less involved for those more familiar with the system processes. The more doctors become educated and aware of these issues, the less requirement from the Architectural Doctor is needed in certain stages.

In other places, there may be a need for more support for the inspections, building solutions, or communications for the patient. And in all of these scenarios, the Architectural Doctor can provide appropriate support. This is why it is detailed earlier in the book that the Architectural Doctor is well-versed in each of these professions, yet might not have the depth or capacity to solve these issues. As an Architectural Doctor, they may not be available for health inspections as a doctor, yet they know enough about the SOAP note procedures and the EHR processes to communicate the relevant details. They are also versed in the architecture and building processes and procedures, so they can discuss these topics with the building and AEC professionals where required.

It also gives them enough insight into how the processes should function and allows them to discuss topics with each professional and the patient.

All of these processes require education, training, and new systems in place for these processes to function correctly.

An Overview of Building Related Health Issues for the Architecture and Building Fields

The chapter quoted from Vitruvius at the start of this chapter shows that topics of health and the built environment are not new. However, two millennia ago, building materials and methods were quite different. That said, Vitruvius's core statement that architects should "have a knowledge of the study of medicine on account of the questions of climates, air, the healthiness and unhealthiness of sites" was critical to comprehend hundreds of years ago. And it's even more appropriate today to state, "without these considerations the healthiness of a dwelling cannot be assured."[141]

In his books *De architectura*, translated as "On architecture" and published as ten books, he mentions another reference to the importance of multi-disciplinary study that can be argued as even more critical in today's day and age:

> "The architect should be equipped with knowledge of many branches of study and varied kinds of learning, for it is by his judgement that all work done by the other arts is put to test. This knowledge is the child of practice and theory."[142]

While architecture is inherently interdisciplinary based on the knowledge required in the math and sciences as well as design fundamentals, the missing piece to this giant puzzle is human and biological health.

It's not expected for the architect to know the in-depth details of these topics, as it is already an extraordinarily challenging and demanding field of study. Yet, not having any context for human and biological health topics excludes a huge part of the built environment puzzle. And that piece of the puzzle is occupant health and wellness.

The Architect & Building Professional - ARxMD Software

As mentioned earlier, in recent years, with the use of CAD systems for building professionals, there has also been the inclusion of Building Information Modeling or BIM with these software platforms. This can also be an excellent way for these software systems to function together between medical platforms.

This Building Information Modeling can include an extensive range of data fields and content as well as metadata of the building itself. The challenge with IFC and BIM is the absence of specific metadata that can include building details, such as the locations of sensors and the building hierarchy of spaces and systems.

Fortunately, over the past decade, the development of more robust building ontologies has emerged, including the Real Estate Core (REC) taxonomy and the Brick Schema. And as I discuss in chapter 11, these two organizations have started to merge these taxonomies to provide a more complete standard for building information that can provide the exact details required for the Architectural Medicine System.

These new taxonomies can allow the inclusion of health-related data that can be exchanged with medical systems and provide large scale data interoperability that has never existed before.

Along with another acronym COBie (Construction Operations Building information exchange), these systems can help Facility Managers (FM) maintain the building systems and the building's health over time. COBie is an international standard for managed asset information, including space and equipment. It provides electronic management to help facility managers maintain the building systems.

The ARxMD building professionals' software interface will provide views they can use to review building issues and record their solutions. These layouts offer details and supportive information to help them understand the health issues and what must be resolved. By utilizing this information, they can evaluate building issues and provide their solutions directly in the software. This way, there can be an understanding of precisely what will be required to resolve the problems and the steps needed to achieve this.

The updated content can be saved to the ARxMD platform when the work is completed. This data can be exchanged and sent to the doctor and the rest of the professionals involved for review and follow up.

These new HL7 connections can allow for future data exchanges, where the building professionals working on CAD-BIM drawings can provide build-

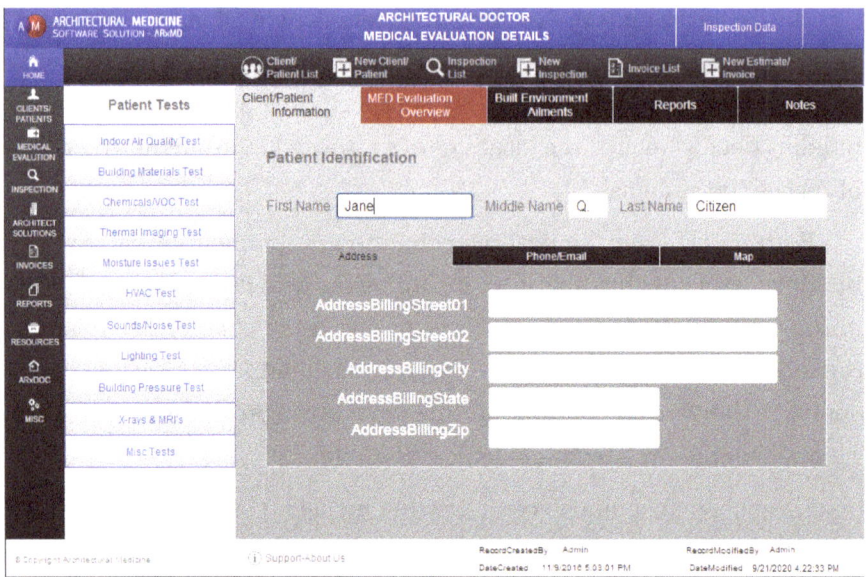

ARxMD interface to record building health data for doctors and healthcare professionals

ing solutions in digital format to be exchanged with the ARxMD software. In the future, these updates can be sent from the ARxMD platform to other professionals for review. And with the new developments of the Real Estate Core and Brick Schema ontologies, the granular details required for managing this extensive data can be maintained and exchanged between medical platforms utilizing the SNOMED, ICD, DSM, and LOINC standards for cross-professional interoperability.

And these integrations between fields bring us to the professional that can facilitate these exchanges for cohesive solutions, which are defined in the next chapter in the role of the Architectural Doctor…

"If you have built castles in the air,
your work need not be lost; that is where they should be.
Now put the foundations under them."

— **Henry David Thoreau**

THE ROLE OF THE ARCHITECTURAL DOCTOR

In chapter 3, I introduced the Architectural Doctor, providing an overview of this new professional. In this chapter, I'm going to get into the details of the role of this new professional and how they will function as an important liaison in achieving the goals of Architectural Medicine. By working with other professionals, they can support the procedures in creating better health and wellness in the built environment.

In the previous chapters, I discussed the roles of the architect, the doctor, the healthy building inspector, and the building informaticist. What's critical to understand about this Architectural Doctor role is that it requires a system to be in place in order to support, monitor, and be a liaison with these professionals — otherwise, there will be fragments of procedures with no clear path to achieve any goals.

The Purpose and Processes of the Architectural Doctor

To revisit the Architectural Medicine System process, the following diagram describes the system and all of the essential professionals involved:

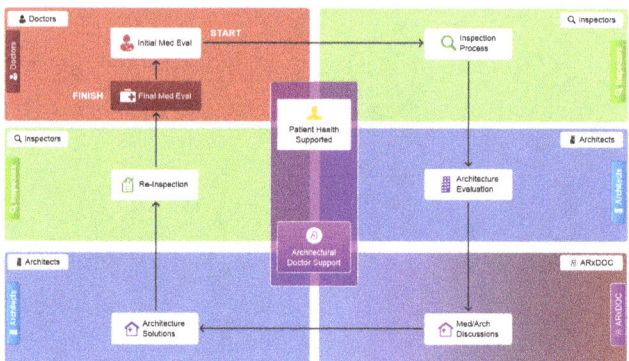

The above graphic shows the roundtrip processes of each professional working together, and as you can see, both the patient and the Architectural Doctor are at the center of this diagram. The role of the Architectural Doctor is to provide support for both the professionals involved and to provide support for the patient as well.

Due to the training of the Architectural Doctor having knowledge in the fields of architecture and medicine, they are able to provide support in each of these steps taken. They can work with the doctor to help in the connections required during initial evaluations, along with the process of working with the Healthy Building Inspector. They can help the doctor with evaluating the value of a building inspection along with subsequent results. They can also provide feedback that would be helpful for the patient if and when issues in their built environment are found.

And because they are well versed in the facets of architecture and construction, they can converse with the AEC building professionals to answer any questions and provide feedback where needed. This will be particularly valuable in the interim stages where these professionals working together is uncommon and unfamiliar territory.

The Architectural Doctor can also provide a bridge between the doctor and the architect when issues need to be reviewed and clarified. This role can also be supportive of the patient, as any building solutions might require more information for the patient to be educated in these processes completed by the architecture and building professionals.

And when the final solutions are updated, the final inspection can be reviewed by this Architectural Doctor to ensure that any details that may need to be discussed are clear for all involved.

Once the final work is achieved, and the final inspection is completed, this new role can provide the support that the doctor may need to help in follow up discussions with the patient.

Keep in mind all of these steps taken are for the benefit of the patient and their health. Having discussions with the patient to involve them and to provide education for them provides a foundation for their health over their lifetime. Over time there can be a long term review of the patient's health recorded in the EHR and CHR, which can include the built environment.

The Architectural Doctor can also help review data for larger scale use of this analysis for big data assessments. This big data can be provided by the collection of anonymous data that has been sorted for analysis by data science and bioinformatics professionals. In doing so, this data can be evaluated between the Architectural Doctor, the epidemiologists, and public health professionals to provide a bigger scope of understanding to provide up to date knowledge on the impact that the built environment has on human health.

The Architectural Doctor – Health, Healing, and Medicine

Earlier in the book, the definition of medicine and healing was outlined, which I'd like to revisit:

medicine (n.)

c. 1200, "medical treatment, cure, remedy," also used figuratively, of spiritual remedies, from Old French medecine (Modern French médicine) "medicine, art of healing, cure, treatment, potion," from Latin medicina "the healing art, medicine; a remedy," also used figuratively, perhaps originally ars medicina "the medical art," from fem. of medicinus (adj.) "of a doctor," from medicus "a physician" (from PIE root *med- "take appropriate measures.[143]

healing (n.)

"restoration to health," Old English hæling, verbal noun from heal (v.). Figurative sense of "restoration of wholeness" is from early 13c.; meaning "touch that cures" is from 1670s.[144]

heal (v.)

Old English hælan "cure; save; make whole, sound and well," from Proto-Germanic *hailjan (source also of Old Saxon helian, Old Norse heila, Old Frisian hela, Dutch helen, German heilen, Gothic ga-hailjan "to heal, cure"), literally "to make whole," from PIE *kailo- "whole" (see health). Intransitive sense from late 14c. Related: Healed; healing.[145]

health (n.)

Old English hælþ "wholeness, a being whole, sound or well," from Proto-Germanic *hailitho, from PIE *kailo- "whole, uninjured, of good omen" (source also of Old English hal "hale, whole;" Old Norse heill "healthy;" Old English halig, Old Norse helge "holy, sacred;" Old English hælan "to heal"). With Proto-Germanic abstract noun suffix *-itho (see -th (2)). Of physical health in Middle English, but also "prosperity, happiness, welfare; preservation, safety."[146]

As *medicine* is defined in the Oxford dictionary as "the science or practice of the diagnosis, treatment, and prevention of disease," it also focuses on "a substance or preparation used in the treatment of illness."[147]

While many associate a drug with a treatment, if you view how the exterior environment impacts your interior environment or your internal health, you might begin to see how important the state of the external environment affects your health.

And this is not only a factor for maintaining good health but for healing and wellness. The Architectural Doctor can utilize this process to focus on health and healing at an extended level, which includes the built environment in this complex equation.

By analyzing the built environment, such as physical components that may be causing health issues, and form factors that could also impact emotional and mental wellness, there can be many other variables added to the analysis that can improve health.

When these facets are revealed and addressed, the "medicine" component of architecture can be seen as an essential component for the patient's health and healing and the health of the general public.

This adds an entirely new set of factors into the medical evaluation that has either not existed previously or has only been a small portion of the doctor's analysis and solution process. Topics such as Social Determinants of Health (SDoH) can also be included as part of the doctor's analysis and included in the overall scope of the patient's health.

The Architectural Doctor can support these steps to add social determinants of health into actionable items to be included in both the patient's analysis and for potential solutions.

Architectural Medicine and the Architectural Doctor

The Architectural Medicine System flowchart shows the doctors' processes evaluating ailments, the inspection when the built environment needs to be evaluated and tested, the connection with architects and builders in evaluating problems, and the prescriptions or an Rx as recipes for healthier architecture for solutions. The overall structure of this process recognizes the importance of whole systems solutions.

During this entire process, the Architectural Doctor can help support the system itself and can also be there to support each professional. By having these integrated steps, the doctor can include building issues in their patient evaluations and work with the inspector, building informaticist, and building professionals to provide solutions.

As these are complex processes, there is an additional facet to support this workflow. The Architectural Medicine Software Solution – ARxMD, offers the option to help facilitate these goals. In the next chapter, I will discuss this topic and go into more detail on the topic of interoperability.

The Architectural Doctor can also help define ailments connected to the built environment and the doctor's evaluations in their analysis. This process will also be new for each professional and profession.

These new systems can fill a gap and provide a bridge between multiple professions that typically do not have an overlap or work together.

The diagrams below illustrate these gaps and provide insights into how the Architectural Doctor can support new integrations.

Current Building Model - Limited Integrations

Limited Communication and often no direct review of building health related issues between the building fields, the health fields, and the occupants (general public).

Occupants/General Public

Architects & the Building Community

Doctors & Health Practitioners

Communication

Limited Communication Between Fields of Architecture and Fields of Medicine

New and Revised Building Model for Health and Wellness

Occupants/General Public

Architectural Doctor — Involved
Architectural Doctor — Involved

Architects & the Building Community

Doctors & Health Practitioners

Architectural Doctor — Involved

Architectural Doctor

This new system of integrating architects and doctors with inspectors and building professionals to create healthier built environments can help ensure that each facet of these developments is interconnected for positive results.

Both architects and doctors have a substantial role in working independently to support the best health and wellness through buildings and medical support, respectively. Yet is there anything else that these two professions and groups can create for healthier built environments?

This question brings up the topic of system processes. Typically, these professions have a form of hierarchical structure, and another change in procedures will include new methods requiring nodal systems for best solutions. A nodal system is one in which collaboration is more fluid and accepted, where different nodes as groups can work together in tandem. Instead of there being an authority group that makes all decisions, the collective group of professionals can work together to provide best solutions for the patient and the public at large. This encourages group participation, and while it doesn't mean that no one is in charge of the processes, it instead is more inclusive to ensure that the many facets and professions can contribute to the best results. It is an important topic to discuss, as the Architectural Doctor's role and this new Architectural Medicine System (AMS) requires new methods and new mindsets in these professions to collaborate together.

The Education, Training, and Interconnective Procedures of the Architectural Doctor

The Architectural Doctor will be required to be educated in both the architecture and medical fields, yet as all this content would be extensive for one person to practice, the focus would be on the integration between these professions. In this way, they can be taught about the core functions of both fields, be informed of the common practices and nomenclature of each profession, and have the ability to communicate and support each professional independently and interdependently. This will provide the necessary support when the doctor needs more in depth of knowledge for their patient relative to the built environment, and the architect needs support to provide building solutions that are focused on the patient's health.

The diagram listed above shows the before and after connections of current and future integrations. By having knowledge of both professions, the ability to ensure integrative solutions are provided, which is paramount. And as these are complex processes, the ability to provide support for the doctor and architect in working together can provide a seamless method to unfold.

The Architectural Doctor's knowledge also includes the ways in which the Healthy Building Inspector and Building Informaticist will function. This includes building inspection procedures, building data analysis, and the digital processes required for each group to provide their piece of the big picture puzzle. The benefits of providing this support for each professional will allow the required steps to become more familiar, and over time, these individual professionals can perform these procedures with more clarity and confidence.

The Extended Facets of the Architectural Medicine System for Procedures and Training

In this section, I'm going to refer to the Architectural Medicine System flowchart in more detail. In chapter 5, I provided an overview of these steps, and in the graphics below, I'm going to dive into these details that were listed as segments AM-1 through AM-4:

Chapter: 11 The Role of the Architectural Doctor

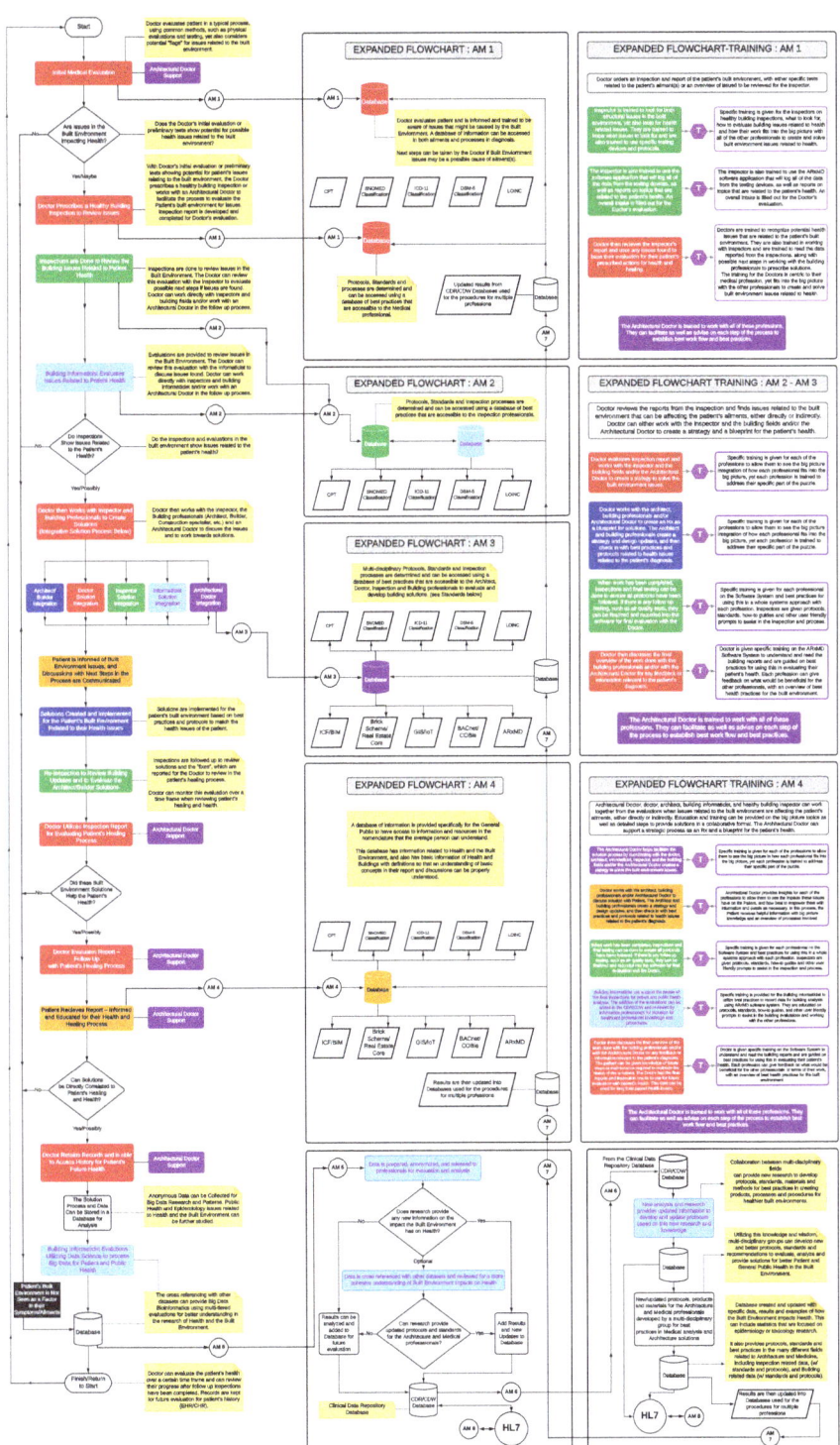

The Architectural Doctor – An Rx for Health & Wellness in Buildings   Part II

The Architectural Medicine System (AMS)
Expanded Flowchart – 1 of 3

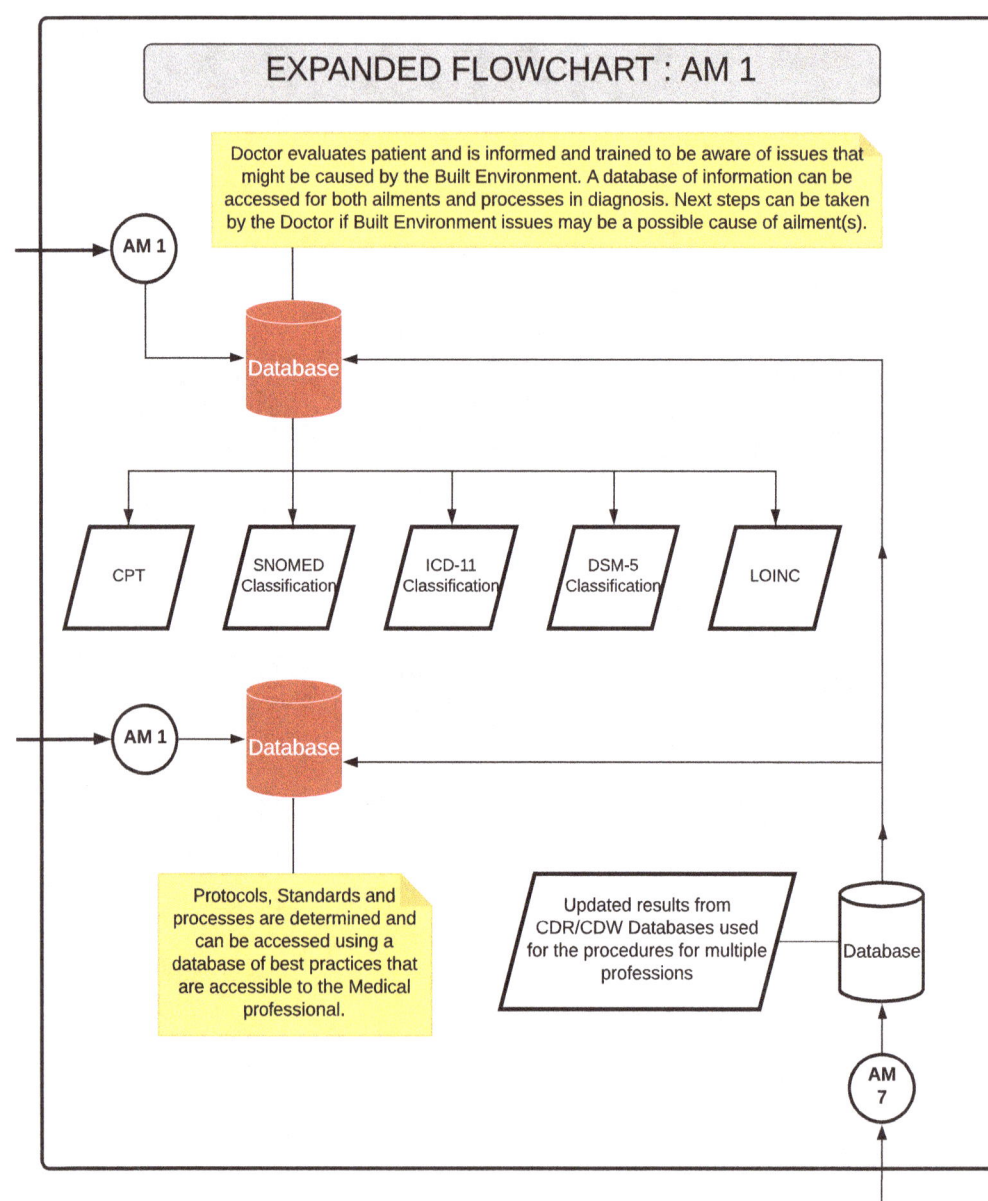

Chapter: 11   The Role of the Architectural Doctor

The Architectural Medicine System (AMS)
Expanded Training Flowchart – 1 of 3

EXPANDED FLOWCHART : AM 1

Doctor orders an inspection and report of the patient's built environment, with either specific tests related to the patient's ailment(s) or an overview of issued to be reviewed for the inspector.

Inspector is trained to look for both structural issues in the built environment, yet also tests for health related issues. They are trained to know what issues to look for and are also trained to use specific testing devices and protocols.

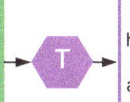

Specific training is given for the inspectors on healthy building inspections, what to look for, how to evaluate building issues related to health and how their work fits into the big picture with all of the other professionals to create and solve built environment issues related to health.

The inspector is also trained to use the software application that will log all of the data from the testing devices, as well as reports on topics that are related to the patient's health. An overall intake is filled out for the Doctor's evaluation.

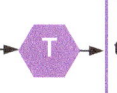

The inspector is also trained to use the software application that will log all of the data from the testing devices, as well as reports on topics that are related to the patient's health. An overall intake is filled out for the Doctor's evaluation.

Doctor then recieves the inspector's report and uses any issues found to base their evaluation for their patient's prescribed actions for health and healing.

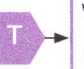

Doctors are trained to recognize potential health issues that are related to the patient's built environment. They are also trained inowkring with inspectors and are trained to read the data reported from the inspections, along with possible next steps in working with the building professionals to prescribe solutions.
The training for the Doctors is centric to their medical profession, yet fits into the big picture with all of the other professionals to create and solve built environment issues related to health.

The Architectural Doctor is trained to work with all of these professions. They can facilitate as well as advise on each step of the process to establish best work flow and best practices.

Expanded Flowchart – 2 of 3

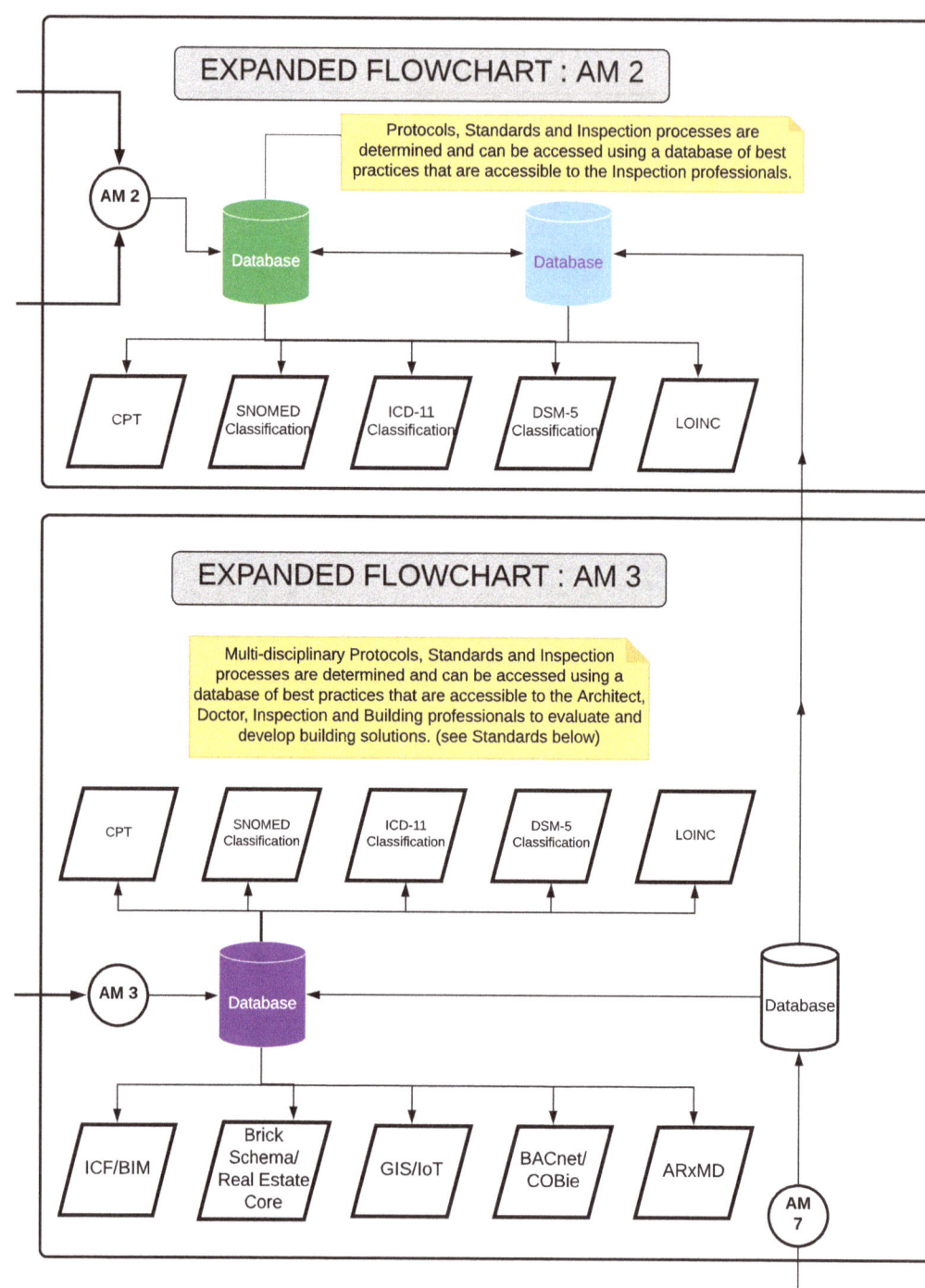

Expanded Training Flowchart – 2 of 3

EXPANDED FLOWCHART : AM 2 - AM 3

Doctor reviews the reports from the inspection and finds issues related to the built environment that can be affecting the patient's ailments, either directly or indirectly. Doctor can either work with the inspector and the building fields and/or the Architectural Doctor to create a strategy and a blueprint for the patient's health.

Doctor evaluates inspection report and works with the inspector and the building fields and/or the Architectural Doctor to create a stategy to solve the built environment issues.

→ T → Specific training is given for each of the professions to allow them to see the big picture integration of how each professional fits into the big picture, yet each profession is trained to address their specific part of the puzzle.

Doctor works with the architect, building professionals and/or Architectural Doctor to create a blueprint for solutions. The Architect and building professionals create a strategy and design updates, and then check in with best practices and protocols related to health issues related to the patient's diagnosis.

→ T → Specific training is given for each of the professions to allow them to see the big picture integration of how each professional fits into the big picture, yet each profession is trained to address their specific part of the puzzle.

When work has been completed, inspections and final testing can be done to ensure all protocols have been followed. If there is any follow up testing, such as air quality tests, they can be finalized and recorded into the software for final evaluation with the Doctor.

→ T → Specific training is given for each professional on the Software System and best practices for using this in a whole systems approach with each profession. Inspectors are given protocols, standards, how-to guides and other user friendly prompts to assist in the inspection and process.

Doctor then discusses the final overview of the work done with the building professionals and/or with the Architectural Doctor for any feedback or information relevant to the patient's diagnosis. The Doctor has the final reports and inspection tests to use for further evaluation and future evaluation with patient's health. This data can be used for long term patient health issues.

→ T → Doctor is given specific training on the Software System to understand and read the building reports and are guided on best practices for using this in evaluating their patient's health. Each profession can give feedback on what would be beneficial for the other professionals in terms of their work, with an overview of best health practices for the built environment.

The Architectural Doctor is trained to work with all of these professions. They can facilitate as well as advise on each step of the process to establish best work flow and best practices.

The Architectural Medicine System (AMS)
Expanded Flowchart – 3 of 3

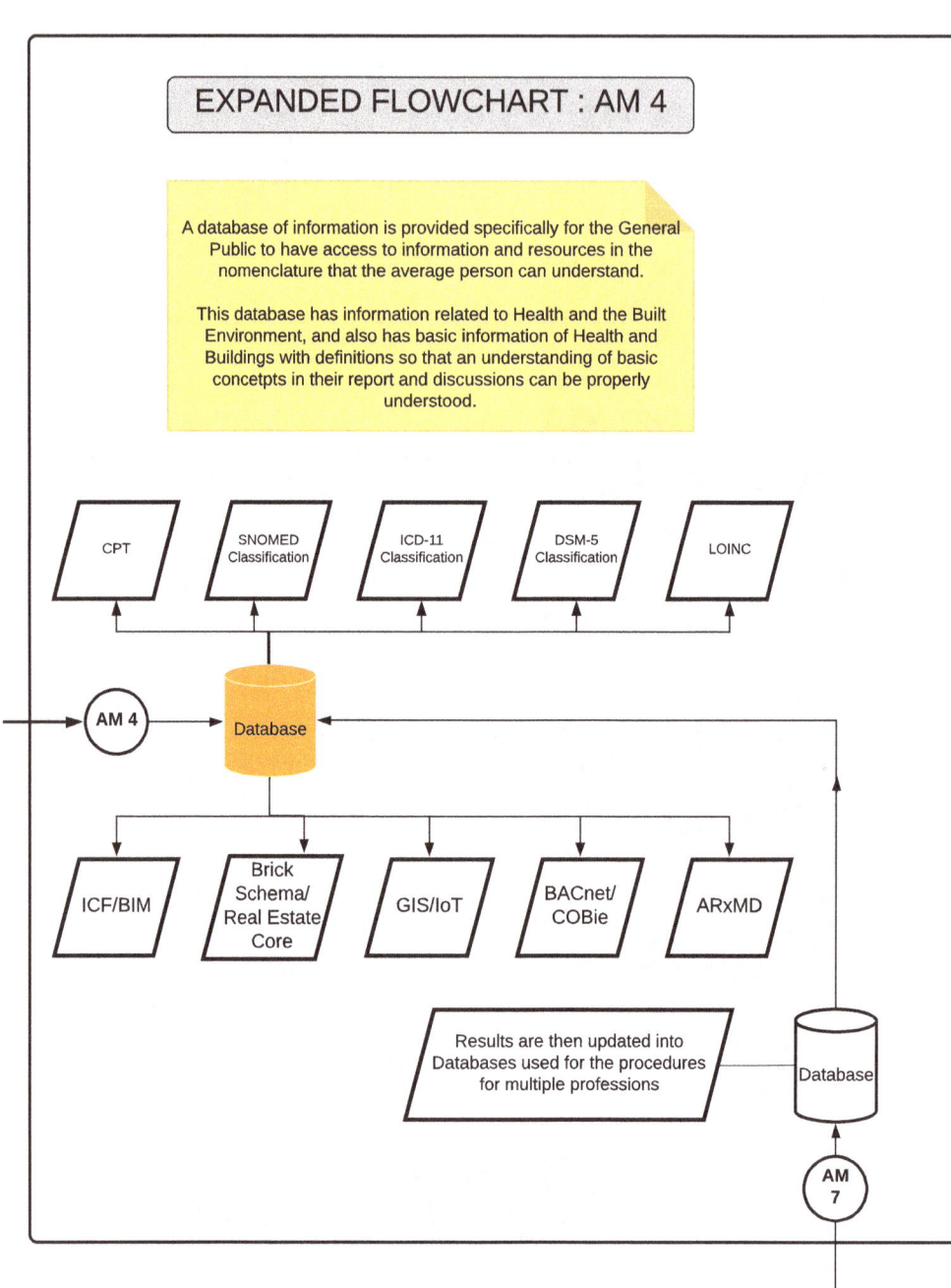

Chapter: 11   The Role of the Architectural Doctor

The Architectural Medicine System (AMS)
Expanded Training Flowchart – 3 of 3

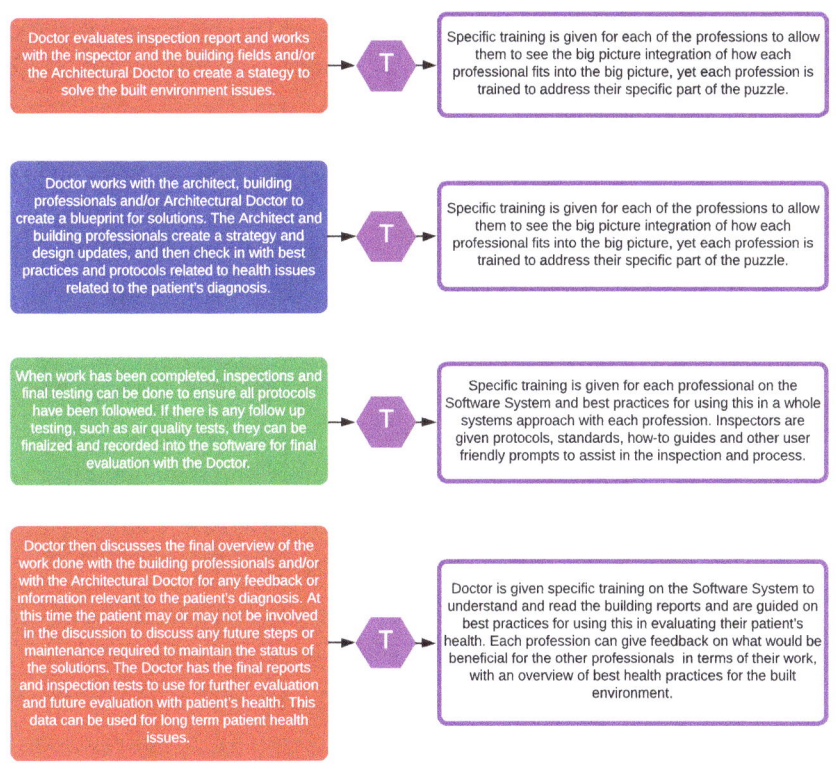

 As a side note, there are many graphics throughout this book and it may be challenging to see all the details. I have provided a link to many of the core graphics in this book for online viewing. They can be viewed using the QR code or at the following link:
https://architecturalmedicine.com/book

I begin these diagrams with the graphic of the entire flowchart of these sections, which have not been presented in whole until now. As you will see, the entire chart listed in book format creates a font size that is extremely small, yet as mentioned previously, I've provided a link to view this chart online.

As can be seen in this extended flow chart, there are systems that can support this integrative approach. These methods, combined with training and the setting of protocols for doctors, inspectors, architects, and builders with a round trip process supported by the Architectural Doctor, can all be created for better health, healing, and wellness in the built environment.

By creating these systems, the doctor is equipped with being able to write a true prescription as an Rx. The origins of the letters Rx originates from the shorthand of a "Recipe,"[148] as the doctors of the previous day and age would write an Rx or Recipe that the pharmacist would then create by putting together a variety of components to form a remedy.

In this manner, an Rx as a Recipe is included in the process of a solution for a healthy built environment, and as such, the term Rx used is defined as the combination of "Architecture" as ARx and "Medicine" as MD to form the phrase "ARxMD" (pronounced arcs – med). Essentially, it is the integration of these multi-disciplinary fields to collaborate and support the concept of health, healing, and wellness in the built environment. And the Architectural Doctor is there to support these procedures as a liaison for all professionals involved.

When viewing these diagrams posted on the previous pages, we can start with the AM-1 detail highlighting the doctor's initial evaluation and the results of this process when potential building issues can be found to impact the patient's health. This diagram references the AM-1 database, which has been cultivated with initial building health knowledge gathered, which is then updated in an iterative format from the data science analysis of building data gathered over time. The AM-1 step supports the doctor's patient analysis and provides guidance in the analysis that triggers a potential built environment connection to the patient's ailment. The expanded flowchart segment leads to the AM-1 training, focused on the doctor being able to recognize potential building issues during the SOAP note analysis.

At this time, the doctor would then request a building inspection to be provided, which leads to the AM-2 segment. This details the training for the Healthy Building Inspector to know how to proceed with a healthy building inspection and to be familiar with working with the doctor in this process. This includes training for the inspector to provide building tests focused on the doctor's request based on the patient's ailments, yet the specifics of the patient are not communicated for privacy purposes.

The inspector is also trained to work with the software, both the ARxMD solution and the common electronic health record. This way, they can navigate different systems to achieve their work and ensure that the information is either sent back to the electronic health record, or if laboratory testing is required, they have the knowledge of these steps and can proceed as needed.

Once the data from the inspection is recorded and any testing data is returned, the doctor will then receive this information. With this new training for the doctor in these methods, the doctor is able to review the reports and either make an assessment for solutions with the building professions or can work with the Architectural Doctor to approve of the next steps.

The flowchart lists the connections to the standards, such as SNOMED, ICD, DSM, and LOINC. This denotes that the proper codes will be utilized for both the medical evaluations and the proper codes for the building inspections. When the Building Informaticist provides more detailed observations, these will also include the appropriate codes to ensure the data is entered properly and able to be exchanged utilizing HL7 FHIR methodologies.

A Color Coded System for Each Professional and Procedure

The database for each professional also includes information about protocols, standards, and processes that each professional will use in their evaluation procedures. Each professional has their own set of procedures appropriate for their work, and as such, is listed in each of these detailed charts in different colors. The red segments represent the doctor and healthcare professionals, dark blue is the architect and builder, green is the Healthy Building Inspector, light blue is the Building Informaticist, and purple represents the Architectural Doctor. There is also the dark yellow color, which signifies the patient and general public.

Each professional can access a database of information that can support their professional processes, yet the content for each is also connected to the cohesive procedures of all professions involved. This allows each field to function independently and interdependently during their work processes.

When the inspection shows issues in the built environment, the next step labeled AM-3 is in effect, and this will require the doctor to be working with an architect and building professional. This is likely the time when the Architectural Doctor can provide the most support, in both helping with communication between the professionals and to provide feedback when assessing the big picture for solutions.

During this process, the architect and builder can receive the project details utilizing the exchange of data using the HL7 FHIR system. This exchange of data can be supported using the ARxMD platform, or when IT professionals are more familiar with the building platforms, the use of an API can provide the proper transfer.

This middle section of the flowchart shows all of the professionals involved in forming a cohesive solution for the patient. This is imperative to ensure all of the details are analyzed, and again the ability of the Architectural Doctor to provide support in this process can become vital when striving for best practices and successful solutions.

The expanded chart listed as AM-2 and AM-3 training provides the education for each professional involved to know what to expect and to provide the solution based on the necessary parameters. As the architect and building professional provide solutions, this data can then be exchanged back to the doctor and Architectural Doctor, and perhaps most importantly, the content of the results can then be provided for the patient.

This information can be presented to the patient either directly using their electronic health record platform or can be communicated by the doctor and Architectural Doctor. The ability of the Architectural Doctor to discuss these issues for the patient's knowledge becomes critical for their awareness of the issues and how they can be resolved.

Once these solutions are provided by the architect and builder, then the approval process will be required from the patient, and eventually, the building solution can be performed.

This brings us to the AM-4 detail, which provides instructions for the inspector to complete a re-inspection after the construction work is finished. This re-inspection is then recorded, and the data is again updated for the doctor to review for their patient. This AM-4 detail is also where the information from all procedures is recorded in the electronic health record for the patient to review. It is also a time when the Architectural Doctor can provide any feedback to the patient or any of the other professionals involved.

In the next chapter, I will go into details of AM-5 through AM-8, which have to do with the analysis of the data, including the benefit of this data being anonymized for the benefit of public health.

These steps of the Architectural Medicine System and the Architectural Doctor can provide a system for each professional, as well as a cohesive set of procedures for all fields to work together. In this manner, an evaluation process can be performed, detailed data can be recorded and evaluated, and solutions can be defined and provided using best practices across many professions. This way, the very large and complex processes can be reduced to smaller steps, and each participant can be provided with their own information to provide cohesive solutions.

Building Operating Systems as Building Management Systems

One of the key developments occurring in this new decade of the 2020s is the development of Building Operating Systems. What's a Building Operating System? If you take time to review the many facets of buildings, you can find decades of Building Management Systems (BMS) or Building Automation Systems (BAS) in use to control the many utilities of a building, especially high rise buildings and structures that require operational productivity, such as industrial structures. Often used interchangeably, BMS and BAS processes allow for machinery and sensors in a structure to be monitored and support the control of building environments, from temperature control and variable air handlers (VAV) to water, lighting, and security controls.

With the advent of the Internet of Things (IOT) and the increase in sensors, from room comfort controls to air quality monitors, these devices have proliferated in the building scene in large numbers over the past decade. And while many BMS processes have been utilizing technology such as BACnet and SCADA over decades, the challenge with these new technologies and sensors has been the availability to add them to previous systems with easy to view graphical interfaces and dashboards. This includes the larger commercial software offerings from Honeywell and Siemens, as well as the systems available for the homeowner, such as the Home Assistant application.

And this is where the concept of a building ontology becomes critical. Technology such as BACnet and SCADA does not easily avail the use of specific building components in the way that these monitoring systems can utilize in non-propriety formats. And this becomes important when adding a wide range of devices that can monitor processes in either real time or over time.

The increase in Digital Twins (DT) for building monitoring has also added to this complexity, as there have been limited ways for these sensors and devices to be added to these DTs to provide a more complete picture of building monitoring.

As such, the need for building ontologies has been recognized, and two main ontologies have been developed to support these devices. The Brick Schema, headed by Dr. Gabriel Fierro, and the Real Estate Core (REC), headed by Dr. Karl Hammar, are both building taxonomies to provide this granularity required for the Architectural Medicine System to be implemented with ARxMD.

This building ontology differs from the IFC standards and Building Information Modeling (BIM) in a specific way. As defined by the Real Estate Core (REC), an ontology can "most easily be thought of as a standard and interoperable schema for building knowledge graphs; it defines the types of nodes you can have in your graph, the types of relations these nodes have with one another, and the types of data values associated with them."[149]

As Dr. Fierro defines on the Brick Schema website, "Brick is an ontology-based metadata schema that captures the entities and relationships necessary for effective representations of buildings and their subsystems. Brick describes buildings in a machine readable format to enable programmatic exploration of different operational, structural and functional facets of a building."[150]

The essence of these ontologies is that they can provide a representation of all building entities, from floors, walls, and rooms to the devices, utilities, and any sensors existing in these spaces. This allows access to their processes and data output. This becomes critical when navigating the concepts of "smart" buildings, where the idea of a smart building is that it is not just a static entity yet changes and alters based on many parameters. In the world of energy efficiency and sustainability, this type of active control, using building monitoring and sensors can help to reduce energy. As buildings use 40 percent of all energy, the reduction of energy use in buildings, especially when considered in a large scale context, can provide huge benefits for the reduction of energy consumption.

This monitoring of energy by use of sensors can expand into topics of health, where indoor air quality and the measurement of particulates, gases, and toxins can become an important factor when monitoring human health. As sensors become more advanced and increase in numbers exponentially, there is a need for this data to be utilized for real-time monitoring. There is also the need for a log of the results of this data over time. To provide this amalgamated interconnectivity, the use of building taxonomies is required for this information to be properly utilized.

Fortunately, these two taxonomy groups have chosen to work together, and as of August 1, 2o22, the groups announced a major harmonization effort between these two smart building metadata standards.[151] These ontologies are also supported by the Building Topology Ontology (BOT), which is a "minimal ontology for describing the core topological concepts of a building."[152]

And when you consider that these building systems have certain operational processes that can be monitored, viewed, and controlled, the idea of this being defined as a building "operating system" is not so abstract. This concept, applied to buildings in cities and with large populations, can become extremely helpful in controlling not only typical building functions for energy efficiency yet also the comfort levels focused on health aspects. This includes indoor air quality, temperature, indoor climate monitoring, and insights into any toxins that may exist within the structure. In addition, when exterior sensors are included in these measurements, there can also be a reference point along with long term data monitoring of the outside environmental conditions. In chapter 13, I discuss some of these topics related to exterior environments in discussions on social determinants of health (SDoH).

This ability to view all the facets of systems in the computing world is called a single plane of glass, or (SPOG), where it can provide a single view of many complex processes. It can be utilized as "a management strategy that looks for ways to manage a complex digital system from a single executive dashboard…to help employees quickly understand the big picture, while also providing them with the ability to drill down and run reports."[153] Not to be confused with the architectural "glazing" nomenclature, this single pane of glass utilized in a building operating system (BOS) can provide insights into building integrity, as well as real-time monitoring for occupant health and well-being.

The Architectural Doctor can also be an important part of these developments, supporting the ability for doctors and health professionals to have greater insights into building health issues and processes to help with the occupant and patient health.

The Architectural Doctor can also be a vital connector in providing these digital solutions for the AEC fields relative to health, as most building sensors in the past have been focused on structural measurements. With the advent of advanced sensors, air handlers can be monitored for airflow characteristics yet also provide parameters relative to health. These sensors can capture real-time data for indoor air quality metrics from temperature and humidity controls to carbon monoxide, carbon dioxide, particulates, VOCs, and many other contaminants impacting occupant health.

The ARxMD Software and Procedures

While building operating systems can provide insights into sensors, devices, and building monitoring over time, there is still the need to have these buildings inspected with a focus on health and wellness. Current sensor devices can provide insights into air quality, such as CO2 and radon monitors, yet there will still be the need for evaluations, for biological issues such as bacteria and viruses. The measurement of VOCs often requires special instrumentation and measurements by building professionals. As mentioned in chapter 7, the healthy building inspector and building informaticist can provide these inspections and evaluations, and as such, there is a need for this data to be exchanged with the doctor and health professionals.

All of these processes can be achieved using the Architectural Medicine Software Solution – ARxMD. By utilizing this software and providing these proper interconnections, the Architectural Doctor can also be there to provide support for the integrations required for these systems to talk to each other.

This includes the coding processes that are either already in place, such as SNOMED, ICD, DSM, and LOINC codes, or can provide helpful service in establishing new codes. These new codes, in addition to current codes, can be included in each of the various integration platforms by using the ARxMD software.

The codes are there for the purpose of expanding the current set of interoperability and would not be intended to replace any current codes. As you can already see in all the above-mentioned systems, there are some codes that exist right now for each platform that relate to some of the built environment issues.

And in places where there are no codes that provide the proper evaluation, testing, and laboratory reporting or standards, the ARxMD codes can fill these gaps and add to the already sophisticated medical evaluations. By including more of the built environment topics relative to the topics of Architectural Medicine, the many gaps that currently exist can be bridged.

Extended Architecture and Medical Processes Require Complex Software Systems

The views above of these extended charts provide for the protocols and training for each step of the process. The Architectural Doctor is there to provide assistance for each of these steps and can be a positive support system for each professional. This way, these new systems are not as challenging for the professionals involved in these new procedures.

As described in chapter 6, the ARxMD software can support these steps and provide familiar systems for each group, yet also provide new protocols to ensure cohesive solutions.

As I have outlined the roles of each professional involved in this system, the ARxMD software can function to support each field in a contextual format. The more complex these processes become, the greater the need for the required advances of these systems.

As these steps are focused on the individual patient, the data sets that can be attained in these building evaluations can also scale up for big data analysis. The utilization of this big data as data science will also require more advanced systems to manage this information for the benefit of the public. In order to support this complexity and allow for proper scalability, in the next chapter, I will review these advanced facets described as part 2 of the ARxMD software solution...

"What I do is the opposite of building walls. I build bridges. A bridge is something that connects instead of separating."

– Santiago Calatrava

CHAPTER 12

ARxMD - THE ARCHITECTURAL MEDICINE SOFTWARE SOLUTION (PART 2)

The previous chapters discussed the many facets comprising the Architectural Medicine System and ARxMD in providing whole systems with a focus on health in the built environment. In this chapter, I will explore the details of this system that can support new integrations with the ARxMD software. A key piece missing in this complex puzzle is the ease and ability for individual patients to receive this documentation about the health of their built environment, along with the capability for this data to be anonymized and included in large-scale, big data analysis.

Without this information, the individual doctor cannot properly support their patient to the best of their ability, and the larger scope of building health cannot be analyzed in terms of epidemiology and public health. This means a large set of data has not yet been included in the public health world for evaluation, and this building informatics could be extremely helpful for future decision-making for societal wellness.

The Architectural Medicine System (AMS) and ARxMD

If you're reading this and find this to be astonishing that such data is not included in the analysis process, I can assure you that there is a good reason. It is a reason that I have learned first hand, and this is due to the deficiency of systems.

The absence of education for doctors and architects in their field related to this topic and a lack of systems provided for these professionals is, in my opinion, the biggest reason why this data does not exist. On top of this, the new professionals that are required to do this built environment testing, the Healthy Building Inspector and Building Informaticist, do not currently exist. Except for a select few doctors and architects that often work together in hospital design, there is very little, if any, collaboration between the fields of architecture and medicine.

And last but not least, the lack of professionals focused on this type of multi-disciplinary research, development, and professional support as the Architectural Doctor and Building Informaticist, also does not yet exist.

Therefore, the many facets that I've listed above have prevented such valuable information and data from being created, gathered, and analyzed, which would benefit and support better health and wellness for the general public.

Software and Systems as "Whole System Solutions"

The term "whole system" can be overused in many parts of the professional world. Sometimes it's merely a buzzword to support sales, and other times it is utilized to promote an overall concept.

Yet, in this case, whole system solutions are not only vital for this process to succeed, they are required. You cannot remove a piece of this puzzle in either the processes or the professions involved, with the result providing a beneficial solution. This is where the Architectural Doctor can truly help provide support for integrative solutions. They can function as a liaison to work with the architecture and medical professionals, the building inspectors, and the many other professions and groups that will be involved based on the circumstances. And while this professional can support these integrations, there still needs to be systems in place to capture, analyze, and readily distribute this data to the professionals involved.

Let me review the ARxMD solution, supporting the methods for each professional to contribute to the whole. The round trip nature of this software solution can be best reviewed starting with the following graphic:

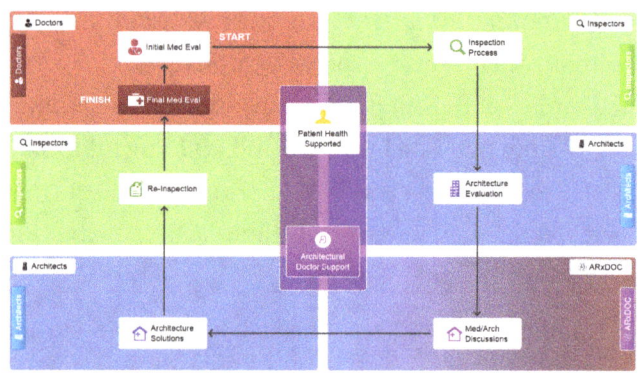

Beginning at the top left quadrant, we start with the initial doctor visit, where the patient comes to the doctor with an issue as an ailment or condition. And it is through this triage of processes, typically called the SOAP note methodology, that the doctor evaluates the patient's ailments to discover the issue.

According to the definition from the National Center for Biotechnology Information of the U.S. National Library of Medicine, the "Subjective, Objective, Assessment and Plan (SOAP) note is an acronym representing a widely used method of documentation for healthcare providers. The SOAP note is a way for healthcare workers to document in a structured and organized way."[154]

During this process, topics related to the built environment, as possibly being a cause or source of the patient issue, do not currently exist in this evaluation method. So, this is where the education portion of the new SOAP note process to include the built environment is required.

Once these new protocols and processes have been added to the doctor's SOAP note methodologies, if there are issues with the patient's health that can be connected to building issues, then the Architectural Medicine System (AMS) can be implemented. And this will include the use of the ARxMD software, either directly or indirectly, that can help provide a real world solution to be implemented.

Just as a doctor will request and prescribe a blood test, MRI, X-Ray, or another standard testing process, the doctor prescribes an Rx as testing for built environment issues in a similar fashion.

As stated above, this process will either be a direct or indirect process, based on the way in which they use their current software systems. One of the benefits of the ARxMD software is the ability to have the software communicate with other platforms, such as a Health Information System (HIS) or other platforms that utilize Electronic Health Record (EHR) systems.

As such, the doctor can utilize the ARxMD solution by placing a request for an inspection as an OBX, which can function with the HL7 technology that will provide interconnections with each software system. This will allow the doctor to do their part of the process, and the next steps will be automatically implemented using the HL7 interoperability for the inspection.

This will occur in a similar manner as other laboratory testing processes, yet instead of there being a request for a blood test or an MRI, instead, it will be a request for another professional to get involved – the Healthy Building Inspector or the Building Informaticist. Using these new evaluation techniques to include the built environment, the doctor can then receive reports on any building issues for their evaluations. With this data, they can recognize potential issues related to their patient's ailments.

For example, suppose the patient has persistent respiratory problems. In that case, the built environment can be evaluated for air quality issues, and the inspector can provide testing in the patient's built environment for indoor air quality (IAQ) problems.

In the top right segment, you can see the inspection listed, which can be the Healthy Building Inspector or the Building Informaticist, or both. Once that data is recorded using ARxMD, the report is filed and sent using the HL7 system to the doctor's EHR or HIS platform. When building issues are found, this is where the architect and building professional enters into the equation.

In the middle right section of the graphic, the architect then receives the issues found in the building. By having this data sent to their ARxMD version of the software or using HL7, the data can be sent to their software platform for review.

Then in the bottom right segment, as a group, these issues are then evaluated, and solutions are then provided by the architect. This group can consist of the architect, doctor, Architectural Doctor, inspector, and informaticist to ensure that all facets of the issues are considered.

At this time, it's critical to ensure that the patient receives proper information about the issues, and the Architectural Doctor can again support this communication to be sure the patient is aware of the pending issues to be resolved.

Once the patient is in agreement with the required work, the architect or builder provides the work in the built environment to resolve the issues. This is shown in the bottom left of the diagram. As they provide these solutions, they will also update the progress in the ARxMD software. Once completed, the reports can then be sent using HL7 processes back to the doctor and the Architectural Doctor for review.

An important part of this process is the re-inspection of the building by the inspector or the informaticist. In the left middle segment, this procedure is then completed, and the resulting data is updated in the ARxMD software and again sent to the EHR or HIS for the doctor and Architectural Doctor to review.

In the top left, this segment is again where the evaluation is recorded for the doctor, with updates recorded over time to monitor the patient issues and updated in the EHR or CHR. This is where the process can be listed as finished or a return to start, as the evaluation process for the patient can be updated over time. Any iterations for their health can be addressed and recorded in perpetuity over their lifetime.

Each Segment Functioning as a Cohesive Whole

Each of these segments has a specific role in the entire process, from start to finish, yet this cyclical motion cannot function completely without each segment working together. It is this nodal integration that is required in order for the process to work. Otherwise, there are too many gaps that would preclude the system from providing proper benefits.

And this is a critical part of the Architectural Medicine System (AMS). Without these integrative processes, the system will not work.

In my opinion, this is why there have not been any professional developments between these fields to help benefit the general public at large. You cannot use ad hoc processes and expect there to be cohesive solutions. Each of these fields are extremely complex and requires proper education, training, and systems to be in place to support these processes.

The Architectural Medicine Software Solution – ARxMD is poised to provide these integrative solutions for each group and to provide a conduit between each group. By including the proper education and training for each professional, especially the doctors, the architects, and the new additions of the healthy building inspectors, building informaticists, and the Architectural Doctor, these systems can work in tandem to provide proper solutions.

And this is just a small group of professionals that can be involved for helpful results. The addition of those in public health, epidemiologists, toxicologists, green chemists, material developers, manufacturers, bioinformatics professionals, and many other professionals that are connected to these topics can all be involved in a larger scope for health, healing, and wellness.

This well-being should not be reduced to a fragment of the whole, as these topics are immersed in the life of the everyday person, and the far-ranging scope should not be undervalued. The built environment impacts all, especially the growing populations that are living in urban areas and spending more time inside buildings. This should not be overlooked, and while it can be viewed as incredibly complex, which it is, this is not a good reason not to move forward in working towards these integrative goals.

It will take some time for this to manifest into systems that are included in these complex modern day systems, yet when they do become part of the professional system, their benefits can be exponential and, in some ways, ironically, immeasurably helpful.

The Use of Big Data and Data Science for Building Informatics

In following up on the expanded flowchart details from the previous chapter, we can now properly review the AM-5 through AM-8 details. These segments provide an overview of utilizing the building inspection and evaluation data for more than just the individual patient, yet to provide data sets for informatics professionals and a clinical data repository and warehouse for public health purposes.

In the next few pages, the graphics show more detail into the expanded flowchart processes. Starting at detail AM-5, the results of the inspections and building evaluations, along with the subsequent follow up visits reported by the doctor, can be anonymized and, with the patient's approval, shared for research. This element of the system is actually an important component of the Architectural Medicine System, as it provides data that can inform updates to methods and protocols, providing best practices in an iterative format.

As mentioned in chapter 7, the importance of informatics relative to building health can be utilized as a critical facet of public health. The built environment does not currently have many metrics that are being evaluated for public health and, as such, can create gaps in healthcare knowledge.

The entry point to this analysis is in segment AM-5, where the anonymized data is prepared for research purposes and provided to the informatics professionals to review. When these analytics provide new information related to buildings and health, this can be included in databases for both the medical and healthcare professionals as well as the architecture and building professions. When research shows a correlation between the built environment and health issues, it can also provide insights for each profession to ensure that updated knowledge is then provided for each profession. This can become a clinical data repository and accessible by each profession to determine changes in education on these topics, providing new standards and protocols moving forward. This cycle can iterate over time and provide a positive spiracycle of events to build upon the impacts of buildings on human, biological, and ecological health. This also supports the dynamic of multiple benefits to the big issues in the world of both climate change and energy efficiency to reduce building energy use. All of these factors can be included for a cohesive view of the human created world that we depend upon for advanced societal functions and benefit human health and wellness.

These data sets can then be utilized in the chart as AM-6, which can provide the available data for other professionals, such as epidemiologists, toxicologists, psychologists, green chemists, manufacturers, and the many other professionals that can utilize these data sets for cross referential analysis.

The expanded data sets can then be included in the building informatic repositories, that is then utilized to inform new practices and protocols in the architecture and medical fields. This is listed as AM-7 on the chart, and when viewing the expanded segments from AM-1 to AM-4, the databases from each is updated utilizing this building informatics repository as AM-7.

This repository is also valuable as a main repository when dealing with other standards in architecture and medicine, which is listed in the chart as AM-8. For instance, the SNOMED, ICD, and LOINC codes are constantly updated in the medical fields, along with updates in the IFC, REC, and Brick Schemas, which inform the interoperability within platforms and between professions. By leveraging the HL7 FHIR protocols, data and standards can be updated for proper exchange. If these code sets are not updated in the building informatics repository, then the exchange of data can become hindered.

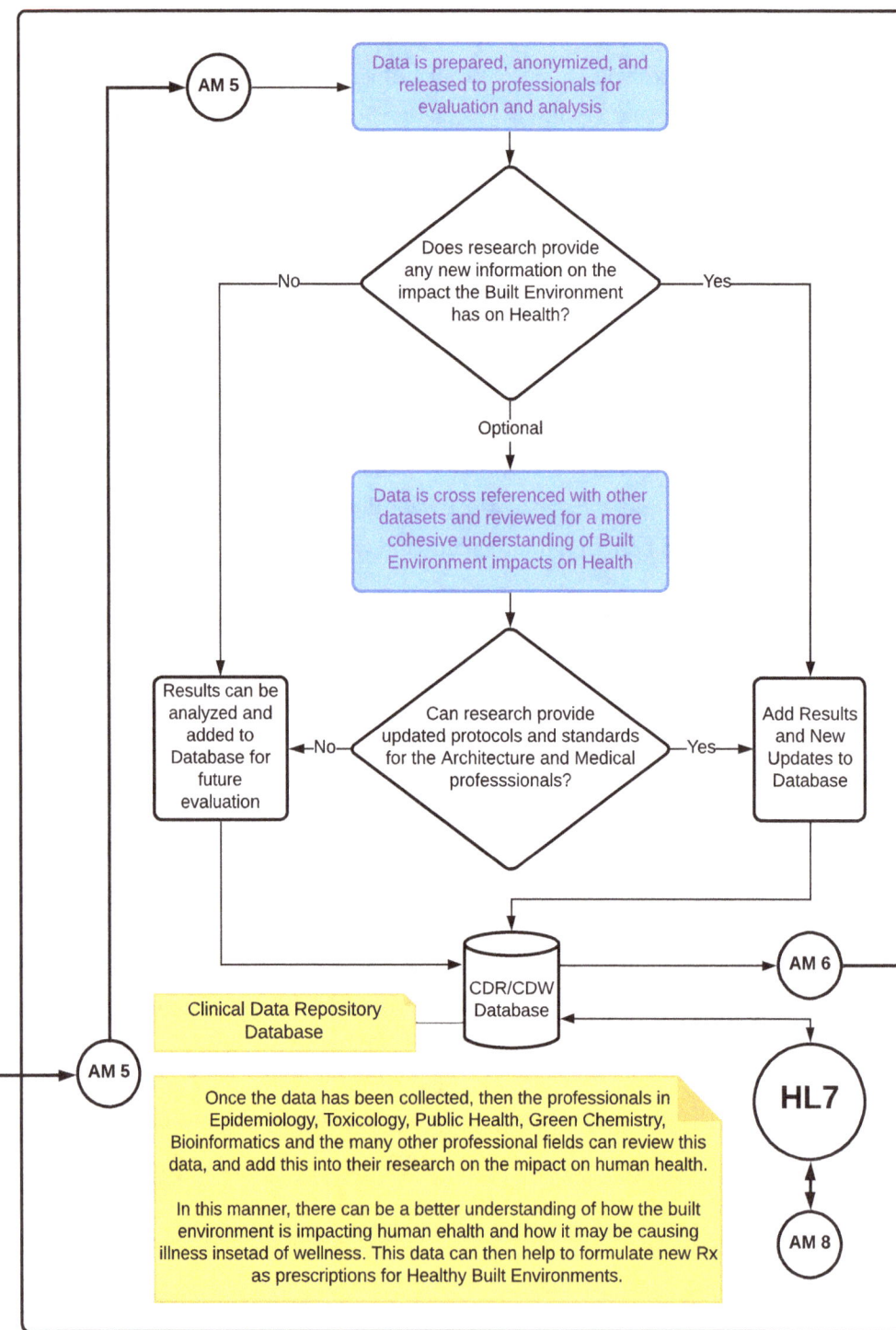

Chapter: 12   ARxMD – The Architectural Medicine Software Solution (Part 2)

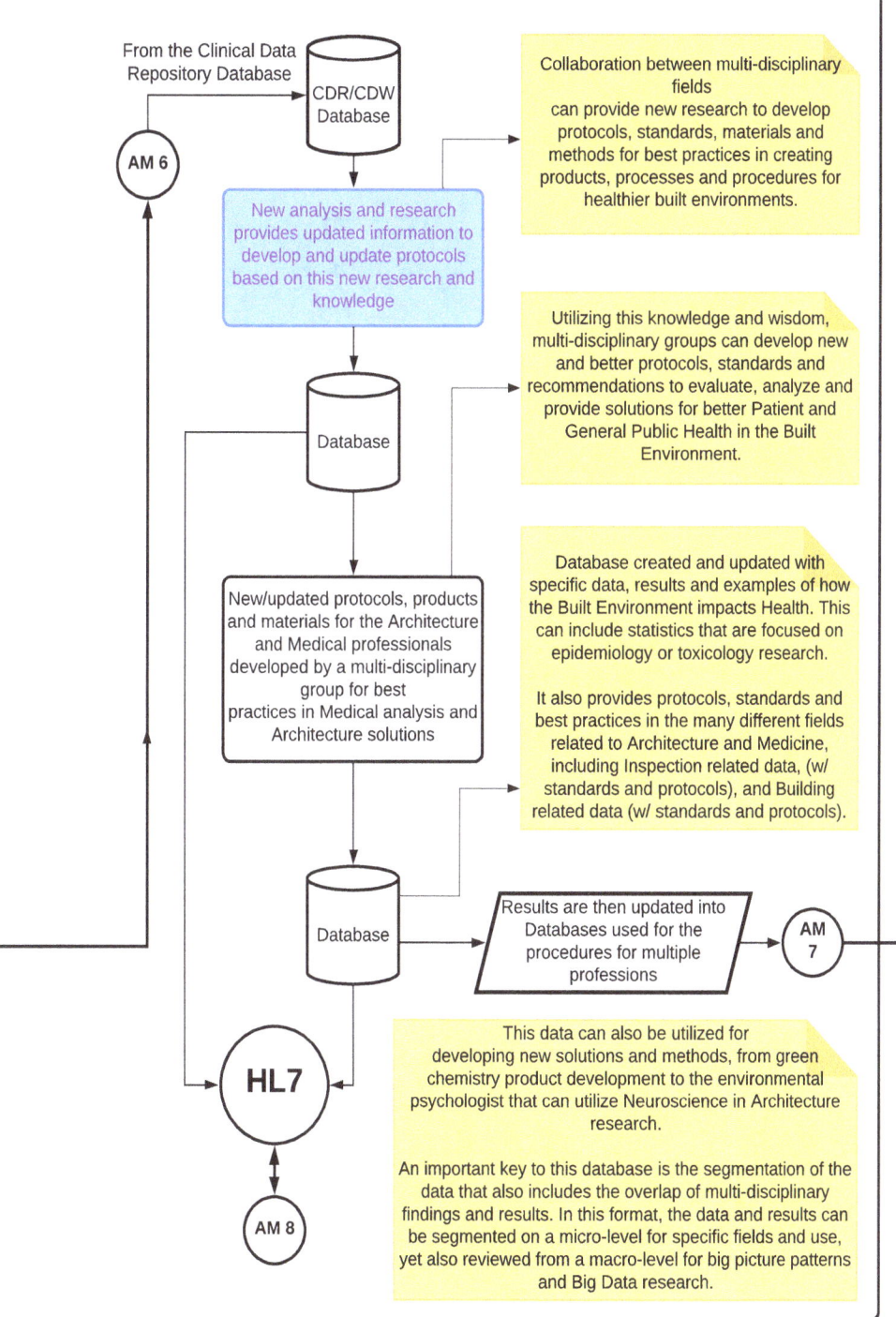

INTERNATIONAL STANDARDS, CLASSIFICATIONS & INTEGRATIONS FOR ARCHITECTURE, ENGINEERING, AND CONSTRUCTION (AEC) FIELDS

ICF/BIM-Information from architectural models can be created for Digital Twins to monitor Health issues in the built environment → **ICF/BIM**

Building information captured from sensors can be defined with detailed metadata for the issues related to Health in buildings → **Brick Schema/ Real Estate Core**

GIS allows for geographic location of IoT sensors in providing location details for exterior and interior building metrics supporting issues related to Physical Health (yet inlcuding other facets of Health) in the built environment → **GIS/IoT** ↔ **HL7** ↔ **AM 8**

The original classifications set for building stadards can be included and integrated into modern systems to monitor building issues and occupant health topics in buildings → **BACnet/ COBie**

The ARxMD software and processes can be included to record, exchange, and provide interoperability between many systems and professions for better health in the built environment → **ARxMD**

Chapter: 12   ARxMD – The Architectural Medicine Software Solution (Part 2)

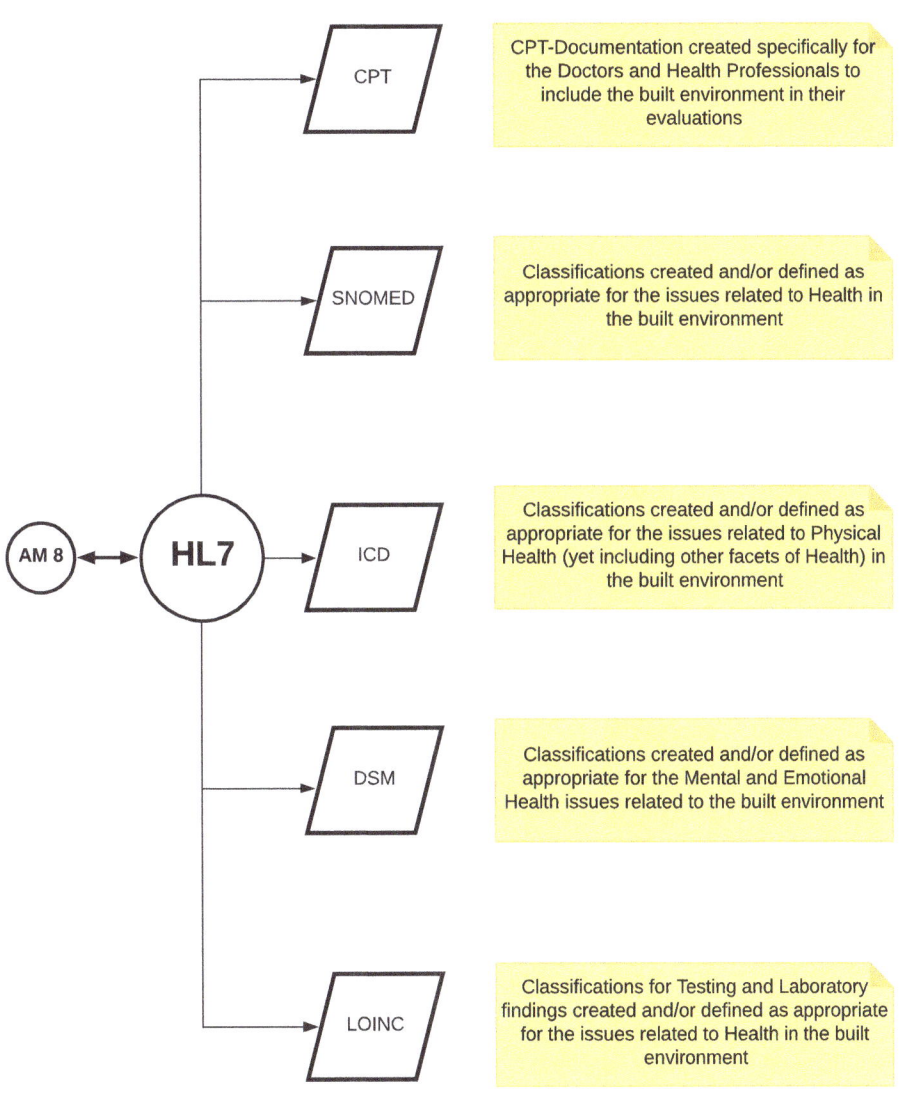

As I've stated throughout this book, the absence of systems can prevent the topics of health in the built environment from occurring. And ensuring that these repositories are properly updated is going to be critical in the future. In this manner, each professional will continue to benefit from the advanced collaborative research and have the ability to exchange data between a wide range of platforms.

The Architectural Medicine System (AMS) Swimlane Diagram

Revisiting the swimlane diagram, the overlap of many professionals working together can show the importance of collaborative efforts, and this requires that each group has the knowledge for their work relative to the whole picture.

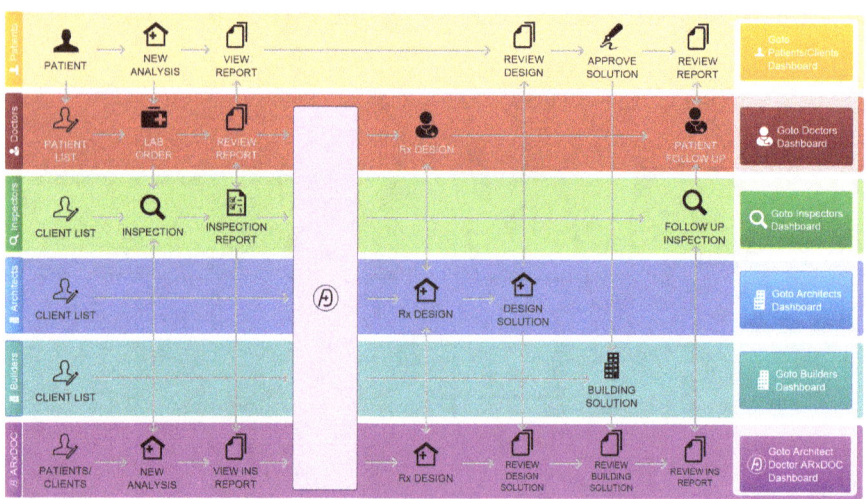

The Architectural Medicine System (AMS) Swimlane Diagram

The subsequent phases include discussions with the patient and these built environment issues, leading to the implementation of the solutions. These problems will then be resolved by designs from the architect and builders and implemented by building professionals.

A follow up inspection will then ensure that the issues were resolved, and if any re-testing is required, it is completed at this time. These follow up reports are then provided to the doctor and Architectural Doctor for final evaluation. These issues and fixes can be discussed with the patient in their current and long-term health evaluations.

Implementing the Evaluations of the Built Environment – The Focus of the Architectural Doctor

Now that this expanded system has been defined, a review of evaluations in the built environment relative to the patient's health is timely. As discussed previously, I described these human health and wellness evaluations in three main facets:

- Physical Evaluations and Diagnosis
- Emotional Evaluations and Diagnosis
- Mental/Psychological Evaluations and Diagnosis

The following is an overview of built environment topics that can cause health issues:

- Indoor Air Quality-Lack of Fresh Air
- CO/CO2-High levels of Carbon Monoxide, Carbon Dioxide
- Radon
- Toxicity of Materials such as:
    - Lead and other Heavy Metals
    - Asbestos
    - Pesticides
    - Volatile Organic Compounds (VOCs)
    - Toxic Chemicals
- Mold/Moisture Issues
- Temperature/Humidity
    - Uncomfortably Hot/Cold
    - Uncomfortably Dry/Humid

- Water Quality
- Noises/Loud Sounds
- Lighting Issues/Lack of Natural Lighting
- Indoor Air Particulates
    - Material Particulates
    - Cigarette Smoke
    - Pollution
- Material Colors – Colors causing negative psychological and emotional responses
- Shapes and forms of structures – Physiologically induced issues/Neuroscience – increased stress
- Reduced exposure to Nature – Lack of trees, water, natural sounds, greenery

The above list can have many different impacts on physical, emotional, and mental or psychological health and wellness, resulting in some of the conditions listed below:

Physical Ailments:
- Respiratory/Asthma (Respiratory ailments)
- Endocrine related issues
- Toxicity issues
- Neurology issues
- Skin disorders

Emotional Ailments:
- Mental disturbances based on certain shapes and forms (see Neuroscience of Architecture, Environmental Psychology, and Architectural Phenomenology)
- Depression

- Neurology issues
- Toxicity issues

Mental/Psychological Ailments:

- Mental disturbances based on certain shapes and forms (see Neuroscience of Architecture, Environmental Psychology, and Architectural Phenomenology)
- Depression
- Neurology issues
- Toxicity issues

At first, there may seem like a similar list of topics for each group of ailments. The case may often be that a doctor, psychologist or therapist, and neuroscientist may see all of the same conditions and have differing opinions and vantage points regarding the physiological results.

This is not to say that there won't be numerous causes of these ailments, yet how many will be diagnosed because of issues in the built environment? When you view these different facets that may be connected to patient health, how can these be determined by the physician or the mental or emotional health experts?

And this is a core reason why this system requires many professionals to work together to provide cohesive solutions in patient evaluations.

These are the many pieces of the jigsaw puzzle that can help professionals provide a whole solution for their patient's wellness.

Dividing the Puzzle Pieces for Evaluation – Putting Them Back Together for Wellness

While the reality is that you cannot separate the physical, emotional, and mental facets in evaluations of the whole person, some steps can be broken down into different pieces of a puzzle to help in the evaluation and diagnosis process. Once these pieces are reviewed independently, they can be put back together for the healing process for optimal human health.

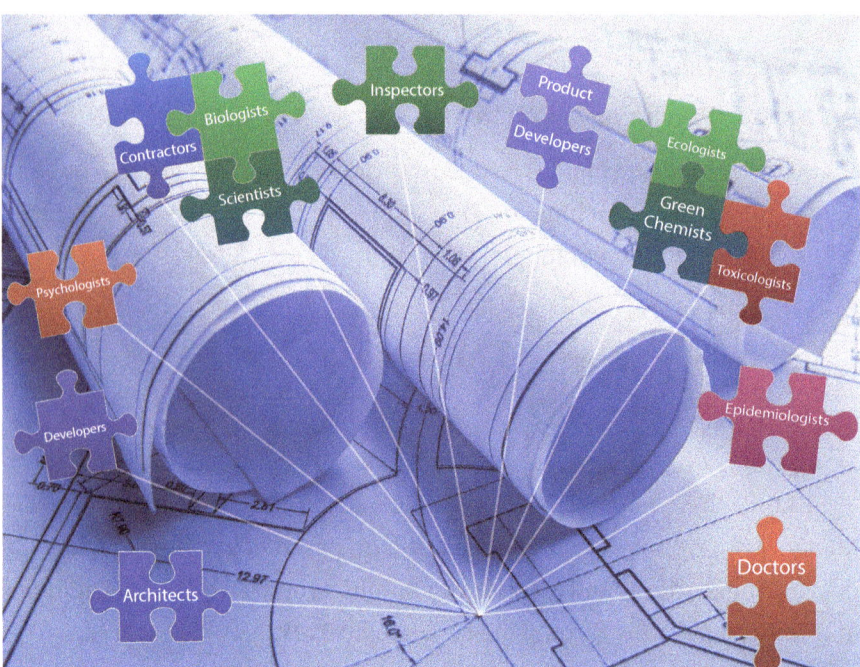

When all of this data is reviewed and analyzed for personal and public health, it can allow for other advances in healthcare that are just beginning to emerge at the time of this writing. This precision or personal medicine directive in the United States has been the focus of "The Precision Medicine Initiative." Precision medicine, also called personalized medicine, "helps your doctor find your unique disease risks and treatments that will work best for you."[155]

In the next section, I will discuss the overlap between the building informatics databases, the medical digital twin, and the building digital twin.

The Interoperability Between the Medical and Architecture Fields – Digital Twins

One of the most interesting developments in both architecture and medicine right now is the development of "Digital Twins."

What is a Digital Twin?

A Digital Twin is a digitized version of a real-world object, whether this is a building or a biological body. The purpose of this is to emulate the building or body for both monitoring in real-time and to provide updates or procedures on this digital twin to monitor and study resulting updates before implementing them in the real world.

The first definition of the Digital Twin was defined by NASA in the final release of the NASA Modeling, Simulation, Information Technology & Processing Roadmap in 2010 as "an integrated multi-physics, multi-scale, probabilistic simulation of a vehicle or system that uses the best available physical models, sensor updates, fleet history, etc., to mirror the life of its flying twin. It is ultra-realistic and may consider one or more important and interdependent vehicle systems."[156]

In their paper " A review of the roles of Digital Twin in CPS (Cyber-Physical Systems)-based production systems, "the authors Elisa Negri, Luca Fumagalli, and Marco Macchi define Digital Twins as the "virtual and computerized counterpart of a physical system that can be used to simulate it for various purposes, exploiting a real-time synchronization of the sensed data coming from the field."

The authors of this definition refer to the possibilities of this technological, real-time process system based on the advent of the Internet of Things (IoT), which proposes to "embed electronics, software, sensors, and network connectivity into devices (i.e. "things"), in order to allow the collection and exchange of data through the internet."[157]

As well, this digital twin can also be a representation of a building's life span, with monitoring and evaluations during the lifetime of the building, and in a similar format, it can also be an emulation of the human body.

With the advances in precision medicine has also been the emergence of the medical digital twin, which I mentioned in chapter 7. The ability for the medical twin to emulate the responses of the body in an accurate format requires accurate DNA data, along with the ability for the digital twin to contain environmental exposures, which can impact the emulation equations.

A research paper published in 2020 discussed the concepts of Building Automation Systems (BAS) utilizing a more responsive building performance process using real-time data through the cloud. They state in their paper, "Buildings Automation Systems (BAS) are ubiquitous in contemporary buildings, both monitoring building conditions and managing the building system control points. At present, these controls are prescriptive and pre-determined by the design team, rather than responsive to actual building performance." In this paper, the authors Caroline Quinn, Ali Zargar Shabestari, Tony Misic, Sara Gilani, Marin Litoiu, and J.J.McArthur state the following, "these are further limited by prescribed logic, possess only rudimentary visualizations, and lack broader system integration capabilities. Advances in machine learning, edge analytics, data management systems, and Facility Management-enabled Building Information Models (FM-BIMs) permit a novel approach: cloud-hosted building management. This paper presents an integration technique for mapping the data from a building Internet of Things (IoT) sensor network to an FM-BIM." [158] [159]

In their paper, they did not mention this as a digital twin, yet the principles are similar and function in a similar manner to a digital twin integrated as a Building Management System.

While the building and engineering fields are developing digital twins for real-time monitoring of structures, those such as the Swedish Digital Twin Consortium aim to apply this concept to personalize medicine by constructing "network models of all molecular, phenotypic and environmental factors relevant to disease mechanisms in individual patients (digital twins); and computationally treat those twins with thousands of drugs in order to identify the best one or ones to treat the patient."[160]

As they state on their website, "one of the most important health care problems is that a large number of patients do not respond to drug treatment. According to a report from the FDA, medication is deemed ineffective for 38-75 % of patients with common diseases. This problem reflects the complexity of common diseases. These may involve altered interactions between thousands of genes, which differ between patients with the same diagnosis."[161]

Therefore, by providing a digital twin in healthcare, diagnostics and testing can be provided before any medications or procedures are presented for the patient, with feedback as to how the patient may respond to treatments.

And the reason why this is such an interesting development with potential for overlap between these professions of architecture and health is as such. In the world of buildings, if you have the ability to provide building calculations and updates on a digital version of a structure, then you can know ahead of time what the cause-effect response might be. These are often defined as Cyber-Physical Systems.

As such, if you have an elaborate digital version of the human body that includes a history of the biological and chemical compositions of a patient with a focus on personalized medicine, then the resulting medical digital twin can provide the doctor with a better understanding of recommendations. The knowledge of how certain procedures and even pharmacological responses can be evaluated before the medications or procedures are provided, can give insights into the results before any procedures take place.

What I propose in this book is that these two digital twins, that of buildings and the human body, can overlap. These overlaps can utilize the data of the building on occupant health, and the resulting impacts of health in buildings can be applied to human health.

This can be represented not just as a report of a building's impact on the occupant yet can be shown as a visual representation of this human digital twin for patient history and health.

The interconnections that software provides in the design, building, and construction monitoring processes can be transferred to the impacts of building health on human and biological health to the human digital twin.

A Brief History of Digital Twins Emerging from CAD and BIM

While CAD has been around for many decades now, the advent of digital fabrication processes with a direct connection between the design model and the procedures to fabricate the components of these designs, has not been around for very long.

There have been certain projects over the years that have utilized these processes, from the work of Zaha Hadid and Patrik Schumacher, who have utilized the digital design process and the fabrication steps using Rhino and Grasshopper, to Frank Gehry and his team utilizing CATIA to design and fabricate the Guggenheim Bilbao. That said, the typical building today is still built with methods that are based on construction drawings built by the on-site crew, even if the plans are digitized.

However, in the past decade, the advent of the digital twin has become more common, not just to provide a path to fabrication from the CAD design but to monitor the life of the building and the many processes that exist in a building during its lifetime. This process of building drawings has evolved with the advent of Computer Aided Manufacturing (CAM) or fabrication. This ability to utilize digital designs to then be manufactured and fabricated utilizing these designs has provided a full circle process, from initial concept and drawing to an end product – all of which is done with computers and robots or CNC machines.

In addition, the progress of BIM – Building Information Modeling has provided the ability for changes in one area of a design to then update other sections of a design so that all interconnections are modified together. This use of BIM can be extremely valuable to ensure that, for example, an update to the location of a wall or stairwell can then update other areas of the design, to make sure that both structural and codes are met to the appropriate standards.

Perhaps in this manner, the building as a living entity can be recognized and reviewed as either being in health and wellness – or not.

By creating a digital version of a physical building, defined as a Digital Twin (DT), the characteristics of the building can be monitored over its lifetime, particularly for Facility Management professionals in larger-scale buildings.

This digital twin is not just a CAD model, it is a living version of the building. As many are familiar with CAD and BIM processes, the intention of these digital drawings is to provide a design overview of the structure and how it is to be constructed. The utilization of the digital twin includes the functions of the building after it's built to provide current construction details of the structure. This is important as many design changes occur during the building process and need to be updated and kept on file.

However, this living digital twin is also utilized for building maintenance, from machinery and functioning components of the structure to the active functions of the building systems, such as air and water quality. Or at least, it can be utilized in this form of facility management that is now possible with the current technological advancements and building capabilities available in this 21st century.

While building information has become more granular over the past few decades, the taxonomy to represent this data has not been as robust to properly map and monitor this data digitally. This is where the Real Estate Core and Brick Schema have entered into the equation as a critical facet. This ontology is required for building information to be provided for Digital Twins for data mapped to 3D spaces as geoinformation or what's known as GIS (Geographical Information Systems). In the next chapter, I will provide more details on this topic as I discuss Geomedicine.

In the medical world, this idea of a digital twin, which emulates the human body to ensure that patient information is not just data in an EHR, but is a living representation of the patient, can have many benefits for both the doctor and the patient. For one, the concepts of personal or precision medicine can become a reality, and the idea of providing research models for health issues can be utilized as a model for how the patient may respond to such health procedures or medications. The use of personal genetic information, emulated on a digital twin, can provide feedback on how these procedures or medications may impact the patient in an accurate simulation.

This can provide a more thorough analysis for a specific patient and not just a theoretical assessment of what might occur for the patient. It can also provide more personalized recommendations, as the simulation can be a way for the doctor to work with the patient during analysis and treatments.

The Potential Overlap With Architecture and Medical Digital Twins

If you are able to view the processes of these two types of digital twins, existing in both the world of buildings and of human digital emulations, there can then exist a potential for overlap between these two for greater health insights. In particular, the results of building evaluations for health, which can then be applied to the patient as an occupant in the building, can show the impacts of this building in a human model.

This information can be applied in a way that can be included in the digital twin of the human body and as such, provide exposure information for the doctor to include in their patient's health analysis. Topics such as respiratory ailments, asthma, chemical exposures, and toxins can be included as potential health causes in the health professional's process. This can provide more in-depth insights into the causes of ailments, as well as the appropriate medical solutions for patient health and healing. After all, if the patient has consistent, long term issues relative to air quality, or exposures to toxic elements, then these details can provide information that otherwise may have never been known. And the resulting medical analysis might have been completely overlooked. This could lead the patient to suffer from a root cause problem that a doctor may strive to resolve with procedures or medications, yet will focus on resolving the effects of these causations and not the root cause itself.

The use of the Internet of Things (IOT), and Smart buildings utilizing sensors and devices for monitoring air quality, toxic gases, and particulates as examples, can provide building maintenance opportunities for healthier built environments.

These topics of building health and the digital twins of buildings and humans requires more involvement and overlap between the building and health professionals. The Architectural Doctor can assist in these integrations, supporting the processes in which these professions overlap, as well as supporting the professionals in learning new methods and procedures.

This requires new research and education for the architect and the doctor, and updates in universities as well as updated systems for each professional, as discussed in this book. It's no small feat to achieve, yet to ignore these potential impacts that can cause health issues has an even greater, long term negative impact. Steps can be taken now to provide helpful benefits for all occupants and patients, while the infrastructure to provide more advanced support between each of these professions can be evaluated and planned strategically.

In this year, 2022, while I'm editing this book, the recognition of building impacts and the required changes have been both obvious and also missing as integrations. In the next section, I will comment on what we've learned or can learn from the coronavirus pandemic and what changes can be made to help resolve issues that have occurred during this timeframe in the building and health fields.

The Coronavirus Pandemic and the Recognition of Building Health

With the ongoing developments of the Internet of Things (IOT), along with Smart Buildings, the ability to monitor not only the building functions but also the building health and subsequent characteristics occurring inside of the building can be monitored in ways that were never before possible.

Digital twins have the potential to span the gaps between architecture and medicine by utilizing the Architectural Medicine System to bridge these gaps. And the gaps include metrics of a building that can cause health issues, from indoor air quality issues and toxic materials to bacteria and viruses that can cause health problems.

The IOT has provided a platform for many types of sensors and meters to measure a wide range of concerns, from carbon dioxide and carbon monoxide to particulates, VOCs, and even pathogens such as bacteria and viruses. Before the novel coronavirus, the topics of lead, asbestos, mold, and bacteria that, for instance, can lead to Legionnaire's disease, were the common types of contaminants building health professionals were familiar with in terms of building issues.

However, with the advent of the novel coronavirus, indoor air quality issues have become much more familiar and have increased building health awareness in the general populous in ways that may predate recorded history.

As such, the topic of building monitors for contaminants has also risen. Over the past decade, smart buildings have included the monitoring of carbon dioxide and other gases as well as particulates, and there are many devices that have been available to track these indoor air topics for the past two decades. However, the ability to send this information to the cloud as a data set, and the ability to monitor larger groups of these devices, especially those in the same building or locations, have created the capacity for a mesh of informatics in real time that has never been realized.

This type of bioinformatics can be extremely helpful in providing real-time diagnostics for better building health and greater wellness in the built environment.

And as these monitors become more common and more affordable with greater capabilities, it has provided a baseline for building and facility management that can provide a large range of building insights in real-time, along with the recorded data to provide informatics over a large period of time.

Add to this the Digital Twin, where these monitors can be viewed in these replications of buildings as digital spaces, and the result is a greater ability to monitor building health in very helpful formats.

This data can be utilized for real-time monitoring of building health, yet it can also be utilized as big data for bioinformatics that can provide insights into the impacts of building health over time.

This long tail or the "long now" viewpoint provided by the Long Now Foundation, created by Stewart Brand, Danny Hillis, and others such as Brian Eno, strives to look at life from a bigger picture view over a long period of time — for them, 10,000 years.[162]

While the current long now might be 10, 50, or 100 years in terms of current human society, each of these viewpoints can provide a bigger picture view for health and wellness, whether this be in 10 or in 10,000 years.

And it is this previously mentioned bioinformatics that can yield public health benefits over time. Through the research of epidemiologists and toxicologists, with information on health related to the built environment, this can bridge the current span between architecture and medicine using these sensors along with the Architectural Medicine System and ARxMD.

The use of this data in a Clinical Data Repository (CDR) or Clinical Data Warehouse (CDW) for data analysis can provide extensive information on health and the impacts of the built environment on human and biological health through building analysis. These processes can allow for data to be anonymized and exported for a CDR or CDW. A clinical data repository (CDR) is an "aggregation of granular patient-centric health data usually collected from multiple-source IT systems and intended to support multiple uses. When a CDR holds data specifically organized for analytics, it meets the definition of a clinical data warehouse."[163]

With these processes in place, this can now include both the architecture and medical professionals viewing and analyzing this information in large data sets, especially with the support of the Architectural Doctor and Building Informaticist.

The extended use of this monitoring and data can become more available to the health and building professionals as it becomes more common in building monitoring systems, as well as available for analysis by those in the public health realm.

And this transitions nicely into the next chapter discussing the topics of public health and social determinants of health (SDoH)...

"We shape our buildings; thereafter they shape us."

— Winston Churchill

PUBLIC HEALTH, SOCIAL DETERMINANTS OF HEALTH (SDoH), & GEOMEDICINE

The history of Public Health is long and complex, yet in viewing these developments, you can begin to gain an understanding of the goals that this historical process has strived to achieve. One of the important facets of learning is the understanding of the trajectory of a subject. Recognizing the history and development of a subject can bring many aspects into clarity in learning the topics being explored.

Chapter: 13 Public Health, Social Determinants of Health (SDoH), & Geomedicine

Public health has been a topic recorded since Hippocrates, yet these matters became more prominent from the 18th to 20th centuries. In the 1800s, public health issues relative to sanitation "occurred simultaneously in several European countries and were built upon foundations laid in the period between 1750 and 1830." As populations in Europe increased, public health garnered more of a focus as there was an increase in "large numbers of infant deaths and of the unsavoury conditions in prisons and in mental institutions."[164]

This timeframe also saw an increase in locations where medical services were provided in locations defined as hospitals and became more common as "voluntary efforts by private citizens helped to create a pattern that was to become familiar in public health services."[165]

This timeframe was also known as an era "characterized by efforts to educate people in health matters. In 1752 British physician Sir John Pringle published a book that discussed ventilation in barracks and the provision of latrines. In 1754 James Lind, who had worked as a surgeon in the British navy, published a treatise on scurvy, a disease caused by a lack of vitamin C."[166]

The Industrial Revolution brought great advances to society from the standpoint of both technological developments and the capabilities to provide more material goods in a scalable format, yet it was also a time when "the health and welfare of the workers deteriorated. In England, where the Industrial Revolution and its adverse effects on health were first experienced, there arose in the 19th century a movement toward sanitary reform that finally led to the establishment of public health institutions."[167]

With many European cities increasing in population by twofold and even threefold in many locations, the population increase also meant a large increase in deaths. This increase was the "result of an increase in the urban population that far exceeded available housing and of the subsequent development of conditions that led to widespread disease and poor health."[168] During the beginning of the 19th century, "humanitarians and philanthropists in England worked to educate the population and the government on problems associated with population growth, poverty, and epidemics." And in the mid-1800s British physician, Thomas Southwood Smith founded the "Health of Towns Association in 1839, and published reports on quarantine, cholera, yellow fever, and the benefits of sanitary improvements."[169]

This timeframe was when Florence Nightingale worked to develop more advanced healthcare processes, which included advancements in hospitals and improvements in building health through her experiences in the Crimean war as a nurse. She was amongst the first to focus on the impacts of health from the built environment and brought awareness to topics that today are common in epidemiology and public health. Her initial public comments from the mid-1800s on the subject of "public health nursing appear in a November 30, 1861 letter to William Rathbone about a 'Proposed Plan for the Training and Employment of Women in Hospital, District, and Private Nursing, 1861.' "[170]

Nightingale's work in initiating better building conditions was also supported by her advanced thinking as a data scientist, in utilizing statistics to support her goals to improve public health. She had skills in mathematics that were "far ahead of her time in understanding the importance of health data. She argued that Parliament should extend the 1860 census to collect data on sickness and disability, and she advocated for the creation of a Chair in Applied Statistics at Oxford University."[171]

Many years later, the "Royal Statistical Society acknowledged her contributions to health data by electing Florence Nightingale to membership—the first woman to be so honored—and the American Statistical Association made her an Honorary Member."[172]

In her later years, she helped the cause of better health processes with her paper "Sick-Nursing and Health Nursing, which was read in the United States at the Chicago Exposition."[173] In 1894 she presented another paper, "Health Teaching in Towns and Villages," written to support the "extension of district nursing in the rural areas of England."[174]

The Poor Law Commission, created in 1834, which explored problems of community health issues, argued that the "expenditures necessary to the adoption and maintenance of measures of prevention would ultimately amount to less than the cost of the disease now constantly engendered." This public health research proved that "a relationship exists between communicable disease and filth in the environment, and it was said that safeguarding public health is the province of the engineer rather than of the physician."[175]

In this manner, the separation of public health concerns of the doctor and medical professionals may have been the divide that eventually led to an absence of the medical profession focusing on health in the built environment. Earlier in the book, I mentioned this division of responsibility and inquired as to who is and who should be responsible for such matters. Perhaps this history shows the time when the physician was responsible for such matters on this level, and moving forward, we can begin to rethread this connection and concerns to health in the built environment.

From this brief history, we can begin to see that health for the public has long been about making the invisible seen, or in today's terms, the ability to identify and measure that which had previously been unknown. For instance, we now know that carbon dioxide, carbon monoxide, radon, and other "invisible to the senses" gases and particulates can cause tremendous health issues and even death. We also know that there are microscopic organisms, bacteria, and viruses, which are invisible to the eye, yet exist and are measurable thanks to the capabilities of microscopes and the pioneers who first learned about these facets of the natural world.

This timeline of public health has brought us to our current day understanding of these natural substances and their impact on human health. It can also provide insights into topics that, in today's world, we may view as common sense. Some two to three hundred years ago, the ideas of sanitation and cleanliness in the environment may not have been so obvious, yet today many would expect this as part of common logic.

I mention this as perhaps, in the future, we may look back at this time when building health is not as monitored and evaluated by health professionals for the patient and public health in a similar manner.

In the next decades onward, there will be a learning curve in how these human created materials, as synthetics, impact human health and well-being. And this facet of health, from both natural and synthetic sources, will bring a larger picture of understanding into clarity, providing future generations insights into public health that we currently do not have.

This includes many aspects of the exterior and interior built environments and how these newer materials and methods are impacting human health. As I discussed in previous chapters about the Architectural Medicine System and utilizing the Healthy Building Inspector and the Building Informaticist, along with the Architectural Doctor, many of these topics can be recognized and resolved in a cohesive format.

And when it comes to the environment and the built environment in terms of public health, one of the popular topics in these discussions is the recognition of Social Determinants of Health (SDoH). In this chapter, we'll delve into this topic, showing how the environment, the built environment, and the exterior world impact human health and what the current status is on these topics.

To start, it's important to discuss the word "determinants." What exactly does this mean?

Definitions of determinant include "an element that identifies or determines the nature of something or that fixes or conditions an outcome," [176] with the word origin being:

determinant

"c. 1600 (adj.), "serving to determine;" 1680s (n.), "that which fixes, defines, or establishes (something);" from Latin determinantem (nominative determinans), present participle of determinare "to enclose, bound, set limits to," from de "off" (see de-) + terminare "to mark the end or boundary," from terminus "end, limit" (see terminus)."

"A determining factor or agent; a ruling antecedent, a conditioning element." [177]

Based on these definitions, the term "determinants" can be defined as that which "defines or establishes the nature of something or that fixes or conditions an outcome."

Social Determinants of Health (SDoH)

Many people involved in public health are aware of a topic called Social Determinants of Health (SDoH). A good definition of this can be found from the World Health Organization (WHO):

> "Social Determinants of Health (SDoH) are the conditions in which people are born, grow, work, live, and age, and the wider set of forces and systems shaping the conditions of daily life."[178]

These social determinants of health can be defined as "the economic and social conditions that influence individual and group differences in health status."[179] This definition includes the "wider set of forces and systems shaping the conditions of daily life," which can point to the impacts that the built environment can have on health.

The graphic by the group goinvo[180], shows the importance of both the built environment and medicine, which together form 18 percent of these determinants of health. In fact, when you view this chart in closer detail, you will see that many of the emotional and psychological factors listed in the other segments can also be included in the topics of Architectural Medicine.

As these topics become more of a focus with health implications, the questions some may be asking are, "what can we do about these relative to the built environment? And how can we apply these academic and research findings to real-world applications to help the general public?"

In this realm, the answer right now varies significantly from location to location. In terms of the ability for health professionals to address many of these social determinants of health, there is a small range of options that are still in development.

However, as this topic overlaps with the medical and architecture fields, this highlights a gap that can be bridged for better health solutions. And this is where the Architectural Medicine System (AMS) has a great potential to fill these gaps and provide better health to a wider range of the population.

What Are Social Determinants of Health (SDoH)?

The U.S. Department of Health and Human Services defines social determinants of health (SDOH) as the "conditions in the environments where people are born, live, learn, work, play, worship, and age that affect a wide range of health, functioning, and quality-of-life outcomes and risks." [181] They group these determinants into five domains; *Economic Stability, Education Access and Quality, Health Care Access and Quality, Social and Community Context,* and *Neighborhood and Built Environment.*

When you review each of these domains, you can see that there is overlap between many of these topics. In particular, relative to this book, are topics related to the neighborhood and the built environment. Other groups are using the revised version of this topic called "determinants of health," such as the goinvo.com group which created the infographic listed below:

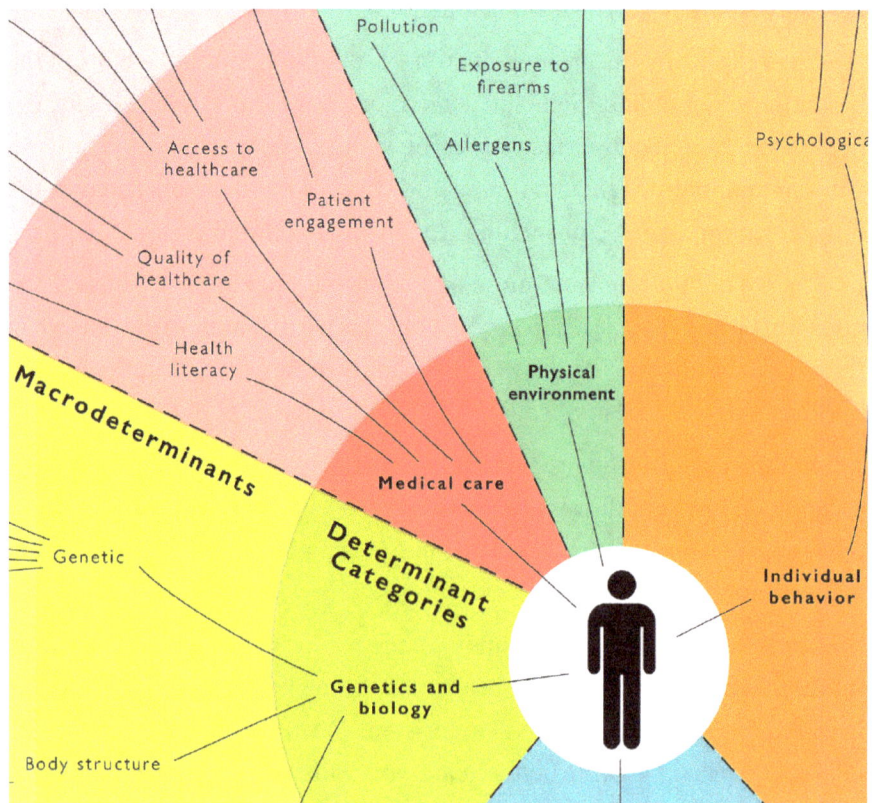

Chapter: 13 Public Health, Social Determinants of Health (SDoH), & Geomedicine

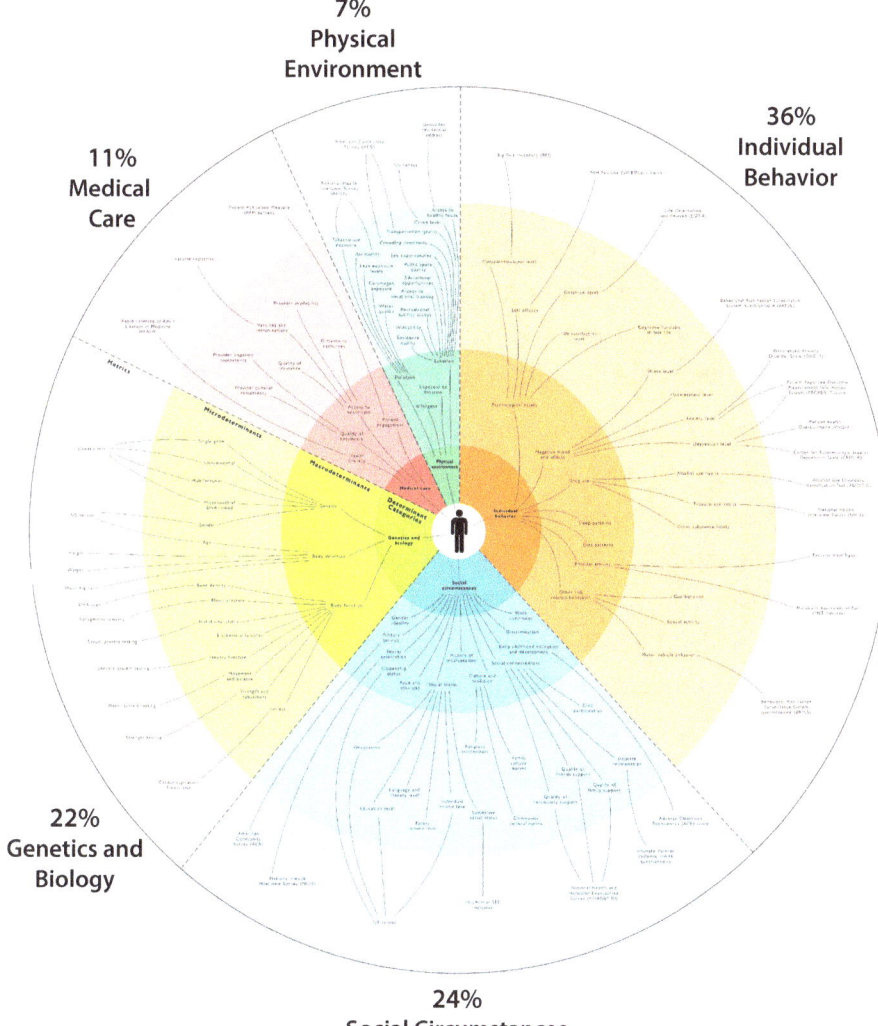

There is a wide range of topics that are included on the determinants of health issues, yet the built environment is a large part of these discussions. Being that the average person spends from 60 to 90 percent of their time inside of buildings, the impacts of this on one's health and wellness becomes even more evident in today's modern world.

The environment in which one lives includes the built environment, as well as the environment in general, such as the towns and cities in which they live and work. This includes the possible issues in this environment that can cause health issues. This is wide ranging, from industrial manufacturing pollutants and issues related to groundwater, to a large range of natural and synthetic chemicals that exist as contaminants. This can also include issues related to older infrastructures, such as lead pipes causing water pollution and older buildings with asbestos insulation.

As listed by the U.S. Department of Health and Human Services, a main goal of the SDoH initiative is to "create neighborhoods and environments that promote health and safety." According to the Centers for Disease Control and Prevention (CDC), the "neighborhoods people live in have a major impact on health and well-being."[182] "Many people in the United States live in neighborhoods with high rates of violence, unsafe air or water, and other health and safety risks. In addition, some people are exposed to things at work that can harm their health, like secondhand smoke or loud noises."[183]

The focal point of these determinants of health is based on metrics that are often challenging to collect for medical professionals. And if the doctor is to gather as much data about their patient's ailments, and few, if any, metrics are taken from their patient's environments, then a large percentage of one's health is not seen nor captured as valuable data for these health assessments.

As one's living environment in today's day and age becomes more complex, with increasing numbers of potentially toxic substances that can impact short and long-term health, there is a large gap in this knowledge that can help determine and define better health that is often excluded.

And this is where the Architectural Medicine System and the ARxMD software have the ability for these determinants of health to be included in the diagnosis process. This data can also be utilized as valuable health metrics and useful tools for health professionals striving to find best solutions for their patients.

This is where a bridge between the fields of architecture and medicine can become a powerful multi-disciplinary force in both determining health metrics and utilizing data points to provide valuable information for the medical doctor and their teams.

But a key question with this topic quickly becomes complex, which is how this data can be captured. Who would be doing this work of capturing the data, and then how will the medical professionals receive this information?

This all requires systems to be in place, along with these two professions working with each other in ways that previously have not existed. This is where the integrations between these fields, along with new processes, procedures, and protocols, become critical. And not just new systems in place for each profession but new integrations that neither group has implemented before.

As outlined in the previous chapters, the Architectural Medicine System can help support this process for the health and medical professionals, as well we the building and architecture professionals. This includes defining the various topics related to built environment issues and their negative health implications. Using methods to define these issues and provide terminology and coding that can be utilized across professions and between different computing platforms is critical to support cohesive systems.

The Importance of Interoperability in Healthcare With Other Professionals

Over the past decade, the Health Level Seven (HL7) organization has been working on initiatives that can support advanced technological developments to support interoperability. The result is the newer integration process discussed earlier in the book called Fast Healthcare Interoperability Resources or FHIR. FHIR is a more advanced standard for healthcare data exchange. To revisit this topic, as defined by HL7, "FHIR is designed to enable information exchange to support the provision of healthcare in a wide variety of settings. The specification builds on and adapts modern, widely used RESTful practices to enable the provision of integrated healthcare across a wide range of teams and organizations." [184]

Because the exchange is based on a Restful Application Programming Interface or API, this means that data can be exchanged between any software platform in a secure process, which is easier to implement into modern day software applications.

And not just health care software, but any software. And this is where modern software applications are able to provide professionals and consumers the capability to record and receive healthcare data in ways that previously were much more complex and often took a longer time to achieve.

An example of this is the Apple healthcare application, which can both send and receive healthcare data between many different healthcare providers and platforms. It is this new standard that the ARxMD software utilizes to provide an exchange of data to the Healthy Building Inspector, the Building Informaticist, and the architecture and building professionals.

In the future, it can include other professionals, such as psychotherapists, that can benefit from the use of this data to help their clients and patients achieve optimal health.

Of course, the data is only one part of these complex systems, and as such, it requires more implementations that will need to be buttressed by the addition of new types of inspections and testing that is also new for the architecture, engineering, and construction (AEC) fields.

These new testing processes will require an important element, and that is the overlap between medical testing laboratories for advanced building analysis testing processes. Obviously, the medical fields have many sets of testing requiring laboratory processes, yet these new testing procedures will require an expansion that will require new training, procedures, and standards. Many of these lab tests may be seen as external laboratory testing processes, which will require new standards for building inspectors and new connections with these medical laboratories.

And one other key component to these new tests is the addition of communication between these doctors and the building professionals, which has not existed previously.

And with these new testing processes, the utilization of the current EHR and Health Information Systems (HIS) can allow for data and laboratory testing results to be readily available. The building inspector professionals will need to learn how their data collection can be added to these systems. As long as the HIPAA protocols are followed using the HL7 connections, even external software systems used by the building and architecture fields will allow these new cross communications.

Along with the utilization of the LOINC laboratory testing codes, these building evaluations can provide proper coding for these new testing processes with a chain of events that can follow the HL7 protocols. For most in the AEC and building professions, these will be new integrations, yet will follow similar procedures that would be required to communicate between many other software platforms using APIs.

When all of these professionals are working together with round trip solutions, the result can be a new set of data for the medical and health professionals, new building related inspection measurements, and new integrations, and in the end, there can be better solutions in the built environment that can then be resolved by the AEC professionals.

These new steps, in turn, can then support better public health and provide new avenues to implement social determinants in health.

The UMLS Metathesaurus and SDoH

When it comes to the topics of interoperability, there is a need to ensure that topics are both included and cross-referenced within the fields of medicine, as well as expanding outside the scope of one field. In the USA, there is the Unified Medical Language System® (UMLS), which spans many different platforms and code bases to provide what they call a Metathesaurus. The UMLS is "a set of files and software that brings together many health and biomedical vocabularies and standards to enable interoperability between computer systems." [185] [186]

For those in the medical fields, this is nothing new, but for those reading this book who may not be familiar with this system, this is an important topic. The reason being is when you have a complex field such as medicine, and there are worldwide standards striving to be provided, you need to have agreed-upon standards.

Right now, the topics of social determinants of health do exist in many of the standard's organizations, such as SNOMED, ICD, and LOINC, yet in order to provide round trip processes that include the built environment and the field of architecture, these topics need to be expanded and developed in multi-disciplinary formats.

A benefit of the UMLS is that it already spans many platforms and can help to provide cross-referencing with the many newer fields that can be included in the work of the Architectural Doctor and Architectural Medicine.

For instance, if there is a closer look into how the built environment impacts patient health, as mentioned throughout this book, SDoH issues will need to be included in the doctor's evaluations, and that will require the need for buildings to be inspected and evaluated.

Being that SDoH is already on the radar of the public health and fields, the next steps would be to ensure that standards are created for these issues in the built environment and how they can be measured and recorded.

The Gravity Project, PhenX, and SNOMED, ICD, & LOINC

In the United States, this is where the work of the Gravity Project can enter into the picture. This organization "exists to serve as the open public collaborative advancing health and social data standardization for health equity."[187]

What I find interesting about this project is the number of social workers and healthcare professionals working together to create standards and codes for SNOMED and ICD, as examples, with the intention to support patient and public health focused on social determinants of health. Their ability and willingness to collaborate and coordinate these complex professions to develop a standard is impressive. I can attest to this high level of professionalism and attention to health developments as I've been participating in several of these initiatives. It has been an impressive group process, and their connections, from grassroots to the higher level government organizations, have provided a great opportunity for SDoH topics to be examined and supported.

By working with groups that range from social workers, physicians, healthcare executives, and software and coding professionals have provided a new code base for SDoH topics.

From a technical standpoint, their work to develop codes and implementation guides (IG) for the HL7 FHIR processes is providing greater capabilities to record and exchange data for SDoH topics.

> "Social Determinants of Health (SDOH) are increasingly being recognized as essential factors that influence healthcare outcomes. This HL7 Implementation Guide (IG) defines how to exchange SDOH content defined by the Gravity Project using the Fast Healthcare Interoperability Resources (FHIR) standard. It defines how to represent coded content used to support the following care activities: screening, clinical assessment/diagnosis, goal setting, and the planning and performing of interventions."[188]

This work provides the following key processes that have not existed to provide successful integrations for SDoH as it "addresses the need to gather SDOH information in multiple settings, share that information between stakeholders, and exchange referrals between organizations to address specific social risk needs, all with appropriate patient consent."[189]

The other facet of this work that caught my attention several years ago was a statement on their interest in providing procedures "to share clinical data to support secondary purposes such as population health, quality, and research." The guide supports the following use cases:[190]

- Document SDOH data in conjunction with the patient encounters with providers, payers, and community services
- Document and track SDOH related interventions to completion
- Identify cohorts of individuals that have a common relationship to another entity (e.g., covered by the same payer)

By leveraging the electronic capabilities of HL7 FHIR and creating implementation guides with new coding, it opens the opportunity for round trip procedures to exist between social work professionals, doctors, and healthcare professionals, and the software and coding professionals to provide whole system solutions for patient and public health.

The next step of these developments, in my opinion, is the arc between these professionals and the built environment professionals to ensure that standards, codes, and procedures can properly inform and support solutions to problems found.

SNOMED, ICD, DSM, & LOINC Integrations With The Gravity Project & PhenX

In the past decade in the USA, the *meaningful use* initiative began a group of developments that have built upon these digital and electronic record processes. Over the past few years, groups such as the abovementioned Gravity Project have worked to develop and implement solutions for topics related to social determinants of health. This includes definitions and terminology that medical and health professionals can utilize to better define determinants of health.

This group has started to define codes that connect the topics of health issues in the environment of patients, including the built environment. In this way, problems causing health issues can at least be recorded, including terms that are included in SNOMED, ICD, and LOINC as proper codes.

This enables a roundtrip process for patients and health professionals in practical formats by enabling the exchange in data, and recording this in the electronic health record or the comprehensive health record.

This dedicated group of health professionals in the Gravity Project have been working to provide both guidelines and codes that have been added to SNOMED, ICD, and LOINC that can be utilized to address these determinants of health.

In October of 2022, they announced that multiple ICD-10-CM codes were approved for implementation by the Centers for Medicare & Medicaid Services.[191]

In terms of the environment, built environment, and housing, ICD-10-CM codes were approved for implementation in 2021. There are several new codes that have been added for current use, including the following:

- New code Z58 Problems related to physical environment
- New code Z58.6 Inadequate drinking-water supply
- New subcategory Z59.0 Homelessness
- New subcategory Z59.81 Housing instability, housed
- New code Z59.811 Housing instability, housed, with risk of homelessness

And as can be seen with the above codes, there are several that are focused on the built environment. These new codes can bring awareness to issues of health based on buildings and the environment, which can help support these interconnections moving forward.

In tandem with this work of the Gravity Project is the PhenX Toolkit. A portmanteau of Phenotypes and eXposures, PhenX "provides recommended standard data collection protocols for conducting biomedical research."[192] A PhenX domain is defined as a "field of research with a unifying theme and easily enumerated quantitative and qualitative measures (e.g., demographics, anthropometrics, organ systems, complex diseases, and lifestyle factors)."[193] As you can see from this definition, there is an overlap with the social determinants of health, which is not by accident.

The PhenX codes have been created to address a number of environmental exposure issues, with some related directly to building issues and building health. The following are examples of codes that are currently listed as LOINC codes:[194]

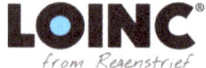

The Logical Observation Identifiers Names and Codes – LOINC browser with PhenX Codes for Environmental Exposures

"This material contains content from LOINC (http://loinc.org). LOINC is copyright © 1995-2022, Regenstrief Institute, Inc. and the Logical Observation Identifiers Names and Codes (LOINC) Committee and is available at no cost under the license at http://loinc.org/license. LOINC® is a registered United States trademark of Regenstrief Institute, Inc."

The following codes focus on topics that the Architectural Doctor can provide support within the medical and healthcare professionals in ways in which are uncommon yet can be extremely helpful.

62534-3   PhenX – environmental exposures – air contaminants in the home environment protocol 061101

62520-2 PhenX – environmental exposures – exposure at work and daily life protocol 060401

62540-0 PhenX – environmental exposures – plastic exposures at work and home protocol 061401

These PhenX codes are from the LOINC catalog, under the "Environmental Exposures" segment of the PhenX listings. The LOINC code "62534-3" is in a questionnaire format that includes a client history process with codes that signify the answers to the many subsets of questions in each segment of the "environmental exposures - air contaminants in the home environment protocol 061101."[195]

This coding from the Gravity Project and the PhenX toolkit can provide initial steps for both the patient, as well as the professionals involved in these evaluations. Ideally, the basic questions would be part of an intake form, with the more advanced questions based on empirical evidence as provided by testing mechanisms that are recognized by the building and testing industries. This way, the subjective answers can provide one set of feedback, while the objective analysis can also be provided for an overall observation that is more complete.

Combining this with the ability for the Architectural Doctor to receive data from the Healthy Building Inspector and Building Informaticist can provide a round trip process using the Architectural Medicine System (AMS). And the data that is collected can be included in the ARxMD software solution, so the many other professionals involved can have access to the results to prepare for best solutions.

Once the health professionals and social workers have systems and procedures to provide a round trip evaluation in their daily practices that include these topics, then more systems can be implemented to support other environmental issues impacting patient health.

The other benefit to utilizing these new codes and systems are the results, which can be analyzed and evaluated by public health and bioinformatics professionals. And as discussed in chapter 12, this can provide a larger scale database of results to be evaluated over time, providing even more insights showing the impacts that the environment has on public health.

Again, this spiracycle of events can provide an evolving metric of information that can provide more robust data sets for each of the professions involved to benefit from over time. The result is an iteration providing new approaches to these topics, and an evolving benefit for training, education, and procedures to be implemented for the health fields.

Beyond Medical Acuity – Social Determinants of Health and PRAPARE

No, I didn't misspell that word above in the title PRAPARE. This acronym stands for Protocol for Responding to and Assessing Patient Assets, Risks, and Experiences (PRAPARE). As defined by the PRAPARE organization, in 2013, "the National Association of Community Health Centers, Inc. (NACHC), Association of Asian Pacific Community Health Organizations (AAPCHO), and Oregon Primary Care Association (OPCA) partnered together to develop, test, and spread a national, standardized, patient-centered social determinant of health (SDOH) assessment tool and companion Implementation and Action Toolkit known as PRAPARE."[196] The objective of the project is to provide a "national standardized patient risk assessment protocol designed to engage patients in assessing & addressing social determinants of health (SDOH)."[197]

The way in which they are striving to achieve this is by "going beyond medical acuity to identify patient risks related to the SDoH, PRAPARE positions health centers and other providers to better understand and manage their patient populations."[198]

As a big part of Architectural Medicine is the Architectural Medicine System (AMS), this approach of providing a process to achieve these goals utilizing a step by step process can help to bridge these gaps of health in the environment. This is another project that can utilize the HL7 interoperability processes to help bridge the gaps in both healthcare and the buildings. In my opinion, the next steps are to involve the field of architecture to become better stewards of these issues and to help resolve building health issues in both remediations for current buildings and revised approaches to new buildings for prevention.

More information about the PRAPARE toolkit and program can be found on their website:

https://prapare.org/

Health Geomedicine, Geoinformatics, Bioinformatics, and a New Map Towards Wellness

Social Determinants of Health are not just about the activity of a community and the events at these locations. They are about the physical, chemical, and possible toxicological facets that include epidemiology topics and the many facets of the environment that can impact the public's health. The inclusion of this data can not only be valuable to the medical professionals for their patients but when collected and analyzed as big data, a larger metric can be evaluated based on these larger data sets.

These larger data sets can inform an even larger group of professionals that can range from those who are manufacturing products and developing construction materials to those who are providing specifications and building codes for these materials and methodologies in the larger construction of towns and cities.

The ability to have this data, showing the impacts of such materials and methods from larger datasets, can provide epidemiologists and public health professionals with tools that can help to provide greater insights and benefits for decision making on a larger scale.

By including these evaluations of health in the built environment and using the standards in a collaborative fashion, such as the UMLS, the codes and standards for including these determinants of health in the doctor's evaluation can be implemented by the Building Informaticist and the Architectural Doctor.

As I've mentioned many times in this book, while these topics of health in the built environment have become more common in research papers, medical journals, and even in sporadic building publications, if there are no systems to implement these into the current systems of the medical and architecture professionals, it is not likely to become a mainstream process within these fields.

This is why the current listings and the creations of codes in SNOMED, ICD, DSM, LOINC, and other standards are so important and can provide a pathway to help bridge these gaps. And any new topics that may not easily fit into current code bases can be created using new standards to ensure that these topics can be implemented into these already complex professional systems.

As I move forward into the rest of this chapter, I will discuss a wider range of topics relative to SDoH, as well as how the built environment issues relate to personal health supported by evaluations by doctors and health professionals.

The Endocrine System and Built Environment Impacts on Health

Earlier in this book, I discussed some reasons why the topics of building health are important, yet with the focus of this chapter on determinants of health, it's pertinent to revisit some of these topics relative to physiology.

With the advent of more exposure to chemicals, both natural and synthetic, in today's buildings, one important topic to pay attention to is the endocrine system. The National Library of Medicine of the U.S. Department of Health and Human Services National Institutes of Health defines the endocrine system as the "eight major glands throughout your body."[199] These eight glands are responsible for creating hormones. These chemical messengers "travel through your bloodstream to tissues or organs. Hormones work slowly and affect body processes from head to toe. These include:"[200]

- Growth and development
- Metabolism - digestion, elimination, breathing, blood circulation and maintaining body temperature

- Sexual function
- Reproduction
- Mood

As the National Library of Medicine states, "if your hormone levels are too high or too low, you may have a hormone disorder. Hormone diseases also occur if your body does not respond to hormones the way it is supposed to. Stress, infection and changes in your blood's fluid and electrolyte balance can also influence hormone levels."[201]

When you consider that health issues such as diabetes and other hormonal issues have become larger health problems in certain regions of the world's population, looking for the culprits and the sources of these issues becomes critical. And in the United States, the "most common endocrine disease is diabetes" and is usually "treated by controlling how much hormone your body makes."[202]

With the average person spending more of their time inside of buildings, the impacts that the built environment has on health should be more of a focus. And the endocrine system is a good metric to explore as a potential canary in the coal mine for potential building health issues.

It's well known in the science and epidemiology fields that certain chemicals and materials cause problems with the endocrine system, yet few doctors have the capacity to expand their evaluations of their patient's health exposures. Including their patient's building exposures and history into their health equations can provide more detailed steps to be taken for both prevention and eliminating the causes of such diseases. This is another example of how the built environment can impact patient health, yet the doctor might not be including these health impacts in their evaluation processes.

GeoMedicine – Geographic Place History and Patient Health Assessments

In Bill Davenhall's paper titled "Geomedicine – Geography and Personal Health", he discusses the topics of personal health and place. And the term "place" in this context is defined as the physical location or geography of where they are located. The term geographic medicine or geomedicine is defined as "a branch of medicine that deals with geographic factors in disease."[203]

Geographic medicine is based on the foundation of the Geographic Information System (GIS). As defined by Davenhall in this paper, "Geographic information system (GIS) technology integrates hardware, software, and data for capturing, managing, analyzing, and displaying all forms of geographically referenced information."[204]

When you add this spatial data to include the built environment, you can quickly recognize the value of such data from an informatics perspective. As Davenhall includes in his article, "GIS allows us to view, understand, question, interpret, and visualize data in many ways that reveal relationships, patterns, and trends in the form of maps, globes, reports, and charts."[205] The use of the geographic information system (GIS), helps to "answer questions and solve problems by looking at data in a way that is quickly understood and easily shared."[206]

Davenhall goes on to state, "GIS has long been used to monitor the health of the planet. With geomedicine, GIS is now being used to monitor the health of individuals. It makes sense, because the health of people depends on the heath of the planet—and that's the basic idea behind geomedicine."[207]

These comments are very much in alignment with Architectural Medicine, the Architectural Medicine System, and the goals of the Architectural Doctor. By utilizing the ability to monitor the impacts of building issues causing health issues, it provides a geolocated inference for medical professionals to use for evaluating patient health.

GeoMedicine, GIS, Clinical Ecology, and Global Health

The topics of Environmental Health, Clinical Ecology, and Geographic Information Systems (GIS) can provide a whole picture view, literally and graphically, of locations to provide health disparities impacting community health. To highlight another quote from Davenhall's article:

> "The strength of modern GIS technology extends well beyond geographically relevant data analysis and powerful data visualization. It excels as a medium that helps inform, organize, and deliver health and human services."[208]

When you provide a health determinant with a specific location, this segues into the topic of Social Determinants of Health. SDoH includes five major segments: *Individual Behavior, Social Circumstances, Genetics and Biology, Medical Care, and Physical Environment.*

When you view the topics of determinants of health, as you can see from the following graphic from the GoInvo group, the segments include a section of the chart that includes the physical environment:[209]

While only 7 percent of the chart shows a direct connection relative to the physical environment, both of the segments "social circumstances" and "individual behavior," 24 and 36 percent, respectively, include the environment as a part of these impacts on health. Topics such as "sleep patterns," "negative moods and effects," "work conditions," and "occupation" can all be included in the category of building health in the evaluations.

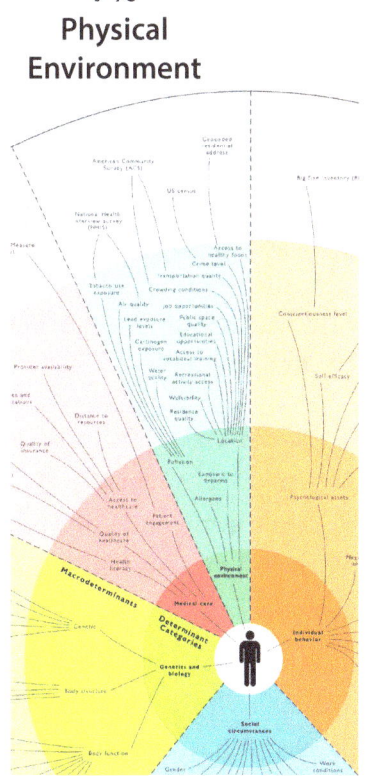

Stress levels are also a major factor in the whole scheme of life. And stress can be included in more than just one segment. There are also different ways in which stress affects health, such as physical stress and mental and emotional stress, all of these factors can be responsible for different negative impacts on human physiology.

As each of these topics can relate to stress, which is the number one factor in the leading cause of death,[210] there can easily be an overlap that can have tremendous impacts on patient health evaluations. As Davenhall discusses in his article, "unfortunately, today my medical record—and probably yours as well—is already a vast collection of clinical facts, observations, test results, and diagnostic conclusions but remains silent about the accumulation of environmental health impacts and risks."[211]

And why?

Why haven't these determinants of health been an inclusive aspect of the typical patient medical records?

My viewpoint, after many years of being involved in this questioning process, is based on the complexity of the medical and the architectural fields. Both professions require a substantial amount of training and the use of systems for their work to be accomplished.

As I learned early on in my direct experience in these processes, if you don't provide a system for these topics to be properly evaluated and included in the current workflows, then there is little that will develop to achieve proper evaluations and inclusion.

For me, this again is why systems, and the Architectural Medicine System (AMS), are so important and why I've spent so much time working to develop these methodologies.

The Future of Geomedicine and Social Determinants of Health (SDoH)

As the typical medical diagnosis must be achieved quickly to "identify a present disease, illness, problem, etc., by examination and observation (of signs and symptoms)," the prognosis refers to "predicting the course of the diagnosed disease, illness, problem, etc., and determining treatment and outcome."[212]

This is an important distinction, as the diagnosis is supposed to identify a disease, illness, or problem, yet what about the causes of this problem or problems? If treatments are striving to provide healing for solutions, yet the cause of the problem, such as exposure to a building issue isn't examined, isn't that going to be counterproductive for best health, healing, and wellness? Again, this is why the inspections of the Building Informaticist and the Healthy Building Inspector are so important for long term health and wellness, as well as quality of life.

Much like the capabilities of lab systems to make clinicians aware of "panic values," GIS can provide the same early warnings to suggest to clinicians that environmental factors need to be explored.

Geomedicine has the potential to transform the way physicians see patients and to provide a more holistic view of the many hidden factors that often defeat achieving successful long-term health outcomes. Referring again to Davenhall's comments:

> "The application of geomedicine, then, is about translating what we know about illness and disease, and what we understand about the role that our various environments play in making us sick (or well), into practical information that allows each of us—physician or consumer—to make better choices about where we live and how we engage with our environment."[213]

From this writing, the takeaway can be an awareness of how this data, provided by these new systems to provide testing results and informatics relative to the environment, can provide more insights into health and wellness based on social determinants of health.

As defined in this book, the use of the Architectural Medicine System, ARxMD, and the building inspections by the Healthy Building Inspector and the Building Informaticist can provide these solutions. The Architectural Doctor's role in this process is to support these systems while helping the professionals involved during these interconnected procedures. This is how testing can be performed and captured for use by doctors and health professionals in a meaningful format for patient health and wellness, along with public health benefits.

One comment in particular that stood out for me during the reading of Davenhall's writing was his comment on geomedicine and the research in the healthcare community. A key component of the long-term work of the Architectural Medicine System is the ability to record and develop clinical data repositories (CDR) and warehouses (CDW). This can allow for building informatics to be included in the healthcare professional knowledge base, yet also requires the utilization of this information to be properly implemented into the medical systems.

Davenhall's comment on this topic is prescient and relative to these long-term processes as he states, "a key element in the growing acceptance of geomedicine will be the exploitation of the body of research produced by the health science community. Also critical will be the ability to build and organize relevant medical content that links place to health conditions, risks, and outcomes."[214]

It is this type of thinking that is critical for the integrative processes between fields to utilize data and knowledge in formats that become built into these professions. And his statement about geomedicine and the importance of this research can be interwoven into the Architectural Medicine System and the goals of Architectural Medicine and the Architectural Doctor in the quotes below:

> "For example, research examining the impact of ambient air quality on cardiovascular and respiratory disease is under way in many nations of the world, and research is confirming that a patient's health is related to proximity to high-volume roadways, an idea being examined using GIS."
>
> "A key element of the acceptance of geomedicine by physicians will be the usefulness and accessibility of this body of research."[215]

There is a substantial body of scientific literature that "describes the impact of geographic location on health problems such as cancer, diabetes, hypertension, and osteoporosis, and the importance of place is becoming better understood. Integrating a patient's place history into existing electronic medical and personal health records is one of the principal roles of today's geographic 'expert' system."[216]

These comments echo the Architectural Medicine descriptions focused on the importance of the integrations between the fields of architecture and medicine and the benefits of these overlaps for public health. The clinical data repository developed by the building informaticist to include building informatics into the extensive medical research can provide another facet of health into the healthcare equation.

As the collection of family medical history helps clinicians look for certain predispositions to diseases, "geographic place will provide the context within which the clinician can assess environmental factors and make judgments about diagnosis, treatment, and prognosis."[217]

As I discussed the ARxMD software solution in chapters 6 and 12, which focuses on capturing, recording, and exchanging this data and information, the next chapter will focus on the use of the standards, protocols and processes that can achieve these results...

"Without standards, there can be no improvement."

— Taiichi Ohno

ARxMD STANDARDS, PROCESSES, & PROTOCOLS

When discussing the processes of these new systems, there are many protocols that will be added to each professional, as well as standards. Otherwise, without any baseline standards, there can be a limited connection to metrics that fall into any usable information to be utilized. Some of these standards already exist, such as codes for the medical and building fields, yet there are new standards that need to be reviewed and analyzed by a new assortment of professionals.

When the doctor requests blood tests, for example, there are certain standards that are defined to help the doctor understand these results. It requires the request for the nurse to provide a blood test procedure and standard, the examination process from the medical laboratory and the Laboratory Information System (LIS), as well the exchange of this data to the electronic health record. Each of these steps requires procedures, standards, and protocols to achieve these complex interactions.

If you review external health issues in the built environment, such as lead in buildings, or topics such as asbestos, there are standards already used by those such as occupational health professionals in the work environment defined by the organization OSHA. These standards can be utilized for the home environment as well as commercial buildings and, as such, provide metrics that are already in place.

What will be new is how a doctor and architect may be prepared to utilize this data, and as such, the emphasis on education and training in the medical and architecture fields, respectively, is essential.

Below are discussions on how each professional can utilize this data and navigate the standards for each profession's part in the solution process.

SNOMED, ICD, LOINC, DSM, IFC, BRICK, REC, and the ARxMD Standards

In this chapter, we will discuss many of the granular topics that are relative to the Architectural Doctor and the many processes of the Architectural Medicine System (AMS). In this book, I've discussed the procedures of each professional and their role in achieving this whole system solution. With the focus on health, healing, and wellness for the patient and populations, there need to be standards in place for each professional to work with to achieve these goals.

A critical part of this whole systems process is the requirement to ensure that data can be exchanged and shared. In the medical fields in the USA, meaningful use initiatives by the government have helped to develop and promote the use of EHRs to help with electronic records and data exchange.

In the architecture, engineering, and construction fields (AEC), the use of IFC, BIM, BACnet, and COBie standards have helped to provide electronic records for both the digitization of blueprints, as well as the ability to exchange this data between systems.

However, unless a design involves a structure such as a hospital, these two standards have very little overlap.

The Role of Ontologies in the Professional World

A word that is critical in every professional field is ontology. The reason being is that an ontology encompasses a "representation, formal naming, and definition of the categories, properties, and relations between the concepts, data, and entities that substantiate one, many, or all domains of discourse."[218] Put more simply, ontologies are utilized to "limit complexity and organize data into information and knowledge."[219]

This becomes critical when discussing the tremendous amount of data involved in both the building and health fields. In the field of health and medicine, ontologies have existed for quite some time and help to provide consistency in medical terminology.

However, in the field of architecture, the development of an ontology has been less developed. In the early 1990s, a group of building professionals created the IFC standard as a way to support the anticipated growth of digitization of drawings with CAD programs. While this IFC standard has been utilized to support the development of Building Information Modeling or BIM, the advent of a building ontology has only started to develop in the past decade. Considering the age-old profession of architecture, this is interesting.

Perhaps this has not occurred previously because of the privatization of data with companies that have developed Building Automation Systems (BAS) and the controlled processes of such automation. Most buildings have become automated with a focus on a single building, and the information of these buildings has not required any shared data or exchange of data between multiple facilities.

Ontologies can help support the standardization of data, and this is extremely important when there is a larger scale exchange of data. Not only the exchange of data within a building and the many systems and products that exist in a building, but the sharing of any data between buildings. This can include the ability for building management to view all building processes in a central location, yet also to view and exchange data between buildings.

When considering the increase in sensors used in buildings that can measure many different facets of a building's processes, this increase in the scale of devices can become problematic if all devices have various languages and data structures.

If this is the case, then the ability to view the data of different structures for reference causes an unmanageable level of data sets that would be almost impossible to manage or view in a centralized format.

And now, when you add the Internet of Things (IOT) as devices that monitor and measure a much larger number of metrics, from temperature and humidity to carbon dioxide, particulates, and VOCs, you can see that the number of devices can increase by ten fold or larger.

As a building manager, the ability to monitor and review these metrics will quickly become unmanageable, and these devices are only increasing over time. This may be a scale that can be handled in small buildings, yet when you consider the immense urban skyscraper and hundreds of units in these high-rise structures, the number of devices can be enormous.

However, the amount of data that can be provided for building evaluations can actually be quite powerful for multiple purposes, including the ability of the building management and occupants to benefit from this information.

Over the past decade, two ontologies have emerged that are now being utilized in the real world: the Brick Schema ontology and the Real Estate Core ontology. And as many standards continue to develop worldwide, there is also a benefit to having a single standard utilized by all groups worldwide.

Fortunately, in August of 2022, these two groups announced they would be working together and merging these ontologies into a single standard. This is great news for the building world and will provide an essential foundation for the architecture profession in the future.

This process is already providing support for metadata organization, such as the Digital Twins Definition Language (DTDL) created by Microsoft, based on the Real Estate Core ontology.

The reason why all of this is important is interoperability and the exchange of data. If this data is to be utilized by building management groups and providing information for building occupants, there needs to be a capability for data exchange.

If you've been following the advancements in the health profession, this sounds very familiar, as the ability to access and exchange data in the United States is not only critical, it is becoming law. This capability for data exchange requires standards that provide software developers and end users the ability to exchange and utilize data sets across many disparate systems.

As these standards develop in the medical fields, this is now occurring in the building sector as well, providing access to data sets across many heterogeneous building components.

While the architecture field has had the BACnet standard and COBie, these standards have some challenges with granular data, which the Brick and Real Estate Core ontologies can resolve. The COBie standard, initially developed by Bill East of the US Army Corps of Engineers, the "Construction Operations Building Information Exchange (COBie) is an international standard relating to managed asset information including space and equipment."[220] And BACnet is a "communication protocol for building automation and control (BAC) networks that use the ASHRAE, ANSI, and ISO 16484-5 standards protocol."[221]

The benefits of a standard such as BACnet is the focus on a system that can allow the communication of building systems for applications such as "heating, ventilating, and air-conditioning control (HVAC), lighting control, access control, and fire detection systems and their associated equipment."[222]

However, these standards could provide an overlap between the architecture and medical fields, especially when connected to SNOMED and LOINC codes, but have had some challenges with defining the many facets of newer building definitions. And this is where the Brick and REC ontology provide this granular building metadata for these solutions.

How?

Well, if you read about BACnet and COBie standards, you will note they are focused on building processes, including Facility Management (FM), to ensure proper building maintenance. Therefore, if you add to this equation health factors and the quality of built environment topics, the result can be more robust data provided by the granular metadata provided by numerous building sensors.

An example of standards used in the medical field is the use of SNOMED (Systematized Nomenclature of Medicine) to define clinical terms, ICD (International Classification of Diseases) for diseases, and LOINC (Logical Observation Identifiers, Names and Codes) for lab results. Each of these three standards will allow those in the medical field to understand clinical terms, diseases, and lab results in a way that is not ambiguous and provides clear communication between several different health professionals.

The Continuity of Care Record (CCR), a standard often used in the USA, provides a process for healthcare professionals to maintain a patient's Electronic Health Record (EHR) over time. The Clinical Document Architecture (CDA), an interchange standard for clinical documents, and the Continuity of Care Document (CCD) provide the CCR data set as a CDA document that is typically using XML encoding. Advances in the electronic exchange of data using HL7 FHIR as a RESTful API can provide a common language of data exchange between the medical and building fields using these new building ontologies.

By utilizing the common standards of computer and network encoding, along with standards used in the medical and building fields, it can provide a transfer of information that is both known and accepted between healthcare and building professionals

The medical industry uses the LOINC standards for testing and laboratory results, and while there are some standards that can be listed in the home and building categories, this is where the ARxMD standards can fill the gaps.

By adding building health standards using ARxMD processes and protocols, the health in buildings procedures can be included in the already familiar systems of the medical and architecture fields. By utilizing the Health Level 7 (HL7) FHIR processes that allow for the transfer of data between systems, this can also be used as a vehicle to transfer data between these health and building professionals.

The Accredited Standards Committee X12 (ASC X12) is a standards organization overseen by the American National Standards Institute (ANSI) and "develops and maintains the X12 Electronic data interchange (EDI)" upon which the original HL7 standards were based.

This Electronic Data Interchange (EDI) is a standard used worldwide by many different systems in numerous businesses to enable the digital exchange of information.[223] As software exchange advances to RESTful APIs and JSON as the format, beyond XML and EDI, these new communication protocols will also need to have a solid foundation of agreed upon standards.

For these different professions to communicate with each in a proper and clear format, there is a need for larger groups of organizations to collaborate on the topics being discussed. And this requires the discussion of new standards of subjects and metrics for each group to agree on.

This interoperability requires the creation, confirmation, and implementation of standards to provide data between these different professionals, ensuring that it retains the meaning and context throughout the processes of the Architectural Medicine System (AMS).

As mentioned, there are a few standards in the SNOMED, ICD, and LOINC standards, primarily focused on social determinants of health (SDoH). These classifications can be utilized when providing an inspection of a certain building location, such as an apartment or a home residence.

In the SNOMED CT database, there are topics related to the environment or geography, which can also be connected to the topics of Social Determinants of Health and Geomedicine.[224]

For instance, the hierarchy of listings for including these two locations in SNOMED CT the listings are providing in the following navigation hierarchy:

> In the "Environment or geographical location," you can select the "Environment" segment, and then "Community Environment," and under the "Residential environment," you can then select "Home > Apartment > Apartment in apartment building" or "Home > Residential Home > Private residential home" as specific categories.

There are many options in segments that can be applied to the health of the built environment to be utilized by the Healthy Building Inspector for classifications during inspections. An example of this is the listing of a "Toxic environment," which is found in SNOMED-CT in the segment of the Environment, under the "Physical Environment" listing and selecting "Toxic Environment." The ID of this segment is:

http://purl.bioontology.org/ontology/SNOMEDCT/285121003

Using this SNOMED CT framework, evaluations can be requested by the doctor and recorded by the Healthy Building Inspector, utilizing the same nomenclature and systems to ensure that the EHR information is updated with the correct specifications.

The next question may be, what defines a "Toxic Environment," and what are the tests and standards utilized to define these "toxic environments?" This is where the ARxMD and Architectural Medicine System protocols, procedures, and standards can be utilized.

By defining specific toxins, subsequent standards can be used as guidelines to record into the EHR systems during evaluations. What can be added to this are the LOINC codes and additional ARxMD codes for standards that do not yet exist in these platforms related to health in the built environment.

Why Are Standards Important?

In both the medical and building professions, there are many standards that each professional has to navigate and understand. The medical field has the SNOMED, ICD, DSM, and LOINC as a listing of common standards, and the architecture fields have ISO, ASTM, IEEE, and IFC as common standards to ensure compliance between products and processes.

> "Information communication is a key component in any system."

And as different organizations create standards, a question that you might be asking is why are these standards important?

Standards provide a way for common practices to be agreed upon. As more systems become integrated across professions, the ability for clear communication is not only helpful but also vital for computers. An absence of the correct syntax will not only prevent clear data exchange; when computers cannot match this exchange of data, they will simply not function. It is imperative to provide these standards for the various professionals working together and for data exchange to be successful. During this book, I've discussed an example of an organization that provides standards: Health Level Seven International (HL7). Founded in 1987, HL7 is "a not-for-profit, ANSI-accredited standards developing organization dedicated to providing a comprehensive framework and related standards for the exchange, integration, sharing, and retrieval of electronic health information that supports clinical practice and the management, delivery and evaluation of health services."[225] In one of the courses I've taken for HL7 integration processes, they provided the following overview of the question of standards:

> "The need for interoperating systems is evident in each part of the healthcare organization. Interoperable systems should share information continuously and automatically through the participating institutions and display the information in a useful way." – HL7 International Training[226]

This is where the term "meaningful use" came into the terminology of the US government to promote and support the electronic healthcare records standards and the use of HL7 to communicate and exchange data between platforms. As this statement is focused on just the medical professions, what will happen when more built environment groups become a part of these solutions?

The Institute of Electrical and Electronics Engineers (IEEE) defines interoperability as "the ability of two or more systems or components to exchange information and to use the information that has been exchanged."[227]

With health topics in the built environment, and as the Architectural Medicine System is implemented between the medical and architecture professionals, the requirements for standards become even more critical. The creation of standards that can communicate with other systems and platforms is also critical. To ensure these information exchange standards are compatible, interoperability standards such as HL7 help bridge these gaps. While these exist in the medical professions, they can be a valuable bridge to connect other fields, such as architecture, engineering, and construction (AEC), in unison.

And as more and more professions and professionals become involved in these whole systems solutions, there is even greater importance for standards to be established for exchanging information and sharing data between these numerous fields.

To highlight the importance of these standards, below is a list of specific data and code formats used as a reference for SNOMED and LOINC. These formats can utilize a code structure common in LOINC using the following example:

Logical Observation Identifiers, Names and Codes (LOINC)

LOINC is a classification for clinical observations. It is primarily used for lab results but can also be applicable to aspects of a physical examination or any other clinical observation. For each observation, the following is specified:

- **Properties** - type of measure, e.g., concentration, numeric fraction, etc.
- **Time** - point in time
- **Sample** - e.g., blood, cerebrospinal fluid
- **Method** - e.g., qualitative, quantitative, and it sometimes include whether it is automatic or manual,
- etc.

For example, the following can be the way that this system uses the ARxMD data recordings using the LOINC format and implemented in the ARxMD software:

Observation for Indoor Air Quality (IAQ) testing:

- **Properties** - type of measure, e.g., concentration, numeric fraction, etc.
    - o **Indoor Air Quality (IAQ) test for sample type "x"**
        - ▪ **Test Code:ARxMD:**
    - o **Measurement using: Machine type "x"**
    - o **Measurement specifications:**
    - o **Measurement Taken(geographical location):**
    - o **Measurement Location(location of device in structure)**
- **Time** – 24 hour recording
    - o 2021-11-01 10:00
    - o To
    - o 2021-11-02 10:00
- **Sample** – Air quality sample:
    - o **Canister used: canister type "x"/**
        - ▪ **Results=**
- **Method** – IAQ type machine "x" with the following results:

- o   qualitative
- o   quantitative
- o   automatic or manual

The above listing can be used as an example of using the LOINC code format for an Indoor Air Quality test for particulates, mold, bacteria, viruses, or other biological factors. It can provide the testing process details, as well as the results.

All of this can be entered into the ARxMD software during the testing process, along with the laboratory results, which can then be entered into the ARxMD software to exchange to healthcare platforms using HL7. The final information can be sent to the Doctor, Architectural Doctor, and others for follow up analysis and evaluations using the HL7 FHIR processes.

As defined by the HL7 organization in the "HL7 Fundamentals Course," there are common interoperability requirements for systems to function. Below is a checklist of steps essential for system interoperability:[228]

- Determine the interoperability requirements (goals, scope, environment)
- Define the applicable standard(s) and artifacts (messages, RPC, document exchange)
- Define the vocabulary and master files or registries
- Specify the communications environment
- Determine how to go from your system to the artifacts and from the artifacts to your system
- Build and document the interface

During the process of the doctor requesting a building inspection, the interoperability list is critical if there is to be communication between these groups. And in order for these steps to be achieved, there need to be standards between professions to enable these integrations.

In the medical field, there are standards that define request exchanges, which occur based on trigger events. These happen after the clinician enters a lab order as the HL7 processes send the order to the appropriate system. With updated standards using HL7 FHIR, the clinician can then enter an inspection order to include testing in the built environment. This can include lab orders for air quality testing and inspections for particulates, mold, viruses, or testing of materials. Other testing, such as water quality, overall building conditions, and many others, such as natural lighting and noise, can be performed based on the patient's ailments. These become part of the ARxMD standards as "lab orders" for built environment standards.

Standards and Protocols for the Medical Fields Related to Building Health

The first group I will discuss are the standards for the doctors and medical fields, as this is the first group on the main Architectural Medicine System flowchart. This system does not require that the doctor is always the first step in this process, yet often the case will be that the doctor will initiate this process.

The current medical processes in many parts of the world using electronic health records use the CPOE, or computerized provider order entry. "Computerized provider order entry (CPOE) refers to the process of providers entering and sending treatment instructions – including medication, laboratory, and radiology orders – via a computer application rather than paper, fax, or telephone."[229]

This process can now include the doctor's request for built environment inspections to provide building analysis relative to the patient's health so that the doctor can utilize this extended information for proper evaluation during their SOAP processes. As discussed previously, the Subjective, Objective, Assessment, and Plan (SOAP) note is "an acronym representing a widely used method of documentation for healthcare providers. The SOAP note is a way for healthcare workers to document in a structured and organized way."[230] This process of inspections in the built environment can be included in the "Computerized Physician Order Entry (CPOE) for Medication, Laboratory and Radiology Orders"[231] and can become a part of the evaluation process for the physician.

With this in mind, the inclusion of built environment standards focused on health must be defined in formats that can be easily exchanged with electronic data with building software and systems.

> "Information interchange is known as functional interoperability, whereas the capacity to understand and use shared information is called semantic interoperability."[232]

As SNOMED CT is structured on a concept-based terminology, the "due to" attribute ("diabetic foot" - "due to" - "diabetes") can be applied to topics impacting health related to the built environment in a similar format. When there are health issues, such as respiratory ailments, the inclusion of the built environment based on this ailment can be configured in the SNOMED CT format as such:

> "Bronchitis"–"due to"–"Environmental > Physical Environment > Polluted Environment or Dirty Environment or even Toxic Environment."

The particulars of these environmental details can be better defined using LOINC codes or ARxMD codes as standards in evaluations. In this way, the built environment can be included in the doctor's assessment and add the built environment as part of their requests for observations or testing. It may also be that a doctor wants to see if the built environment is causing issues related to their patient's health, so they can provide a better treatment plan for both short and long-term health.

Some of these issues are related to determinants of health, yet without proper testing, these building health issues can not be factored into the health equation. And this is where the Healthy Building Inspector, the Building Informaticist, and the Architectural Doctor enter into the picture.

International Integration for Healthy Building Standards

A great opportunity for these standards to be developed and accepted are groups such as the ASTM Committee E31. This group supports Healthcare Informatics and "develops standards related to the architecture, content, storage, security, confidentiality, functionality, and communication of information used within healthcare and healthcare decision making, including patient-specific information and knowledge."[233] ASTM International is a "globally recognized leader in the development and delivery of voluntary consensus standards…used around the world to improve product quality, enhance health and safety, strengthen market access and trade, and build consumer confidence." Formed in 1898, and founded by Charles B. Dudley, Ph.D., the American Society for Testing and Materials (ASTM) changed its name in 2001 to ASTM International.[234]

These standards organizations are pivotal to providing any changes in systems, and when dealing with many different professions, especially when they are not as familiar with collaborating, this is of particular importance. Another organization supporting the wide ranging healthcare issues is the Cochrane Library. Their mission to "provide accessible, credible information to support informed decision-making has never been more important or useful for improving global health."[235] As defined in their mission statement, "Cochrane is for anyone interested in using high-quality information to make health decisions. Whether you are a clinician, patient or carer, researcher, or policy-maker, Cochrane evidence provides a powerful tool to enhance your healthcare knowledge and decision-making."[236]

The benefit of these organizations, whether they are focused on standards or improvements to procedures, are the worldwide contributions from many people interested in global solutions.

Standards, Protocols, and Procedures for the Healthy Building Inspector and Building Informaticist

The second group that requires protocols and standards are the building inspectors, that will be providing these observations and recording these evaluations. Perhaps these individuals will be from the typical building inspection field. Yet as mentioned previously, the measurements and testing for human health are rarely on the list for common building inspections, except for topics related to some air quality and certain substances such as lead and asbestos.

Therefore, the Healthy Building Inspector and Building Informaticist will need to include new testing processes, protocols, and standards to learn and follow. These new inspection processes will also require new communications that include standards to ensure proper functions between health professionals, which is a new facet of interaction for these professionals. These new inspections will have processes that may include medical laboratories, which will also be new for these building inspectors and laboratory professionals. And again, new standards are required for interoperability.

Let's take a look at some new inspection standards focused on human health and wellness in the built environment that will be required:

- Indoor Air Quality
- Interior Particulates and Gases
    - Unhealthy particulates
    - Carbon Dioxide
    - Carbon monoxide
    - Natural gas leaks
    - NO (i.e. – cooking areas)
- Exterior Particulates and Gases
    - Industrial area pollution
    - Factories and manufacturing pollution
- HVAC Systems Based on Human Health Measurements
- Materials and Potential Toxic Substances
- Insecticides and Pesticide Residue
    - Airborne in HVAC systems

- o   Particulates
- Unhealthy Temperature and Humidity levels
    - o   Mold issues
- Noise and Sound Quality Issues
    - o   Exterior noise
    - o   Interior noises-building and population issues
- Smells and Aromatic Issues

Each of these topics requires a process and standards that are either measured on site, or captured for laboratory testing. The addition of worldwide standards for these advanced tests in the built environment will improve evaluations for public health and wellness.

Environmental Psychology Evaluations

Another factor in evaluating health and wellness in the built environment is the environmental psychology facets, which are often ignored and can be more challenging to provide metrics and standards.

The field of environmental psychology has several evaluation processes that can be included in these inspections, yet if the inspector or informaticist is neither trained nor familiar with these evaluations, this will be challenging to have in the inspection process.

What would be helpful in these inspections would be the addition of an environmental psychologist to evaluate these built environments for a more detailed evaluation of patient health. The doctor can flag this additional inspection process in the initial SOAP evaluation, mainly if the issues include neural or psychological problems that might show potential issues on this level.

Therefore, the inclusion of these processes should come from psychological professionals and utilize the DSM-5 specifications related to built environment issues.

This focus is new to most building professionals, and even this evaluation approach may be new to those in psychology fields. However, when you consider that the average person spends 60 to 90 percent of their time inside buildings, not including this in the evaluation process seems to be a significant missing piece of the health evaluation puzzle. Some of these measurements may be challenging to provide in terms of metrics and data. Including psychological professionals in this process can help determine metrics useful for patient health.

What this looks like in the future may change, yet several statistics can be included right now that have measurability for useful purposes. These are discussed in chapter 16 in the segment on the Neuroscience of Architecture.

Standards, Protocols, and Procedures for the Architectural Doctor

As you may now see with more clarity, these processes require complex systems with complex integrations and many professionals working together. The Architectural Doctor can provide support for the process and integrative support between these professions to achieve these goals.

Sometimes the Architectural Doctor will also be required to spend time with the patient as the general public, as many of these processes will require overlap and advanced communications. Since many of these processes will require going to the patient's home or built environment, this can also be challenging for the patient to navigate. Many people are not very familiar with how buildings function, and adding evaluations to the place they call home can be stressful.

The Architectural Doctor can be this liaison to help the patient, yet also help to support the integrations between professionals. The medical doctor, for instance, may understand the facet of the patient's health issue yet may not be well versed in the inspections and architectural solutions. Therefore, to help the medical doctor in the process, as the Architectural Doctor is well versed in the architecture and medical fields, clarity can be provided when issues need to be addressed. This can also be the same for the building professionals and the inspectors, who might be comfortable with the construction portions of the equation, but are not versed on the health implications.

Due to the Architectural Doctor being versed in both fields, they can help bridge the gaps and provide proper communications where required. And as they are familiar with each profession, they can help advise on the standards needed to achieve these procedures. They can help facilitate the process, with each group providing their feedback and the view of the patient appropriate in this system of solutions.

Each profession has its specific terminology, which can be intimidating and confusing for the layperson. Yet, the individual professional will not always have the time to discuss each component. Having someone as a rosetta stone who can translate each professional vernacular can provide better communication for each group involved. The Architectural Doctor can provide these connections for better communication and support.

The Architectural Doctor does not have to be a doctor or an architect. Because they are trained in each profession, they understand each professional's main procedures and functions. This way, they know enough about architecture and health, as well as the professional processes, to give them insights into each part of the big picture equation.

And this complex equation requires a method to join all of the pieces into a cohesive whole. This brings us to the next chapter, Bringing it all together...

"Knowing is not enough; we must apply.
Willing is not enough; we must do."

— Johann Wolfgang von Goethe

BRINGING IT ALL TOGETHER

Now that I have outlined the many puzzle pieces and defined the Architectural Medicine System flowchart, in this chapter, we'll talk about how all of this system can function for cohesive solutions. Achieving these integrative solutions will require many facets in the medical and built environment fields to collaborate in new ways.

This will require new approaches, such as the Architectural Medicine System, and new mindsets for cohesive partnerships. By utilizing new standards discussed in the previous chapter, groups that have never worked together can provide new procedures and define protocols for best practices.

Integrating the Fields of Architecture and Medicine – How Do All of These Topics Fit Together?

In chapter 4 on Integrative Architecture, I discussed the two triads of the building puzzle. This first triad includes green, sustainable, and healthy building, which are listed in the following diagram as Energy, Ecology, and Health, respectively. The second triad includes the Physical, Emotional, and Mental or Psychological facets of Wellness.

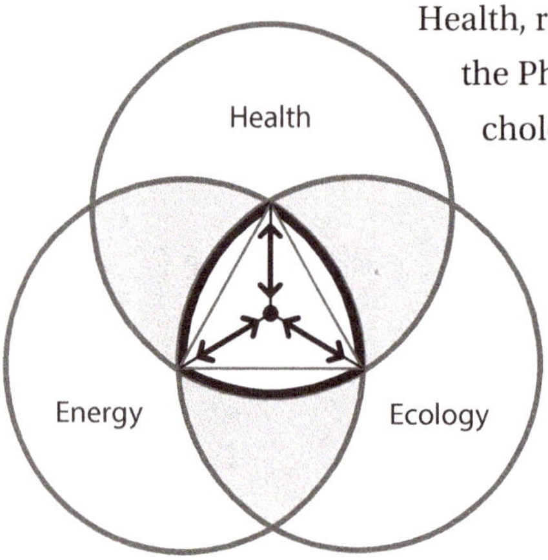

When placed together, this double triad of "Energy, Ecology, and Health" and "Mental, Physical, and Emotional Wellness" are interconnected to support the vitality of human thriving.

This is what can define a strong foundation of a building – rooted in recognition of having Ecological respect for the planet's natural ecological systems, the optimal creation and use of Energy for efficiency, and the focus on ensuring the Health of all occupants as well as planetary health.

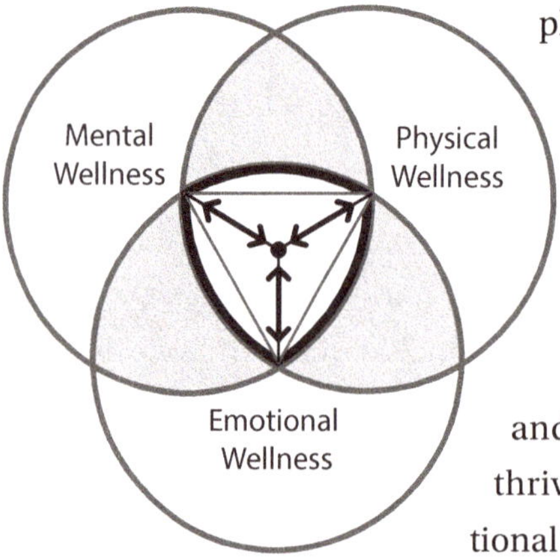

These roots of supporting life can then create a strong base to allow and support the foundation of human thriving for mental, physical, and emotional wellness and well-being.

Chapter: 15 — Bringing It All Together

The Double Triad of Architectural Medicine – Health and Wellness in the Built Environment

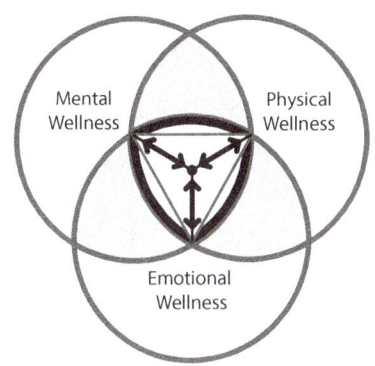

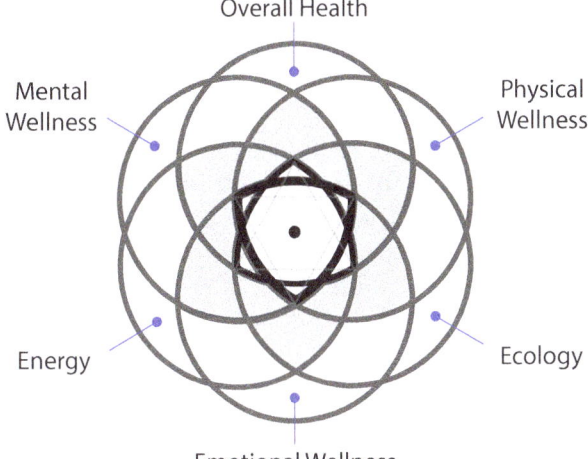

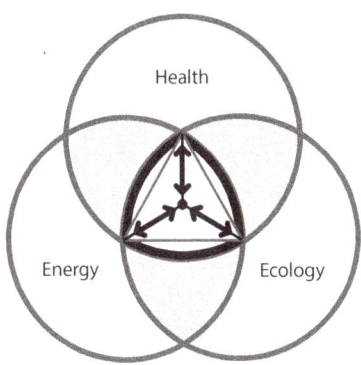

The Intersection of Energy, Ecology, and Health in the Built Environment

Health/**Healthy Building**

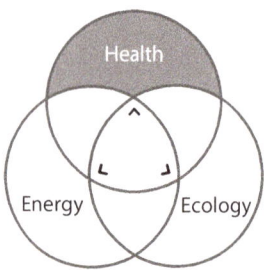

Issues related to physical health, removing toxic materials and improving occupant health.

Groups and organizations with a Health focus in the built environment include:
Healthy Building Network, Bau Biologie and Biophilia

Energy (Efficiency)/**Green Building**

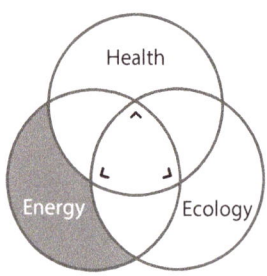

Issues related to optimizing Energy use, sourcing more sustainable energy options, striving to reduce pollution, and working to reduce carbon footprint.

Groups and organizations related to this Energy focus include: Architecture 2030 and the US Green Building Council (USGBC)

Ecology/**Sustainable Building**

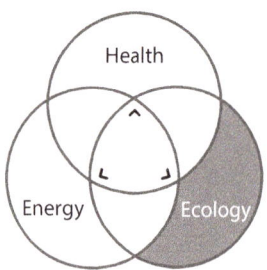

Recognizing and designing for the Ecology, creating more sustainable solutions with materials and methods. Considering Life Cycle Assessment (LCA) in all designs.

Groups and organizations with an Ecological focus in the built environment include:
Biophilic Design and
the Permaculture Institute

Chapter: 15 Bringing It All Together

An Overview of Mental, Physical, and Emotional Wellness in the Built Environment

Physical Wellness

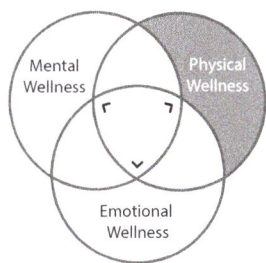

Are you surrounded by stagnant, polluted air? Are there chemicals and chemical smells in your space all day? Are getting enough sunlight? Is your body being cared for and allowing for topics such as ergonomic functionality? Are you around constant stress? What is this impact on your physical wellness and your immune system?

Mental Wellness

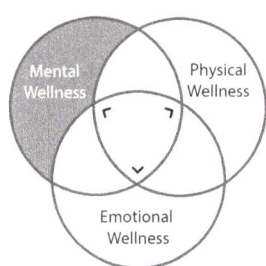

Do you have the ability to think clearly? Is the space you're in comforting for your mind or chaotic in sights, sounds, and thinking as well as sensory stress? How does this affect your mindset? What impact does this have on your ability to concentrate, on your mental wellness, and on your immune system?

Emotional Wellness

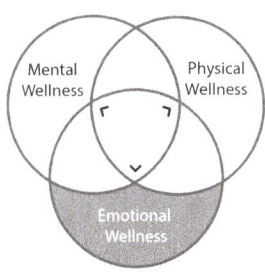

Are you surrounded by loud noises and a chaotic emotional environment? How does this affect your nervous system? Are the sights, sounds, smells, and sensory inputs impacting your emotional wellness? What impact does this have on your stress levels, your emotional wellness, and on your immune system?

The Double Triad of Architectural Medicine: Health and Wellness in the Built Environment

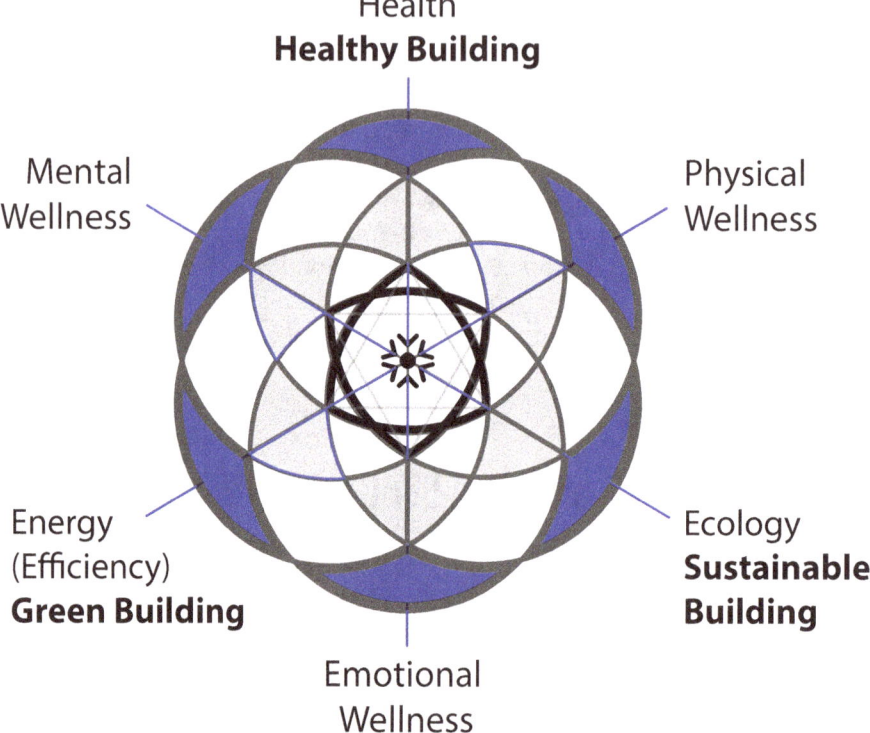

This group of graphics shows the progression of these six topics, connected as triads, and then each triad placed together to form an integrative, cohesive whole. To be clear, there are many overlaps between these six topics, yet it's also important to recognize that currently, healthy building is mostly focused on physical health, while physical, emotional, and mental wellness includes the health and well-being of the entire human experience.

These overlaps are not only closely defined, but they can also be missing in many approaches in the building and medical professions and can cause gaps in supporting optimal human health. This book has delved into each of these depths that are required by professionals for proper evaluation in the built environment. Yet to not include all of these topics when supporting patient and population health is, in my opinion, a miscalculation.

In my book Architectural Medicine, I provide more in depth explanations of these topics independently. Yet, a key focus of Architectural Medicine and the Architectural Doctor is to ensure that all of these topics are considered together. By factoring all of these together, it ensures that each of these six subjects are integrated into the future of architecture and the built environment. In this manner, the many facets of the puzzle pieces for optimal living can be calculated into these big picture equations.

By putting all of these pieces together in the jigsaw puzzle of the built environment, *architecture* can become *medicine* for preventive health and provide nurturing environments for human health and wellness.

These models of integrated designs can provide a pathway toward wellness, similar to an Rx for health and a blueprint for health and wellness.

The Architectural Medicine System, ARxMD, and the Architectural Doctor – providing an *Rx for health and wellness in the built environment.*

The Overlap of Digital Twins in Architecture and Medicine

As mentioned earlier in this book, new advances in building data modeling ontologies have spurred the developments of the Digital Twin in the building fields. Being able to use these building ontologies, the physical objects of the building can be denoted and described as data and included in 3D spaces. This can include data of not only objects but of processes and sensors. And while building automation systems have existed through BACnet for decades, the ability for these systems to be described and communicate data in real-time, or almost real-time, using modern day APIs has not been easily accessible.

Microsoft's Digital Twin offerings on the Azure platform as a PAAS are an example of these advances having real world impacts to monitor and provide building statistics. Their Digital Twins Definition Language (DTDL), based on the Real Estate Core (REC) and the recent merging of the Brick Schema, can provide a physical representation of a building as a virtual copy with a timeline of building functions.

And with the developments of Digital Twins in the medical realm, it can allow doctors and health professionals to monitor, evaluate — and as future developments allow — provide the ability for testing as simulations to be done on the digital twin body. This can provide analysis of various pharmacological responses for evaluations before they are given to the patient. As the DNA of the person is embedded into the medical digital twin, the DNA of the building can be provided for the building digital twin, and any alterations, changes, and timelines of issues can be monitored and recorded for an understanding of future performance.

In earlier chapters, I reference the DNA of Buildings and Cities as being critical for understanding the future developments of architecture. Yet, in this manner, it can also provide insights into the future performance of buildings and cities.

When the big data of a building through a digital twin can be overlayed with the medical digital twin of a patient, the amount of data that can be updated for patient health can be enormous and, subsequently, exponentially helpful to provide insights for health professionals for their patients.

These digital twins, as an overlap between the architecture and medical fields, can provide an emerging field of medical informatics and building analytics that has never existed.

And the benefit of using the ARxMD software setup is that each portal is customized for each professional and can provide these integrations and data informatics. In this manner, the architect and building professionals have customized fields for their work, while the doctor, inspector, and informaticist have fields and layouts appropriate for their work. There are standardized fields that each professional can view, yet only the specific data for their use is exchanged between the various platforms.

Nodal Systems - A New Metaphor for Integrative, Cohesive Solutions

When all of the facets are considered and included in design solutions, it can be akin to how a tree functions as a whole, where the root systems, the trunk, and the branches all function together. A tree has an integrated support system, where the roots support the trunk and branches with stability and nutrients. In contrast, the branches convert sunlight into energy through photosynthesis and distribute this back to the roots and the rest of the tree for health. The trunk provides a functional transportation system to bring the nutrients from the roots to the branches and the energy of photosynthesis to the roots, as well as the stability of the tree for structural integrity.

This model of symbiosis, where the interdependency of the many facets can support the whole of the organism, can be a model for integration — whether this is an individual human or the entire planet's ecological health.

The roots of a tree can support the branches for vitality, health, and optimal performance, which is then returned to the root systems from energy produced through photosynthesis for ongoing nutrition for the entire tree's health.

With professions becoming more specialized and depth of research becoming deeper in each subject, this can cause a silo process that causes separation from information and knowledge. As such, the term silo is used to represent this metaphor of a professional that is segregated from other professions and professionals. The silo analogy, if you are not familiar with this term, is taken from the farm silos that provide storage for grains and other crops. This is important in the world of agriculture to ensure that these crops are kept from spoiling until the time is ready for them to be distributed. However, this analogy in the professional sense is not a positive, and too often, these silos prevent collaboration. This can also lead to a lack of valuable knowledge from being distributed to society.

In contrast, the analogy of the tree as a metaphor for a nodal configuration provides a metaphor for collaboration, and that of professionals working together for mutual

Farm Silo denoting the metaphor of the professional silo, with limited interconnectivity and lack of the exchange of information.

benefit. By converting the farm silo of deep research into the tree root system, where this depth of knowledge is an analogy of a deeper dive into subject matters, the knowledge does not have to remain in the depths of academia and research. Instead, the

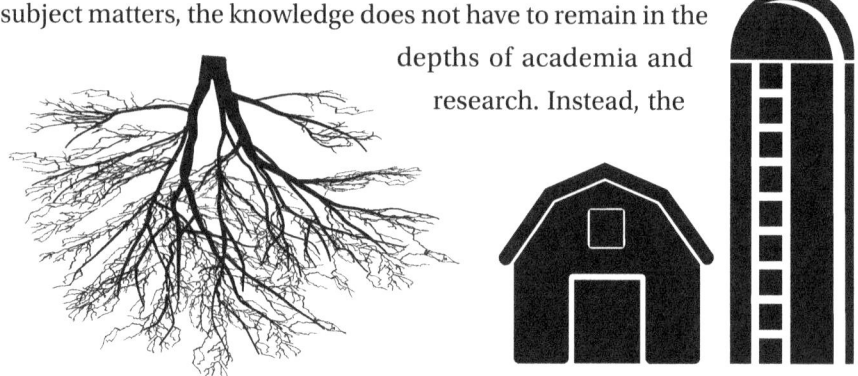

The old metaphor of a farm Silo in contrast to the new Nodal systems of plants and trees. The key to this new metaphor is the option to share the deep data of the roots with the rest of the tree and branches for the beneficial interconnectivity and exchange of information.

roots are connected to the trunk, which provides the transportation of these nutrients to a tree. As an analogy, the trunk can be seen as professionals that can disseminate this information and provide integrations amongst other professionals, such as that of the Architectural Doctor and other integrators in the professional world. These various professionals can be viewed as the branches of the tree, as those who utilize this information as knowledge in practical formats. In this manner, the information becomes knowledge that is applied to benefit society.

This complex dynamic of different professionals working together to support a cohesive goal is also comparable to the high-level athlete who can perform at their optimal by having the support of their mental, physical, and emotional health. It takes multiple professionals to support this athlete and requires a large knowledge base supported by deep research and distributed by coaches and consultants for optimal performance.

Chapter: 15 — Bringing It All Together

A common format in creating the potential of these goals is to have several diagnostic features customized for each athlete. A customized training plan is required to reach the athlete's end goal of blossoming and reaching their potential to flourish. This requires a strong foundation and roots of support, a solid base as a trunk to achieve this health and well-being, and a support team can branch out to utilize numerous topics in synergy to help them achieve their goal.

These graphics of a silo, roots, branches, and a trunk can emulate this analogy, providing a visual as a new metaphor for collaboration. These new systems require not just new approaches, yet new mindsets in collaboration between new professions. Another takeaway from these diagrams is the similarity of these roots and branches to that of the nerves and nervous system.

If you expand on this metaphor and recognize the strength of the roots and branches expanding outward, yet then returning to a connector for proper communication, you can easily see the similarities of this image as nerves and neurons. And as this is the format in which bodies communicate and even process data — in the image of the neurons of our brain — this metaphor can be supported by how nature itself functions.

While this may not be a common analogy in the world of architecture and medicine, such support can be provided through the architecture, building, and healthcare fields. And a game plan to achieve this goal can be provided in the format of a similar blueprint, simply applied in a different manner with all professionals working together. Instead of the goal being an athlete attaining their goals, the end goal for the built environment is for the inhabitants to flourish in their lives as individual patient and as public health.

Creating a strong support system in the format of the built environment allows for the spaces in which people work, play, and live to provide the foundation of support to achieve these goals – whether a trained athlete or someone striving to reach their potential in any modality. This focus on social determinants of health (SDoH), a recognition of location benefits through geomedicine, and an integrated platform of professions working in collaboration for public health can be attained in a similar manner.

Just as the athlete has support in the form of coaches, diagnostics, and personalized information to provide the best methods for them to succeed, this can be designed into one's life through the architecture they spend time within.

And like the solid roots that provide strength and vitality for a tree, this can provide a foundation of support in a healthy manner in the same way a building's foundation provides support for the entire structure. Like the branches that provide energy through photosynthesis to support these roots and the entire tree, the building's design and functionality can ensure that the foundation is kept solid and strong. And all of these systems in place can then support the structure's inhabitants to ensure that they are supported, protected, and nurtured for good health.

As such, it's not just the materials and the methodologies of the structure that can support optimal health. It's how the space affects, impacts, and influences your life — mentally, physically, emotionally, and spiritually.

Architecture and the built environment have a considerable impact and influence on one's everyday life, so much so that it may be unrecognized and even ignored. For many, it has become so commonplace to go to a place for work, and to become so accustomed to their own built environment of their home, that these concepts may be overlooked.

This does not infer that these aspects of life need to be constantly analyzed, yet if one is seeking improvement, good health, and striving to achieve positive health goals, these are factors that one's life is built upon. Ignoring such matters would be akin to a contractor building on a foundation that has not been appropriately analyzed for structural integrity. And to simply build without considering how this foundation will support and hold the rest of the building is a recipe for disaster.

Nodal Systems – From The Old Silo Analogy To Cohesive Roots, Trunk, Branches and Neurons of Data Exchange

These new nodal systems of functioning between professions, and utilizing the deep research of data scientists, researchers, and academic knowledge can be applied in formats that promote wisdom. The removal of the silo, replacing this instead with the benefits of a root system, provides deeper gains of knowledge and can then be utilized by many working professionals in practical formats. This also mimics the branching nature of neurons and the synaptic nature of the data exchanges of our brain. Nature itself functions in this manner and benefits from an interconnected system of processes and actions.

From the old metaphor of a farm Silo to the new nodal systems of plants and trees. This new integrative metaphor can also be viewed as nerves and the nervous system. The roots and branches can be reversed to overlap, and the trunk can be seen as the transmitter. Our brains function with a similar data exchange process. This new format can be described by utilizing the representations of a tree and neurons as a way to envision these interconnected processes.

We as humans have much to learn from the natural world and from each other, and as new professionals function in these nodal formats, the benefits in the future are synergistic methods of interoperability.

In the process of achieving a goal in which one is striving to succeed, you would not ignore these essential foundations in achieving high-performance goals.

And so, why would these fundamentals of the built environment be ignored in one's everyday life?

To not examine this foundation would be to build on the grounds that could not support the building. It would therefore create a circumstance where, later on, as the building is developed and more floors are added, the scaling up would not be supported, and all could come crashing down.

Our human health and wellness require a strong foundation to be built upon to grow and stay healthy.

At this point, there is enough content discussed in this book for you to digest how complex these topics can become and the myriad steps required to achieve these goals. One of the key developments that has encouraged me through the years, especially when all of this can be so complex, is the successful development of the Integrative Medicine field. While not a separate field in medicine, it has defined a new way of functioning for the typical medical doctor's procedures and has required new training, education, and new processes to be included for the doctor and health professionals.

Over the past several decades, these integrations have become more embraced by doctors and patients as methods to provide goals of better health and wellness.

It has not been a smooth and easy road, nor an easy process, and it continues to develop and grow in universities, hospitals, and the common doctor's office. But the purpose has not been to find the easy path but to explore the path towards the best health and well-being, and this is not always so clear and simple. This process requires that new modalities and different procedures are considered and factored into the health equation, which is often unique for each person. There is not always a formulaic process to follow, yet even with this being more complex, the demand for these new processes has increased over the past 20 to 30 years.

However, the work that medical professionals have achieved on this path over the past several decades has provided new solutions that have helped many people to achieve and maintain better health and well-being.

Reverse Engineering the Problems with Forward Thinking Design

By viewing some of the gaps that currently exist between the architecture and medical fields, there can be a "Reverse Engineering" combined with a "Forward Thinking Design" process that can show a path toward solutions.

For many people in the world, the letters PRND are seen almost every day in English speaking countries as they are the letters on their car's dashboard. They stand for Park, Reverse, Neutral, and Drive, and it is fitting that this view has become a mantra of everyday driving.

These four letters can also be a reminder of the process of creating better solutions where issues exist and can be utilized in the following format.

A good approach to solving issues is to begin by slowing down and placing our processes in "Park" mode in order to begin the evaluation process. When you can stop and review what the issues are, it can provide greater insights into the problems you are dealing with. It's extremely helpful during this "Parking" time to begin evaluations and to look back at how the current scenario came to be. How was the current problem created? What were the processes that led to these problems?

In this manner, we can then look back or go in "Reverse" to view and look backward to see how the current problem had been created.

At this time, by viewing the steps that created the current problems and placing this process into a "Neutral" view of thought process, it can help to review the past and these steps with an open mind. And when this can occur, with an honest reflection of how the problem was created, then a large percentage of the problems can be viewed with more clarity.

At this time, a fresh and honest view can then provide insights into the problems, and the creative process for solutions can be placed into "Drive."

This is where the forward movement can create new solutions, but instead of them being solutions that might cause more problems or are utilized without the wisdom and knowledge of how the initial problems were created, new solutions can be designed for whole system solutions.

Whole system solutions are created when you can understand how the many pieces fit into the big jigsaw puzzle of the problems that you are solving. If you do not view the larger picture and how each piece impacts other parts of the puzzle, the result can be a solution to one problem and the creation of more problems — sometimes worse than the initial issue.

Viewing the whole picture, you can create a new approach to solutions that consider the many issues of how the problems were created and how new solutions can support the issues – without creating more problems in the process.

P RND — Park-Reverse-Neutral-Drive

This process of pausing, reviewing, evaluating, and then designing can be a methodology for creating better solutions as whole system solutions.

This specific reminder can also be utilized to reflect on the importance of R and D (RND) in Research and Development.

> "By including the many facets of issues, and their short and long-term impacts, it can provide a procedure that can help to prevent problems in the future, while solving current problems."

And because some problems are unknown, this same process can be utilized when there are more design solutions required.

This agile and circular process can become a spiracycle in an upward and positive format.

Architectural Medicine System – Reverse Engineering the Solution with Forward Thinking Design

The reverse engineering portion is to view what the end goals are and then work backward to a place where we are today to move forward. And that moving forward can be supported by "design thinking" such as that of healthy Hospital design processes and by those such as Dr. Diana Anderson, Dr. Andrew M. Ibrahim, and Dr. Bon Ku, who are pioneering the design process as medical doctors. The book *Health Design Thinking: Creating Products and Services for Better Health* by Dr. Bon Ku and Ellen Lupton is a great example of doctors providing architectural solutions from a medical standpoint.

Another great example of pioneering work is that of Dr. Diana Anderson as the *dochitect*. As both a medical doctor and architect and a feat few would even try to achieve was recognized as a recipient of the 2018 AIA/AAH U40 List of Healthcare Design's Best Under 40. Her book, *The Dochitect's Journal: A collection of writings on the intersection of Medicine and Architecture,* provides insights into this world of these professions functioning together for better built environments.

Another standout is Dr. Andrew M. Ibrahim MD, MSc, of the University of Michigan's Surgery & Architecture and Chief Medical Officer at HOK, a global design, architecture, engineering, and planning firm.

I highly recommend following their work, and they each can be found on Twitter:

- Dr. Diana Anderson – @dochitect
- Dr. Andrew M. Ibrahim – @AndrewMIbrahim
- Dr. Bon Ku – @BonKu

By involving doctors in the built environment design process, it can provide more insights into solutions, and over time this can iterate to better design solutions inside and outside of the hospital setting.

Integrative Medicine and Integrative Architecture

The expectation that these new changes in evaluating the health of the built environment will also take time, yet cannot manifest without an integrative approach.

As Integrative Medicine has become a focus on best practices between modern medicine and traditional medicine, there is an opportunity for Integrative Architecture to do the same in the building world.

In chapter 4, I discussed the topic of Integrative Architecture and how this process can help build bridges to support healthier, greener, and more sustainable building solutions. And in this manner, each of these topics eventually supports the health of the ecology and biology of the planet. As we begin to recognize our own human biological needs and requirements and see the deeper connections between our biological and ecological health, these topics can become more familiar to the average person.

And when this awareness of biological and ecological health is more readily recognized, then actions toward focusing on these topics can become more commonplace.

In today's world, many of these interconnections have been forgotten or ignored, and it may take some time to re-evaluate and reconsider to see the importance of these decisions. This may take some time to develop, yet we are also going against the clock in some ways, as the scale of our human interactions with planetary health has become more impactful at a quicker rate.

If we are to find solutions, we need to do so in a different manner in how these problems were created. There is a well-known quote discussing this topic, which is often attributed to Albert Einstein. While I cannot find any concrete evidence that this was indeed Einstein, it does outline a higher level of thinking required to address many of the current day problems in the following statement:

> "We can't solve problems by using the same kind of thinking we used when we created them."

Solutions to modern day problems must use a different methodology than the origination of the problems themselves. As many issues have often been created in a silo or as individuals or groups in an insular format, one of the keys to providing whole system solutions is in working together.

These new solutions must transcend the origins of the problems, and a helpful approach will be to solve them in a nodal format instead of a hierarchical, siloed approach. This was outlined earlier in the chapter on the replacement of the silo and the use of the new nodal system based on the functions of a tree or plant. Our nervous system also functions in a similar manner, so there can be great benefits when thinking about scalability as well.

Integrative Systems to Help Support Emotional and Mental Health in the Built Environment

As defined in earlier chapters, the Architectural Medicine System is intended to ensure that the Architect, Doctor, Inspector, Informaticist, and the Architectural Doctor all work together for cohesive solutions.

This includes the Architectural Medicine Software Solution -ARxMD, which can integrate the processes of evaluations, and inspections, of the built environment. This can provide a platform to record building issues that are found and report these building issues for solutions to be created by the architecture professionals. And the final inspection and evaluation steps can provide a round trip system to ensure, from start to finish, this cycle of processes provides positive results.

With a focus on working with the healthy building inspector with building health related issues, these inspections can also help to support other health professionals, such as psychologists and mental health professionals.

By including factors in the built environment that may pose health issues, such as the mental and psychological impacts of lead paint, these building topics can be included in mental health evaluations to provide better support for health professionals to provide more cohesive solutions.

After all, if a psychologist can understand that there may be physiological issues impacting their patients' mental health issues, then the solution process can include other health professionals to provide more complete solutions. Yet right now, the inclusion of built environment topics, defined as social determinants of health, are not commonly included in a health professionals evaluation process. And so, it is not only the medical doctor that can benefit from these systems in providing physical health ailments, yet also the health professionals focused on mental and emotional health and well-being.

The Architectural Medicine System flowchart can also pertain to those focused on mental health. The psychologist can also utilize this building information as helpful guidance for steps to take for their patient's best health. When the six segments of the Architectural Medicine System cycle are reviewed again, this time, the doctor in the top left corner can actually be recognized as a psychologist, psychiatrist, or other mental and emotional healthcare professional that can benefit their patient with such building health knowledge.

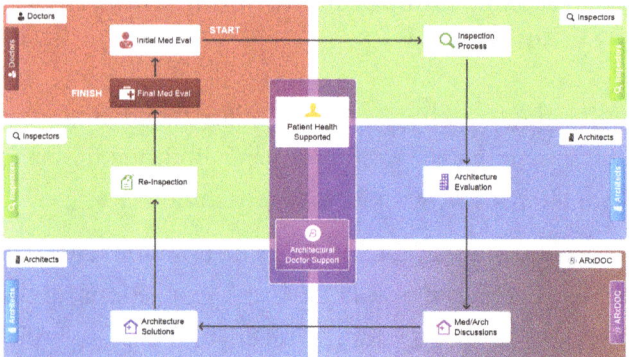

In chapter 16, I will comment on the use of neuroscience in architecture and how this can be utilized for health evaluations in the built environment.

Chapter Summary – The Importance of Whole System Solutions In the Future

At the start of the book, I provided a graphic that showed an absence of connections between the fields of architecture and medicine, and through each chapter, I have provided detailed steps in how these fields can overlap for the benefit of patient and public health.

Chapter: 15 — Bringing It All Together

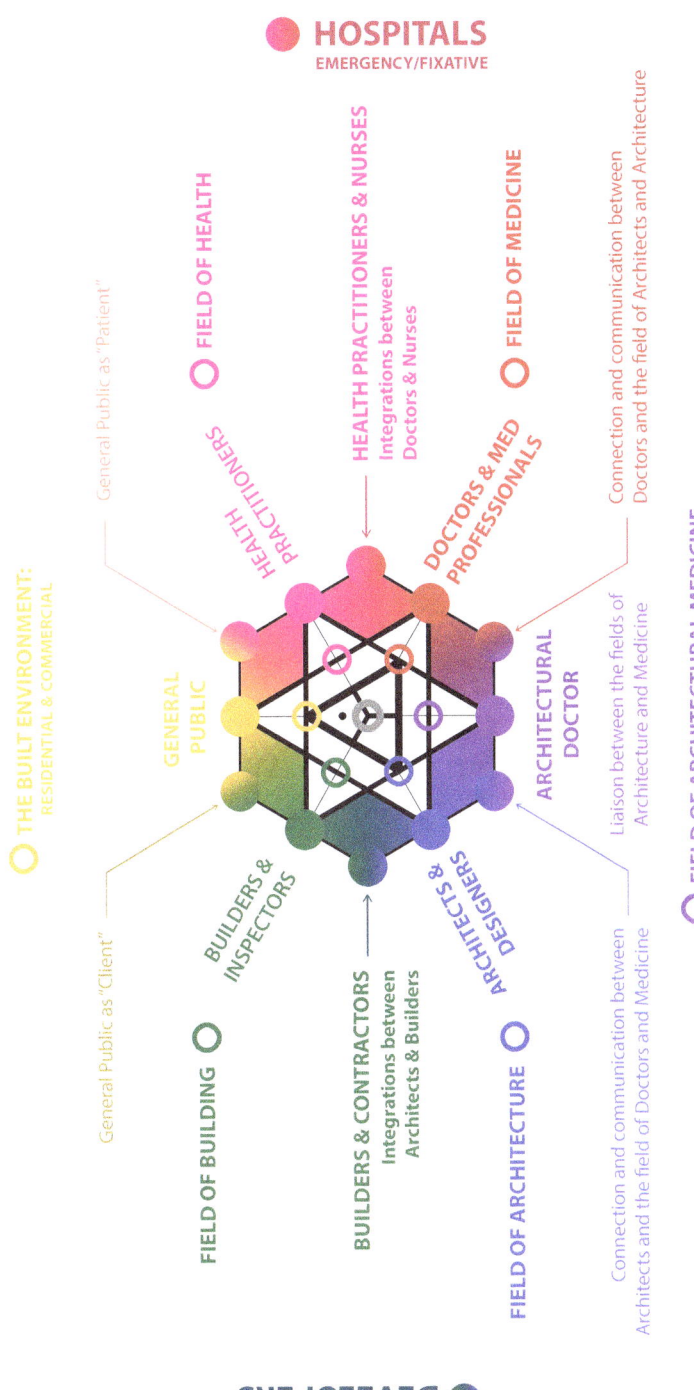

An important part of these new nodal processes means that new professionals will work together in ways that have never before existed. And when this is achieved, new viewpoints can provide different approaches toward cohesive, inclusionary solutions. This can help provide new results while striving to prevent new problems from being created at the same time.

New Integrated Building Model for Health and Wellness

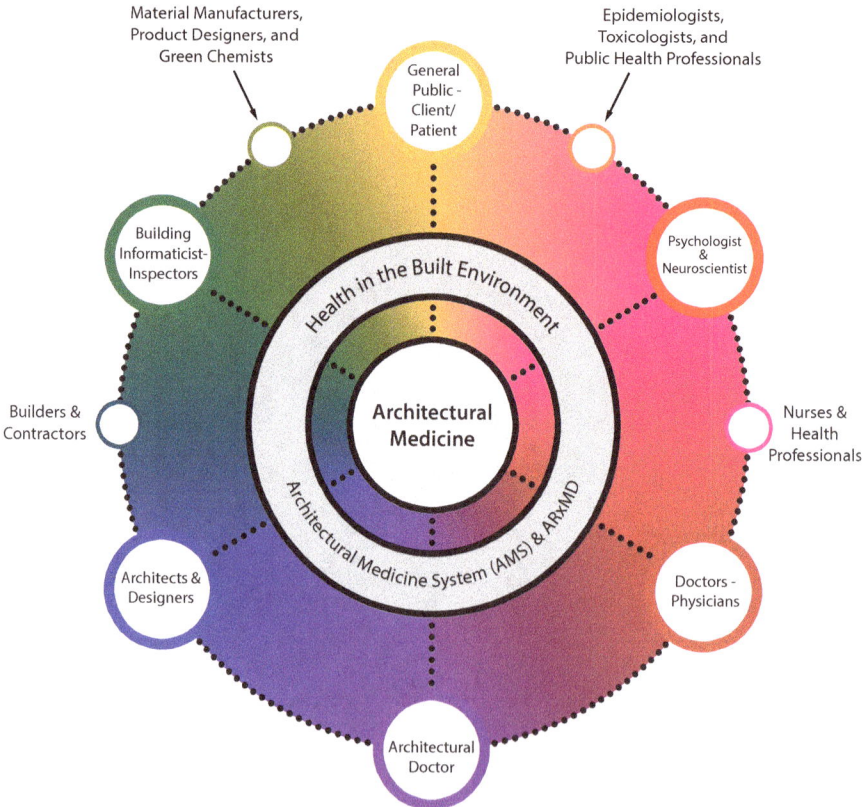

These integrations include new topics such as Environmental Psychology, Architectural Phenomenology, and Green Chemistry to include a wide-ranging set of viewpoints as ways to provide whole system solutions. From issues related to toxicologists and epidemiology professionals to psychologists and neuroscience professionals, the question of how they fit together highlights the importance of multidisciplinary, integrative solutions.

And, of course, the main goal of all these professionals working together is to understand the importance of finding solutions for the patient as the general public. With integrative systems working together between the building and health professionals, cohesive solutions can benefit the public at large.

This may take some time for these integrations to develop, yet small steps in working together can provide exponential benefits, and as such, the more work done now to establish these integrations, the better our current and future generations will be.

As we venture into the 21st century with the topics of health, well-being, and quality of life at the forefront, this approach requires another facet of creating lifestyles for humanity in a more nurturing format.

And this is exactly what I'll discuss in the next chapter...

"If I were asked to name the chief benefit of the house, I should say: the house shelters day-dreaming, the house protects the dreamer, the house allows one to dream in peace."

— Gaston Bachelard

NURTURING ARCHITECTURE FOR A FUTURE OF WELLNESS

Another component of the Architectural Doctor's work can include the steps needed to support emotional and mental wellness in the built environment. The choices of design are wide ranging, and while there may not be a formula for all designs for health and wellness, there are some characteristics of designs that can support well-being.

Some of these design factors are being explored using neuroscience, where evaluating responses to specific designs can be monitored using fMRI or functional magnetic resonance imaging. This process measures real-time brain activity by detecting changes associated with blood flow. It's already been determined that images with sharper and more angular designs, along with materials with harder surfaces, have a response in the brain center located around the amygdala. In a later section of this chapter, I will cite the science that rougher images show an increase in activity, defining the fact that physiologically, the brain is experiencing stress. As such, it will increase stress in the physical body. Even if the person is not showing signs that they are stressed, these brain scans show that the body is responding in a manner that triggers the fight, flight, or freeze responses in the brain center.

Contrary to these harsher, sharper images with a rough material texture, images that are more curving and have a softer texture do not have this negative physiological response. These curving shapes and forms showed no activity in the brain center, thereby providing a more comforting design experience that does not induce stress.

This is important research, as it can show the impacts of design elements and prove that there are certain designs that can increase stress physiologically. This can also define that there are designs that can reduce stress and support a more comforting, nurturing environment for humans to be more relaxed. The images that did not trigger a stressful response are curving forms and softer textures as design elements. They show that these forms and textures can provide more nurturing, and reduce stress for better health and wellness.

This research is opening the capabilities between science and the arts. When this knowledge is utilized in the creation of architectural designs, the results can support well-being and provide less stress for the inhabitants.

The Architectural Doctor can utilize this research to educate the architecture and building fields and help patients address design issues in their built environment to support their well-being.

In earlier chapters of this book, I discussed the emotional and psychological impacts of the built environment on human health. In my other book, Architectural Medicine, I spent a few chapters discussing these topics, as they are essential to evaluate when creating truly healthy architecture for the whole person. These topics include how the built environment impacts physical health and emotional and mental or psychological wellness.

When it comes to the impacts on the body, the physiological effects include the emotional and mental aspects of good health, not just the physical influences. But architecture and medicine are complex, and as such, no simple formula can be provided to fit all facets of people and life. The role of the architect and doctor is to ensure that science is utilized and the use of the arts is implemented for health, healing, and wellness.

Architecture that is more than healthy building, is architecture for the whole person — physically, emotionally, mentally, and spiritually.

And architecture for wellness has to include the whole person, and medicine for wellness has to include the many facets of a person's life, which consists of the environments in which they live – either natural or those developed by humans.

Parametric Architecture and Curving Designs for Good Health

One of the facets of architecture I have not discussed is based on design styles and approaches to design. I've done this on purpose, as the topics of design can often become formulaic, and many can get stuck on the design equation as a mantra.

> "It seems so obvious to me that we feel at home in spaces that are curving." [237]

The quote above is from Elora Hardy, a woman who runs an organization that designs bamboo structures and many different natural elements that she works with in Bali. Her story is interesting because she is not an architect, yet had experienced the world of fashion in NYC with well-known designer Donna Karan.

I have included her quote and work in this book because her approaches to creating the built environment are based on non-formulaic approaches. Instead of designing structures that are based on historical representations of architecture, she asks how the body may move through spaces in a similar format that fashion and clothing fit the body.

Utilizing the unique qualities of bamboo, it is a sustainable product that is quick to grow and can provide incredibly valuable sustainable building solutions. What's more, the materials can provide a way of designing structures more in alignment with the natural world, and more fitting to the natural ways of the human form.

We often forget that humans are not just living in nature; we are nature. We often forget that our bodies are curving shapes and forms. And as such, the more curving and flowing designs are, the more in tune they are with the human form.

> "It's just fun to think, okay, there's probably a good reason why they've always made a chair like that, or a door like that. There's probably a good reason why that's usually the way it is. But what if it wasn't? What else would it be? It's an ongoing process of just trying to reinvent the universe in a way that it didn't exist before." — Elora Hardy

Designs for Health - The Future of Architecture and the Architectural Doctor

One of the aspects of the Architectural Doctor, which has not been discussed in this book until this chapter, is the potential for the Architectural Doctor to provide design support for health in buildings from the start.

Instead of focusing on unhealthy issues, the future capabilities of the Architectural Doctor and Architectural Medicine can utilize new knowledge. In the future, using the wide range of new knowledge between architecture and medicine from building informatics can support the development of healthier architecture from the outset.

Instead of focusing on the issues causing a lack of health, this knowledge can be applied to new architecture to support wellness initiatives. By utilizing the knowledge pooled from this work and the big data and bioinformatics of the Architectural Medicine System and the ARxMD software, the fundamentals of evidence-based design can support new designs for thriving. Between the two fields of architecture and medicine, there can be valuable knowledge to apply as building wisdom.

It also adds to the question of architecture and looking at designs from a new viewpoint. Most architecture today is rectangular in form and can be defined as box-like in shape. The flat walls, mostly at 90-degree angles, define most structures with little to no curving profiles.

To be fair, the reason is based on the history of buildings, primarily developed using straight timber logs and using materials that would function well in linear and planar formats.

However, as our technology advances and the fabrication and manufacturing provides improvements in capabilities for different shapes and forms, what designs would better reflect structural integrity and better health and wellness?

Why Parametric Architecture? Why Are Curving Designs Important as Nurturing Designs?

If you look around, wherever you are, you will likely see two types of designs. You will either be looking at the buildings that humans have created or you will be looking at nature and nature's designs. Each will have different approaches to designing and building, yet perhaps you've never thought of these two worlds of design before in a comparative format to each other.

If you view the architecture humans have created, you will often see a common design theme. And that theme is more along the lines of boxes or rectilinear architecture. If you look at the designs of the natural world, you will see few box-like structures as rectangles and, instead, lots of curving forms. Even if you view trees, you will see that some of the tree trunks are about as much of a straight line as will exist, but the many other parts of the tree will have curving forms and shapes. The massive amount of designs in nature, from animals, insects, plants, and the curving forms of the earth, are filled with free-form shapes. That's why organic architecture is stated as such — mimicking the curving forms of nature.

> "And so a question that comes up so much when we're trying to find the right curve or the right shape, or the right level within a building is — What would nature do?"
>
> — Elora Hardy

If you even take a moment to look at your own human body, you will see many curving forms, from the spheroid shape of your head and eyes to the many curving parts of your body. Both internally and externally, the shapes and forms of your body are primarily curves.

And there's a probable reason for that, which you can at least recognize if you are not sure of nature's design origins. Buckminster Fuller pointed out this reason in his discussions on tensegrity: the strength of materials is at its highest when in tension. His geodesic domes are an excellent example of this. And as Donald Ingbar wrote about two decades ago in an article titled "The Architecture of Life, " your cells' design also mimics this geodesic design, including tensegrity on the cellular level.

But you don't need to recite the design strategies of Fuller and Ingbar to help support these design clues. If you've ever taken a piece of paper and tried to stand it on edge as a flat plane, you will quickly see the lack of strength inherent in this design format. However, if you crease the paper into a triangular configuration, you will soon see that triangles provide a strength that a flat plane cannot. And then, if you increase these triangular forms into a curving plane, you will see that the strength of this design will allow the paper to be placed on the edge and stay upright.

And in this manner, it behooves humans to learn how to utilize less planar forms and more curving forms based on material strength. This can also allow fewer materials to be used, which means less negative environmental impact.

> "If you erase the word "house" from your mind, and going away from a sense of four posts and a roof… if you approach it from a clean slate , it's really fun to just think…, what kind of shelter does nature want for us."

These quotes of Elora Hardy are from the Apple + plus "Home" series, season 1, episode 3. The series highlights unique homes, and each episode discusses each homeowner's design approach. What I find particularly interesting about the series is that, while it does focus on the unique qualities of the materials and methods, the story of their home is often focused on the nurturing qualities that these architects and designers, as homeowners, have created.

Home is often about nurturing — a space and place for your physical well-being and your soul. There is no design equation that can provide these as blueprints.

Yet there are design elements that can support these nurturing designs, whether they be curving shapes and softer forms or reducing materials and substances that can cause physiological harm.

From the contaminants as toxins on the physical body to the curving forms to decrease negative emotional, mental, and physiological impacts, there can be an Rx in the built environment for better health and wellness.

Curving, Parametric Designs and Moving Forward in the World of Architecture

To be clear, this is not a criticism of human architecture for criticism alone. In fact, most of these new design methodologies of a parametric format have not been readily available in the world of construction and building until recently.

Not until the mid-1990s did these designs begin to appear worldwide, except for the rarity in structures such as Frank Lloyd Wright's Guggenheim in New York City or the Sagrada Familia by Antoni Gaudi in Barcelona.

But there is more than just structural strength in these curving designs providing benefits. There is also the value of visual cues to provide less danger.

This can be shown from the neuroscience research of Moshe Bar, whose team showed that when there are curving forms, the brain center responsible for fight, flight, or fear, is less triggered.[238]

And yet when there are more angular forms, especially those with sharp edges, then the brain center can be triggered, and a fear response can exist.

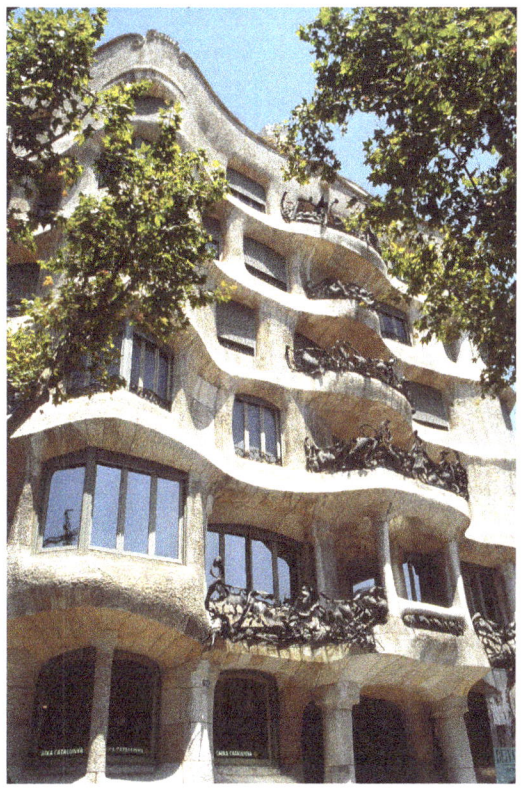

Antoni Gaudi, Casa Milà, Barcelona – 1998
Photo by author

This is particularly interesting, as this fear response can provide physiological stress even if the person is not feeling this way or aware that they are stressed. This means that the human body can be under stress in particular environments and designs without even being aware of such impacts.

This physiological response can be an enormous aspect of stress in one's daily life, particularly with the increase in time spent around and living inside buildings. Since stress is the number one factor in death in today's modern world, the capability to remove stressors can help reduce these aspects, reducing dis-ease and contributing to a better sense of well-being.

And it is this type of design understanding, on both a visual and physiological level, that can contribute to the knowledge of the designs of tomorrow for wellness.

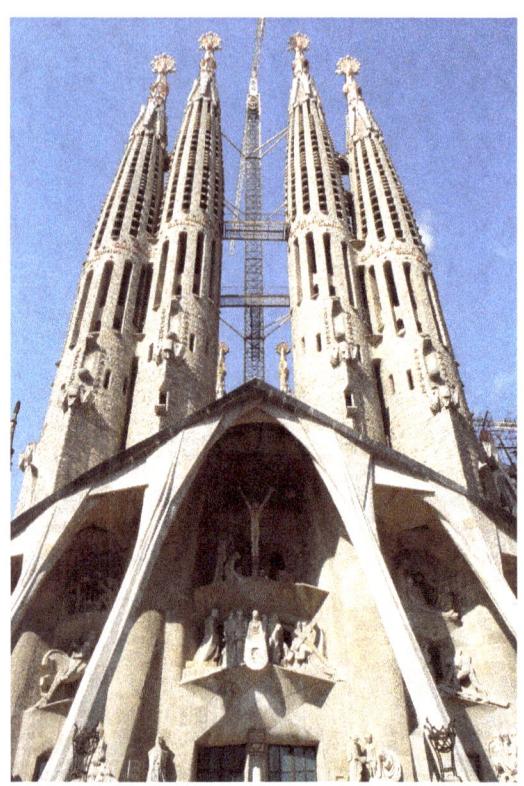
Antoni Gaudi, Sagrada Familia, Barcelona – 1998
Photo by author

Parametric designs in architecture have increased over the past two decades worldwide. The newer design capabilities of CAD systems, combined with digital fabrication and manufacturing processes directly from these digital drawings, have allowed many of these new shapes and forms to proliferate.

It is a new era in architecture, and these new shapes and forms for many may be unorthodox. Yet as I've mentioned earlier in the chapter, the box-like forms that we have become accustomed to are actually the strange shapes on this planet. Organic forms define planet Earth, and perhaps the emergence of these forms that we live and work within may provide a resonance back to the natural world that we are connected to as human beings. We, as human beings, are nature. Perhaps these new forms will create a resonance to support planetary health and all of its inhabitants, and human created developments will then support better human health as well as biological and ecological well-being.

Nurturing Designs Can Lead to a Healthier Society

There is no doubt that in places with a preponderance of crime, stress increases, and there becomes a lack of quality of life. Viewing this in the opposite way, one can ascertain that environments with fewer stressors can lead to a better quality of life.

And in places that provide a better quality of life, this can lead to less crime and violence, which can provide less stressful places for the masses. In doing so, this stress reduction can provide better short and long-term outcomes and support more capabilities for wellness.

> "I try to give people a different way of looking at their surroundings. That's art to me."[239]— Maya Lin

One of the ways to achieve this is to design places that support human nurturing, with architectural spaces externally and internally that support better health. This can be a mix between better physical, emotional, and mental health, all of which can be implemented with better design choices in the built environment.

A part of this understanding can be gleaned from the word origins of nurture:

nurture (n.)

c. 1300, norture, "upbringing, the act or responsibility of rearing a child," also "breeding, manners, courtesy," from Old French norture, nourreture "food, nourishment; education, training," from Late Latin nutritia "a nursing, suckling," from Latin nutrire "to nourish, suckle" (see nourish). From mid-14c. as "nourishment, food."[240]

And the origins of the word nourish can be found in the following etymology:

nourish (v.)

c. 1300, norishen, "to supply with food and drink, feed; to bring up, nurture, promote the growth or development of" (a child, a young animal, a vice, a feeling, etc.), from Old French noriss-, stem of norrir "raise, bring up, nurture, foster; maintain, provide for" (12c., Modern French nourrir), from Latin nutrire "to feed, nurse, foster, support, preserve," from *nutri (older form of nutrix "nurse")[241]

As can be seen in these word descriptions, nurturing and nourishing is the process of providing nutrition for good health and for proper development. Perhaps this nourishment and nurturing, provided by initial feeding from the mother, is one of the reasons why many reference the earth as "mother," providing the nutrients for life and well-being.

nurture (n.)

1: Training, Upbringing

2: something that nourishes : Food

3: the sum of the environmental factors influencing the behavior and traits expressed by an organism

nurture (v.)

1: to supply with nourishment

2: Educate

3: to further the development of : Foster

nurture is a synonym of nourish—both are derived from the Latin verb nutrire, meaning "to suckle" or "to nourish."[242]

nurture

b. In extended use: the careful fostering, cultivation, or encouraging of something.[243]

The Oxford dictionary takes this definition further into the extent of development by stating the process of cultivation and the encouragement of something with careful fostering.

The above definitions highlight "training, education, and fostering," all three supporting a healthy life in the same way a table with three legs can provide a solid foundation. All of these definitions focus on the combination of offering proper development and growth, with a focus on cultivation to achieve optimal potential.

And with these conflations of meanings, Architectural Medicine and the Architectural Doctor strive to achieve optimal health and wellness.

This is not an easy process to formulate, and as such, there is a need for many facets to be considered. It requires the sciences and the arts to work together in a symbiotic format. These multi-disciplinary methods will require overlap between fields that have never collaborated before and new fields and professions to fill the gaps to achieve this collaboration process.

The lack of formulaic processes may cause unease for many. Yet, as such, it provides an opportunity for creating new processes and systems, such as that of the Architectural Medicine System (AMS).

In so doing, we can collaborate in the likes that have never been observed in recorded history, which can provide new opportunities for positive change.

It's reported that Einstein is quoted as saying, "insanity is doing the same thing over and over and expecting different results." Again, I found uncertainty as to the origin of the quote. It does sound plausible for Einstein to say for one simple reason — its truth speaks wisdom. Doing the same thing over and over and expecting a different result is what we are doing if we are not making changes to the way we live on this planet.

And so, to deter these problems from creating more challenges, there is the need to review these problems in earnest and then work together as a cohesive humanity to find solutions. It requires us to view life as a whole, with the goal of whole system solutions for optimal health and wellness worldwide.

There are no shortcuts to this process, so let's get to work…

Creating Blueprints for Wellness

To follow up on this topic of creating healthy architecture from the outset, the knowledge that can be applied to current and future architecture can be extensive.

In order to create architecture that is focused on nurturing, it is essential that designers have a greater understanding of human psychology, as well as a better understanding of human physiology.

This is due to the fact that humans are impacted in many different formats, especially when it comes to the senses. Therefore, if there is a greater understanding of these impacts on physiology due to sensory experiences, these insights can provide deeper meanings of architectural shapes, forms, and the many facets of design.

And this is where the Neuroscience in Architecture developments can provide fascinating insights into the next worlds of architecture. These insights literally offer a view into human physiology never before possible. It is also another bridge between the fields of architecture and medicine that can provide developments to help support design solutions in powerful and meaningful ways.

Creating blueprints for wellness requires a focus on the built environment that includes the work of the architect and creator of environments, along with the wisdom of medicine to provide health, healing, and wellness.

When these facets are implemented into a cohesive whole, the results are whole health. And when there is total health, then wellness and quality of life are possible.

For this is an architecture that can support a better future for humans, and humanity at large, to achieve human thriving. With a focus on design and building that considers all of these facets before sitting down at the proverbial drawing board, it can provide generations to come with the built environments that can support their best health.

While this may sound like an excellent approach to the design-build practice, it will require changes in how architects and doctors think and new training, education, and systems to achieve these goals.

Utilizing the topics discussed in chapter 4 on Integrative Architecture, focusing on green, sustainable, and healthy buildings, this can be combined with the focus on optimal health and wellness — physically, emotionally, mentally, or psychologically.

A new viewpoint on architecture and renewing the way designers and the masses view architecture will also help provide new forms, such as parametric architecture and curving designs. It is, however, not the pure responsibility of the architect and doctor alone. They need the public's support to demand these changes and require institutions around the world to support these changes and updates in the built environment.

NeuroArchitecture and NeuroScience in Architecture

In the *Architectural Medicine* book, I discuss the topic of emotional and psychological or mental wellness relative to the built environment using examples of NeuroArchitecture or Neuroscience in Architecture. Whether you define it as Neuroscience in or of architecture, either defines the same criteria: measuring the way the brain responds to shapes, forms, and designs.

By utilizing fMRI systems methodologies, studies show that the physiological impacts of shapes and forms can be measured and can also help provide insights into the body's responses to design elements. For example, someone may view a shape or design and not have much conscious thought about these design forms, yet physiologically, the body may respond. The brain center, in particular, the amygdala, is a metric of either a calm feeling or a stressful scenario. This is known as the flight, fight, or freeze process, and the amygdala provides this feedback in measurable formats.

A fascinating aspect of this neuroarchitecture research is that some people may not feel stressed seeing particular shapes and forms. Yet, their physiological response is recorded as such by the amygdala. This brings up questions on how the mind may be ignoring such stressors in their lives, including the built environment's impacts on their experiences.

This opens up a whole world of unknowns that we can explore to understand better human experiences, especially those that can be impacted by stressors and the processes of decreasing such stressors.

As mentioned in a previous paragraph, studies done by neuroscientists show that when people were shown pictures of sharp, pointed designs and hard surfaces using fMRI processes, these scientists could indicate that the brain center was triggered, showing increased stress levels.[244]

The physiological responses of this research show the impacts of the environment on stress levels, and as social determinants of health increase in scope along with geomedicine, the future of this research is sure to be fascinating.

This is certainly of interest for future studies if we as humans strive to provide better solutions to decrease these stresses for longer lives and more quality of life.

Wellness Centers and the Benefits of Nurturing Architecture

In the *Architectural Medicine* book, I devoted a whole chapter to the topic of a "Wellness Center." And to extend this to another level, I will state that in this book, the concept of a Wellness Center should also extend to one's home. The home can be experienced as a Center and place for people to gather.

Having a Wellness Center can be extremely valuable to a community providing a location where people can achieve and maintain good health. It can offer a service to focus on creating and maintaining good health, while depending on the hospital for times when it is required.

A wellness center for communities can provide a place to focus on wellness and well-being and provide a template for healthy living. This is opposed to each person being required to try and find this wellness in a world that does not support nor echo such in life.

If your health is reflected to you in a hospital or by visits to doctors when you are sick, what type of mindset will you have for the rest of your life? When have you truly seen positive examples of good health and wellness in your life? And as such, how do you think this impacts how you view life?

Psychologically, by having positive reflections of wellness and places and spaces that echo and support this mantra, you can then be provided a blueprint as a template for well-being.

Being surrounded by places and living in spaces that provide comfort and nurturing can provide you with a mindset that is not only healthy but provides you with options to live your life in more healthy formats. It doesn't have to be perfect, nor do you always have to be thinking about health and wellness. But if you don't have any models in your life to achieve these goals, and be provided templates as pathways towards these goals, then you either have to find it on your own or redesign the wheel to achieve the end results.

That seems neither sensible nor wise as an approach to living, and while you don't have to strive for perfection, you can find that others have provided templates for good living.

That sounds like a blueprint for wellness that is both wise and sensible and can provide you the options to customize these blueprints to create your own life with the goals of well-being and quality of life.

An Rx for health and wellness in life, as well as in the built environment, can support this well-being. As buildings need a solid foundation for structural integrity, we too, as humans, require a solid foundation to live a life built on health and quality of life. It won't simply happen without any effort, and as well, it may be wise to focus on these ideas to provide wellness centers for community and public health.

And following this mindset of an Rx as blueprints or templates for wellness, this transitions into the next chapter on the future of Architectural Medicine and the Architectural Doctor...

> "I will not follow where the path may lead,
> but I will go where there is no path,
> and I will leave a trail"
>
> — Muriel Strode

WHAT'S NEXT FOR ARCHITECTURAL MEDICINE AND THE ARCHITECTURAL DOCTOR?

As I've written throughout this book, the process of creating architecture that supports better health and wellness has at its foundation three important processes. The first is to realistically and honestly evaluate the built environment and its impact on human and ecological health. The second is to utilize these evaluations to properly ascertain where things can be made better. And the third is to repeat this

Chapter: 17 What's Next for Architectural Medicine & the Architectural Doctor?

process and iterate, as I define as a spiracycle over time to continue to make things better.

However, in order to achieve these goals, there is a critical need for evaluations, which require data and scenarios in which to evaluate. As big data and analytics provide bioinformatics, there can be great insights gleaned from these evaluations. Yet the processes required to provide this data, including the Healthy Building Inspector, the Building Informaticist, and the Architectural Doctor to support these processes, is still missing in the building process.

It also requires the medical professionals to recognize the impacts of the built environment and how to include this in their patient's health evaluations. And then last but least, it requires the architects and building professionals to include these health variables to become not only added to their design and building solutions but embedded as critical design elements that drive their building solutions.

This is again where the Architectural Medicine System (AMS) can provide support, and the ARxMD software can be utilized for processes to proceed.

While there is much work to be done to achieve these processes, there is also great promise that can result from these multi-disciplinary, integrative processes for current and future architectural designs.

Technology for Humanity

There is little doubt that technology has provided humanity with tremendous capabilities, yet as the old but true saying goes, "with great power, there is a need for great responsibility." This is another quote that, when reviewed deeper, seems to have different opinions as to the origins. While I cannot properly cite this quote, it stands on its own as an important component in life.

In the previous chapter, the topics of nurturing were combined with recognizing that we as humanity have decisions to make in the goals we are striving to achieve. It's either health and wellness for the planet and humanity, or we head into more destruction.

At this time in the world, this great technological power is not being treated with the great responsibility that it merits. Now, to be clear, I'm an advocate of technology, if the purposes and processes are to benefit humanity. While this statement can vary depending on the person stating this, the intention of this statement is to say that technology is a tool, and every tool has benefits and detriments.

The tools of technology can provide better solutions to many of the world's problems, that is, the problems that humans must navigate. The same technology may also be a detriment to the other creatures and organisms that we live with on planet earth, and this is not very wise.

As technology is a tool – from a fork to a supercomputer – there are benefits to how these tools are used as well as detriments. The use of these tools is determined by those using this technology and the mindset of those making such choices in using these devices.

For me, the focus on mindfulness and awareness is not just a buzzword. It is a mindset that can provide support and helpfulness for the masses or can be used as a weapon against the masses. Which choice is determined and decided by those using these tools highlights the importance of a healthy mindset.

While these topics may sound far from the decisions made by the Architectural Doctor and those choosing to follow the ways of Architectural Medicine, they are, in fact, very close to the processes in this world that require decisions to be chosen for beneficial developments.

Technological developments have never been as powerful as they are now, and if you are reading this in the future, then that time is your "now" as well unless, of course, some catastrophic event has occurred to delete the current technological process. If this did occur, the possibilities of this book remaining are also in question.

Future technological developments require a mindset and ethical choices that are based on striving to provide helpful solutions, and in this process, the steps taken with these technological solutions can provide and offer tremendous help to the masses. When utilized with topics such as the

Chapter: 17 What's Next for Architectural Medicine & the Architectural Doctor?

Architectural Medicine System (AMS), the benefits can be better health for the populations.

The utilization of ARxMD – the Architectural Medicine Software Solution can provide real-time answers as well as a long tail of solutions for humanity moving forward. This can be achieved when individual benefits are provided, as well as the exponential benefits of the big data that can be analyzed and evaluated.

While this book is focused on the Architectural Doctor and the processes of Architectural Medicine, there is also a bigger picture view that includes human psychology that must be addressed.

With many technological advances continuing to provide positive solutions for the health of humans, there is also an important topic that must be included in this discussion. And that is the mindset and ethics that humans have and will require moving forward into the future.

A New Mindset, Along With New Systems on This Planet

In the year 2000, I began writing an article titled "Building the Bridge Not Yet Built." It was focused on the viewpoint that many of the issues in the world caused by human beings were due to a lack of big picture viewpoints on the impacts that humans have on the planet.

This topic, while not new, had been written after several decades of my living on this planet and feeling unsure as to how solutions could be provided. The biggest issue was reflected back to me during a presentation given by one of my mentors, the architect Bosco Büeler based in Switzerland. During one of his talks that he gave in the USA in the late 1990s, he spoke of a canyon in Switzerland that was bigger than the grand canyon in the United States. When he spoke of this canyon to the audience, you could hear the questionable responses and the look of surprise and confusion on the faces of the audience. No one thought there was a canyon as big as the Grand Canyon, and certainly not a canyon of this size located in Switzerland.

But the canyon that Bosco was referring to was the gap between different thought processes of people, and how people in Switzerland and other parts of the world thought in different formats. These differences in opinions and thoughts of the world are sometimes greater than the gaps that exist in the physical world, such as the Grand Canyon.

These large gaps exist all around the world and include the very nature of human thinking, which includes many different viewpoints. When it comes to issues in the current day, the number of viewpoints and varying opinions is almost equivalent to the almost 8 billion population on this planet.

In the world of architecture, there are many who don't see any problems with how the current built environment is produced and find no reasons to make any changes. And yet we know from scientific data that we as humans are causing environmental issues that are based on human impacts, and not just a cycle of the world's climate.

But even if you disagree with the data, are you so sure that the current ways in which humans are impacting the world are so positive? Aren't we supposed to be stewards of the planet? If so, how on Earth can you justify that our current ways of treating the natural systems of the planet are acceptable?

And even if climate change is not accepted nor believed, how is it ok to have landfills, and garbage dumps, and the excesses of the material world with no recycling processes to support regeneration as the natural world itself functions?

If we are so advanced as a humanity, how is it that our technological advancements cannot emulate the simple functions of nature?

Shouldn't our advancements as a human race be more advanced than what nature can achieve?

From the 1970s to the 90s, this climate change was known as global warming, with scientists providing caution to the fact that human impacts on the planet were both heating up the globe, as well as causing issues such as the decrease in the ozone layer based on products created by humans.

In December of 1985, Carl Sagan provided feedback and warnings on global warming and climate change at the United States Senate. His words were more a matter of fact than a warning. His practicality, combined with his concern for human impacts on the planet, was a big part of his life's mantra and an important voice in the scientific community: [245]

> "The power of human beings to effect and control and change the environment is growing as our technology grows, and at present time we clearly have reached the stage where we are capable both intentionally and inadvertently to make significant changes in the global climate and in the global ecosystem.
>
> I'd like to close by just saying a few words on the kind of perspective that this problem and related problems pose to us. Here is a problem which transcends our particular generation, it is an intergenerational problem, if we don't do the right thing now, there are very serious problems that our children and grandchildren will have to face. It is, alas, a global problem.
>
> I think that what is essential for this problem is a global consciousness, a view that transcends our exclusive identifications with the generational and political groupings into which by accident we have been born. The solution to these problems requires a perspective that embraces the planet and the future because we are all in this greenhouse together."

Somewhere in the 1990s, the term climate change emerged and took over from global warming as a definition, mostly defining these same issues. And while the name changed, the warnings of global warming did not change, even if many in the world do not agree. The challenge is that many often do not agree because it negatively impacts their way of living, and for some, they don't want to make changes to how they live.

This means there is a gap between the way different humans think, which refers to the Bosco Büeler story in previous paragraphs, truly is a greater divide than the huge gap that we call the Grand Canyon in the southwestern USA.

And why is all of this important for Architectural Medicine and the Architectural Doctor? Keep in mind that up to 40 percent of all the energy used in the world is from the production, building, and maintenance of buildings. Yes, I wrote that correctly – 40 percent.

That's the bad news.

The good news is that we can choose our energy sources and decrease these negative impacts by exponential factors, by focusing on the type of energy used by buildings and by providing more efficiency in these processes. Yet to find solutions to these issues, you first need to acknowledge that there is an issue to start with. Once you start with this knowledge, then you can work towards a solution. But no solutions can properly be resolved without acknowledgment first.

So this is what humanity must do first, and moving forward, we can work together as a global humanity to provide solutions. Keep in mind that energy production and pollution processes impact health in powerful formats. This is why I've stated earlier in chapter 4 and in later chapters, that you cannot separate the energy, ecology, and health issues of the built environment.

I state global humanity on purpose, as we also need to become aware that we are global citizens, and as such, we cannot provide solutions for just our local places. However, if we do not provide local solutions, then we certainly cannot impact the global population. You can see this interconnectivity is both an independent and an interdependent process. You cannot separate the local health from global health. Our population of humans, nearing 8 billion during this time of writing, requires that we act both locally where we are, with a global mindset in considering the impacts that our choices have on the entire planet. As I listed in chapter 3, in November of 2022, the planet's population is projected to reach the 8 billion milestone, which is the month that this book is being published.

This is admittedly not going to be easy, yet if we don't do this, there will not be a choice, and instead, the choice will be made for us by the planet. Nature's ecological systems are itself complex processes. Yet, in the mindset of many humans, the natural world is primitive. This is a big mistake and will

Chapter: 17   What's Next for Architectural Medicine & the Architectural Doctor?

either be learned by humans to make beneficial choices, or will be forced upon humanity based on consequences.

The natural systems can only handle so much change created by humans before nature itself has negative connotations. Nature exists in a balance, and when human behaviors and decisions ignore this balance, then the consequences will be nature requiring itself to find this balance again. This will likely be a negative impact on life for humans as we know it.

What I think is important to state is that nature itself is not against humans. It is not nature versus humans. Nature is not trying to defeat humanity, nor is it against humanity. Yet if humans go against the very nature of natural systems in balance, and actively work against this balance, then nature will need to act accordingly to regain that balance. And it is in this manner that humans may see nature against humanity, but this is both a false pretense and an incredibly ignorant view of the balance of nature.

What's also of note in this commentary is that, too often, humans have forgotten that they are not only living in nature; they ARE nature.

You, as a human being, are not only a part of nature, but your body is also nature. Your cells and organs are all made of natural materials. Your hair, skin, and nails are silica, your body consists of around 70 percent water, and the very nature of your body is a composition of materials made of the elements in nature from which you are built.

You are not separate from nature; you are nature, literally.

So, if you are to live against nature, you are actually living against the very nature of your nature.

And this is really an inconvenient truth and a disappointing failure of humans to both recognize and utilize as a teaching opportunity for us all. We should have been schooled about this at a very early age, even before we are taught language and math and the many other subjects that are wonderful about learning and knowledge.

This is not at all to say that we shouldn't learn about the ABCs and the subjects of math, science, history, and the arts. It is to state that before we are educated on these important subjects, we should first be educated about our own humanity and what it means to be human. And if this can't be decided upon by the masses, we should at least be taught the essence of who we are as not only living in nature, but also a part of nature in our natural bodies.

In my opinion, I believe that if we are taught this from an early age, many of the problems that humans have created, in terms of the destruction of the natural world, would be resolved. As no intelligent being would destroy the very nature that it depends upon for life, nor would it destroy the very nature of itself.

And so, as we move into the 21st century, we as humanity have a lot of work to do, and one of these core teachings is to remind humans that we are part of nature. To protect the natural world is not something of a commodity to choose or not choose to preserve, but it is literally a matter of life and death to conserve for health and wellness. In the world of wilderness training, there is the rule of 3s. These rules are not set in stone nor complete, but they are general rules for most scenarios when in survival mode. These rules change for different scenarios of survival, yet many of them can be utilized as guidelines. That said, by viewing these, one can receive a sense of what's required in life as a baseline for living on this planet. They are listed in the following order, as you require the proper order of these rules for survival: [246] [247]

- You can survive around 3 Minutes without air (oxygen) or in icy waters
- You can survive around 3 Hours without shelter in a harsh environment (unless in icy water)
- You can survive around 3 Days without water (if sheltered from a harsh environment)
- You can survive around 3 Weeks without food (if you have water and shelter)

It makes absolutely zero sense and logic to not recognize this and to not make changes that conserve and preserve the very health of the environment and ecological systems of the planet. Just as it makes zero sense and logic to

Chapter: 17 What's Next for Architectural Medicine & the Architectural Doctor?

poison ourselves and expect health and wellness to be the result.

Obviously, this book is not about the health and wellness of our ecological systems, but I do have a forthcoming book on this topic titled *Symbiosis Global – Nature is the Most Advanced Technology*. It is my hope to have this published in 2023.

What's critical to state and to capture from the above statements is the following. By focusing on the health and wellness of our environments, to provide the necessary elements for not just survival, but for thriving, we can focus on the critical steps to take to ensure that we can provide this health for humanity. In terms of the built environments, we also must recognize that our buildings impact not only our health, but the health of the planet. And the more you delve into this topic, the more you see that the boundaries that separate humans from the planet are actually nonexistent. You can't separate the topics of ecological and environmental health from human and biological health.

Our human health and the health of the planet are one and the same. And the quicker we can recognize this and design to live with the planet, the quicker we can find a rebalancing of the planet's health along with the wellness of humanity.

Green Chemistry, Biomimicry, Biophilia as Signals for a Better Future

Throughout this book, there have been the downsides of health impacts from the built environment, yet there are some positives as well in these evaluations. One benefit is the many groups that have been developing over the past several decades to address these problems seeking solutions.

Three examples of these developments are:
- Green Chemistry
- Biomimicry
- Biophilia

Green Chemistry

The concepts of green chemistry have emerged from professionals who recognize the toxicity of many chemicals and have chosen to focus on solutions to these issues for human and biological health. Dr. John C. Warner is one of the founders of green chemistry.

He co-authored the seminal book *Green Chemistry: Theory and Practice*, which first described the "Twelve Principles of Green Chemistry." He is among a growing group of professionals around the world who are creating and developing green chemistry to support the replacement of dangerous chemicals, while inventing new approaches to chemistry for better health and wellness.

Dr. Warner is President, Chief Technology Officer, and Chairman of the Board of the Warner Babcock Institute for Green Chemistry, which he founded with Jim Babcock in 2007. According to Warner and Babcock, green chemistry is defined as "a revolutionary approach to the way that products are made; it is a science that aims to reduce or eliminate the use and/or generation of hazardous substances in the design phase of materials development. It requires an inventive and interdisciplinary view of material and product design."[248]

Following up from her book *High Tech trash*, Elizabeth Grossman's *Chasing Molecules* has a much more "potentially" uplifting view on solutions to the issues of technology as waste.

The often insoluble scenario of dealing with the production of technology can leave even the heartiest of optimists in a puzzle, yet this is where the promise of green chemistry could provide solutions for humanity's future.

Green Chemistry follows the "principle that it is better to consider waste prevention options during the design and development phase than to dispose or treat waste after a process or material has been developed."[249]

For a technology to be considered Green Chemistry, it must accomplish three things:[250]

- It must be more environmentally benign than existing alternatives.
- It must be more economically viable than existing alternatives.
- It must be functionally equivalent to or outperform existing alternatives.

Based on the Warner Babcock Institute, Green Chemistry presents industries with the opportunity for growth and based on the estimate that only "10% of current technologies are environmentally benign; another 25% could be made benign relatively easily. The remaining 65% have yet to be invented! Green Chemistry also creates cost savings: when hazardous materials are removed from materials and processes, all hazard-related costs are also removed, such as those associated with handling, transportation, disposal, and compliance."[251]

The benefit of green chemistry holds the promise of "environmentally benign alternatives to current materials and technologies," which can be "systematically introduced across all types of manufacturing to promote a more environmentally and economically sustainable future."[252]

As Architectural Medicine is focused on health in the built environment, this also includes the impact of the materials and objects that compose these buildings.

The twelve principles of green chemistry address a range of ways to reduce the environmental and health impacts of chemical production, therefore reducing the negative health implications, supporting good health, and preventing disease and illness.

Therefore, when materials and products are developed and manufactured to have less negative impact on the environment and health, they can support good health and wellness in all environments.

As I have mentioned, Architectural Medicine recognizes the importance of both environmental and ecological health, as this cannot be separated from the overall health of humans and the biology of the planet.

Biomimicry

Popularized by Janine Benyus in her book *Biomimicry: Innovation Inspired by Nature*, Biomimicry is defined in her book as a "new science that studies nature's models and then imitates or takes inspiration from these designs and processes to solve human problems."[253]

The Biomimicry Institute, created by Benyus, defines this as an "approach to innovation that seeks sustainable solutions to human challenges by emulating nature's time-tested patterns and strategies. The goal is to create products, processes, and policies—new ways of living—that are well-adapted to life on earth over the long haul."[254]

As a key component of Architectural Medicine is indeed architecture and the built environment, the more that the designs, engineering, and systems of the built world can be in tune with nature's systems, including, of course, human health, the less potential there can be for disease and the greater capacity can exist for health and well-being.

By utilizing the wisdom of nature and implementing nature's core design lessons into current and future architecture, there can be many benefits for the health of humans as well as the many other organisms that live on planet Earth. This means that designing using these Biomimetic approaches can provide good health for humans, as well as the ecology of the planet. This, in turn, can support short and long-term health for all living organisms in the natural and built environments.

The term biomimetics was "coined in the mid 1900s by the American Otto Schmitt who developed the concept of 'biomimetics.'"[255]

After he developed the "Schmitt trigger by studying the nerves in squid, attempting to engineer a device that replicated the biological system of nerve propagation, he continued to focus on devices that mimic natural systems and by 1957 he had perceived a converse to the standard view of biophysics at that time, a view he would come to call biomimetics."[256]

In 1969 Schmitt used the term "biomimetic in the title of one of his papers,"[257] and soon after found its way into the dictionary.

Chapter: 17 What's Next for Architectural Medicine & the Architectural Doctor?

> "Biophysics is not so much a subject matter as it is a point of view. It is an approach to problems of biological science utilizing the theory and technology of the physical sciences. Conversely, biophysics is also a biologist's approach to problems of physical science and engineering, although this aspect has largely been neglected." — Otto Herbert Schmitt[258]

As Janine Benyus, co-founder of the Biomimicry Institute, states, "the core idea is that nature has already solved many of the problems we are grappling with. Animals, plants, and microbes are the consummate engineers. After billions of years of research and development, failures are fossils, and what surrounds us is the secret to survival."[259]

This approach can provide solutions in the current and future world that addresses the issues of biological and ecological health before, during, and after the design process is developed — from the small house and largest skyscrapers to vehicles, airplanes, and the everyday products used in life.

In essence, it is learning from the wisdom of nature's designs to then apply this knowledge and wisdom to provide solutions to the human created world.

Biophilia

First used by Erich Fromm to describe a "psychological orientation of being attracted to all that is alive and vital,"[260] in 1984, Edward O. Wilson introduced and popularized the hypothesis in his book, Biophilia, as "the urge to affiliate with other forms of life."[261]

The term biophilia means "love of life or living systems"[262] from the prefix *bio* meaning "life, life and, or "biology," and *philo* meaning "loving, fond of, tending to."[263] Wilson uses the term in the same sense when he suggests that biophilia describes "the connections that human beings subconsciously seek with the rest of life."[264] He proposed the possibility that the deep affiliations humans have with other life forms and nature as a whole are rooted in our biology.

Utilized in architecture, Jana Söderlund and Peter Newman define biophilic design as a "sustainable design strategy that incorporates reconnecting people with the natural environment."[265]

In the documentary *Biophilic Design-The Architecture of Life*, Stephen Kellert starts that Biophilic Design "may be seen as a necessary complement to green architecture, which decreases the environmental impact of the built world but does not address human reconnection with the natural world."[266]

Biophilia discusses and questions how our Architecture impacts our multi-faceted human lives and the importance of nature for our wellness and well-being.

As quoted above, the term biophilia is used to "describe a psychological orientation of being attracted to all that is alive and vital,"[267] which is an important facet of the psychological health discussed in terms of the built environment.

As I have discussed, while the physical aspect of human health is more common with buildings, such as sick building syndrome and toxicology, there is also the facet of how the built environment impacts psychological health.

And designs that embrace the natural world and provide access to nature have been recorded since the early 1980s with Roger Ulrich's research study, "View through a window may influence recovery from surgery."[268] [269]

This research pioneered the field of Evidence-Based Design, which continues to provide a deeper understanding of how important nature is to health, healing, and wellness.

These developments may have started in the hospital setting, yet they show the importance of such design elements, those such as Ulrich and a growing number of designers utilizing these methodologies continue to show these design benefits inside and outside of the hospital setting.

As we move into the future, utilizing this knowledge as wisdom can be applied to all architecture for better health and wellness in the built environment.

Chapter: 17 What's Next for Architectural Medicine & the Architectural Doctor?

The Future of the Architectural Doctor

One of the key takeaways from this book is that the next steps are not only complex yet require collaboration between many different professions. It is my hope that once the main fields of architecture and medicine begin to work together toward integrative solutions, then the many other fields and subfields will also become part of the solution process.

This includes the fields of psychology, public health, epidemiology, green chemistry, and biomimicry to name just a few professions. The reason why this would be so valuable is that when there are many different professionals viewing issues from their specific viewpoint, then they can provide a new angle of thought on an issue, and in this manner, can also provide new solutions. These interconnections can also provide a better understanding of complex puzzles and can ensure that one solution doesn't cause multiple other problems.

As the world becomes more complex, it requires more complex thinking to ensure cohesive solutions. This process is not only indicative of the times, but a revision to many previous models that have existed in the professional world. These older hierarchical processes have their place, yet the newer nodal modes of working together can provide the interoperability that the complex future will require. The benefit of utilizing this nodal format is based on equanimity of inclusion, yet it also provides a networked solution process that can include the many complex components of the current and future systems of the world.

With almost 8 billion people living on this planet, there is a need for healthy systems to be provided, if healthy people are part of human goals.

The future of health and wellness for humanity will require the built environment in the health evaluation process, and with the increasing time spent indoors, the result will require the medical and architecture fields to spend more time focused on building health. The Architectural Doctor will be a key component of these integrations and an important part of these integrations. By providing support to each of these already complex professions, education and training will become paramount for each group to be well-versed on these topics. And the importance as a liaison to help integrations between these professionals will be critical for these complex processes to function in healthy formats.

The use of the Architectural Medicine System and the Architectural Medicine Software Solution — ARxMD, as blueprints for these interconnections can be supported as an Rx for health and wellness in buildings.

In the next chapter, I will discuss some thoughts on the future of the Architectural Doctor and Architectural Medicine in a larger context...

"A profound design process eventually makes the patron, the architect, and every occasional visitor in the building a slightly better human being."

— Juhani Pallasmaa

SOME THOUGHTS ON THE FUTURE

As I've written in the previous chapter, the question of "what's Next for Architectural Medicine and the Architectural Doctor" can morph into this chapter titled "some thoughts on the future." While there is an overlap between these two topics, I've chosen to define each one independently. The reason is that what might be next, could or might overlap in the future, yet some of these are merely ideas. The previous chapter focused on some details that can be used to achieve the goals of Architectural Medicine and the Architectural Doctor for health and wellness in the built environment. This chapter includes topics that may or may not be next steps, yet possible as eventual goals in the trajectory of a future focused on health and wellness.

In this chapter, I'd like to dive into some of these ideas and provide some possibilities of what the future can hold, specifically oriented towards wellness in the built environment as well as the health and wellness of our planet.

After all, as there are active discussions about traveling outside of our oblate spheroid, we call Earth, what types of built environments will be created outside of this planet? What kinds of topics are going to be important to discuss if and when we travel to outer space? And what types of built environments are we going to need to create to visit and potentially live on other planets? But more importantly, how can we provide built environments on this planet before confidently leaving to explore other exoplanets?

To be fair and honest, if you know anything about topics related to "space architecture" or outer space travel, you already know this topic is being addressed and is not new. In fact, there are educational programs and professional designers and architects that are already working on these solutions and have been for decades. So, while the subject is not new, public awareness of these topics might be new for many.

To be clear, I'm not going to get into details on space travel or the architecture on other planets. What I will plan to discuss is the importance of thinking about these topics and how they can introduce deeper thoughts into architecture on planet Earth.

A Failed Experiment Is Not a Failure

And this brings up the topic that is a reflection of this statement, which is to say again that some of the topics of future architecture and the architecture of space are not new.

However, it does bring up a topic that I believe has been misrepresented, especially by those in the general public.

In the late 1980s and 90s, an experiment was held that I believe does not have enough attention paid to the results. And that topic is the Biosphere 2 experiment, held in the state of Arizona in the United States. According to the article in Science News titled *Brave New World of Biosphere 2* by Dan Vergano, "constructed between 1987 and 1991, Biosphere 2 was originally meant to demonstrate the viability of closed ecological systems to support and maintain human life in outer space."[270]

I recall this project quite succinctly, as it was for me of great interest. In the late 90s, I actually traveled to Oracle, Arizona, to visit this site. Mainly, my travel to this location was of interest due to the architectural experiment, yet some years later, I realized it was an even bigger project than I first realized.

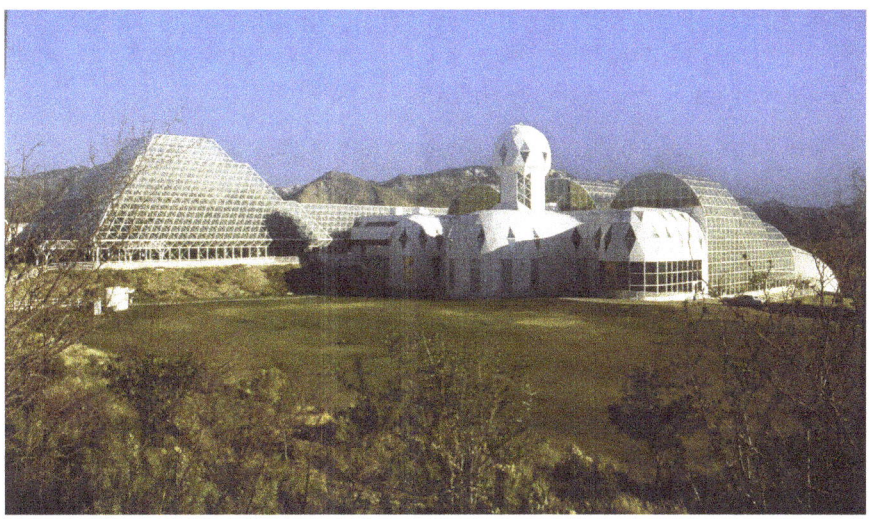

Biosphere 2 – Oracle, Arizona 1998. Photo by author

The premise of Biosphere 2 was to emulate Biosphere I — the Earth. And in this realm, the project was both a failure and a success.

I recall this topic because our family had discussions about this during dinners in the late 80s and early 90s, when this was discussed on the news and written about in the papers all those years ago. And my father, in particular, commented that it was a big failure.

On the other hand, I had thoughts of this as a big success in terms of the architectural achievements and what was being explored, as was never before attempted on this scale.

Many saw this as a failure based on the fact that, after only a short few years, the original team had to leave the premises, which was seen as a failure.

There were several issues that led to the perceived failure, from the experimental experience to the business side of the venture. As stated on Wikipedia, "Biosphere 2 was only used twice for its original intended purposes as a closed-system experiment: once from 1991 to 1993, and the second time from March to September 1994. Both attempts, though heavily publicized, ran into problems including low amounts of food and oxygen, die-offs of many animals and plants included in the experiment, group dynamic tensions among the resident crew, and outside politics and a power struggle over management and direction of the project."[271]

Yet years later, I did recognize that my father was correct, yet also incorrect, in the assessment of this venture. And this was based on the premise of the experiment itself. The experiment did not prove a disappointment because those who entered the experiment had to leave due to the above mentioned reasons. Instead, the experiment was a tremendous success in proving how valuable the planet, or Biosphere I, really is.

What I'm stating is that in the few times humans have tried to emulate the processes of nature, they have not succeeded. And this does not show a failure in my mind, as much as it shows how incredibly sophisticated and complex the natural world really is.

If you still think that nature is primitive, then all you must do is simply view the Biosphere 2 experiment to see how untrue this is. If you take the time to review this experiment, you will find that millions of dollars were spent to emulate the systems and functions of the planet. A large team of very intelligent and capable people were involved in the design and implementation of this project.

No, this was not a failure. It was a successful display of how complex and sophisticated the natural ecological systems on this planet really are.

Instead of seeing these experiments in negative terms, we should instead, in my opinion, recognize the amazing qualities of this planet and have reverence for the natural ecological systems we call planet Earth.

Instead of seeing this as a way to verify the tremendous sophistication and value of the natural systems of the planet, many humans merely see these experiments as failures. Yet the real failure is the inability to recognize and learn how valuable the planetary systems of nature are. And instead of seeing how valuable the planet is and how difficult it is to replace, most instead focus on these experiments as lacking success.

The best results we can recognize are how valuable the natural world is and how irreplaceable it is. This, to me, would be recognizing these experiments as being successful, if only to show the value of Nature.

Looking Backward – Moving Forward

Using the Biosphere 2 experiment as a valuable expression of the worth of the planet, it can place a human mindset of reverence for what we have and take measures to ensure that we protect this valuable commodity. Of course, it's not a commodity, yet in today's world, if you don't talk in this manner, then many who are making decisions for us all often have no interest in conservation and preservation.

No amount of money can replace nature, and if this is not learned – and quickly at that – the end result will be catastrophic.

While the above comment is dystopic, what can be taken from this is the opposite, which is to say that if we can revere the planet's natural systems, and take care of them, then the results will be beyond what any money could ever provide.

The Need for More Experiments in the Built Environment for Better Health and Wellness

And that brings up one of the key problems with buildings, which is that they last a long time, or perhaps should last a long time. However, with the expenses and longevity of buildings, few choose to make decisions on unproven materials or methods. And so that means that more buildings are built in the common format, and fewer experiments are done to strive for better solutions.

This provides a cyclical problem that does not have any ending, and so we continue to build in ways that provide limited solutions to these issues. As I've mentioned in other segments of this book, this cyclical process can be represented by a spiracycle, in that it is either spiraling up in a positive format or downward in a destructive format.

The Biosphere 2 experiment was an extremely important experiment to undertake, because it challenged not only the building methodologies and systems that are required to provide these "biosphere" conditions, yet it provided processes to measure and evaluate over time.

It is my sincere hope that many of the universities, governments and a wide range of businesses can work together in earnest to explore and experiment with newer approaches or refine current and previous methodologies that can help provide solutions to these problems.

This includes the study and research to find newer materials and methods, as well as to optimize our current materials and methods for a future that can reduce the negative impacts on the environment, increase our energy efficiency, and provide these materials and methods to promote and support better health.

Without these approaches to support these solutions, it will be even more challenging to provide the confidence that many others will make when they choose remediations and newer building projects.

This is a big mistake, in my honest opinion, as we cannot expect changes by not making changes. And with building projects costing so much to begin with, who is going to start making these big changes that can help to reduce our negative impacts on the planet, people, and the many life forms that share this planet with us?

True WHealth

It may be hard to fathom this statement, as money can provide so much for people, yet the reality is that money will have no value at all without the support of the planet's health and wellness.

You can have billions or trillions, yet none of this will have any meaning at all without a healthy planet that provides a healthy ecological system. Even if you could build another Biosphere, for example, Biosphere 3, or perhaps leave this planet to Mars or an exoplanet, the fact is that we don't know of any other planet that can provide the "whealth" that this planet provides right now.

A portmanteau of *wealth* and *health*, the term *whealth* can be a reminder of what is valuable in life – good health.

Sure, perhaps we can find an exoplanet in the future that we can venture to and explore. In fact, I think this is a wonderful prospect that future generations can look forward to. However, if it means we have to leave this planet right now or even in the near future, how will we get there? We have just started our explorations into space, and even if we could travel to another planet, Mars would be the only option right now based on the amount of time it would take to travel as well as the potential for a livable scenario.

And that would mean that it would take seven to nine months to arrive to the planet Mars. And according to NASA, this seven to nine months is if we were to launch from Earth at the proper time that the Mars orbit would be in alignment based on the travel trajectory.[272][273]

Not only would it take this long to get there, but on arrival, we'd have to create an entire ecological system that does not exist there right now. This is no small task and is even questionable to be able to achieve with our current technological capabilities. After all, even with all of the resources to create Biosphere 2 on planet Earth, none of these resources currently exist on Mars. And if we cannot reproduce the biosphere here on planet earth, to do so on another planet without any of the resources we already have here is quite a bit of wishful thinking.

> "It is no measure of health to be well adjusted to a profoundly sick society."[274] — Jiddu Krishnamurti

As Krishnamurti stated, conforming to a sick society is itself an unhealthy process, and as humans have created and developed magnificent accomplishments, if they are not supporting the health of the planet and society, then it would be wise to contemplate these developments.

The incredible architect Nader Khalili did provide a genius building process called superadobe, which can provide the development of structures using long bags that can be filled with sand-like materials, of which Mars consists of. And these long sandbags, filled up and layered in horizontal rows to create a building, are only a facet of the building process that would be required.

As posted on the California Institute of Earth Art and Architecture (CalEarth) website, the organization was founded by Khalili in 1991, and his work spans several decades with the following listing some of Khalili's achievements: [275]

> "In 1984, Lunar and Space habitation became an integral part of his work. He presented his "Magma Structures" design, based on Geltaftan System, and "Velcro-Adobe" system (later to become Superadobe) at the 1984 NASA symposium, "Lunar Bases and Space Activities of the 21st Century." He was subsequently invited to Los Alamos National Laboratory as a visiting scientist. Starting in 1984, he presented papers and was published in several symposiums and publications including those of NASA, and the "Journal of Aerospace Engineering" for which he was awarded by the American Society of Civil Engineers. Khalili was a member of the team of "Lunar Resources Processing Project," along with the Princeton based Space Studies Institute, McDonnell Douglas Space Systems, and Alcoa."[276]

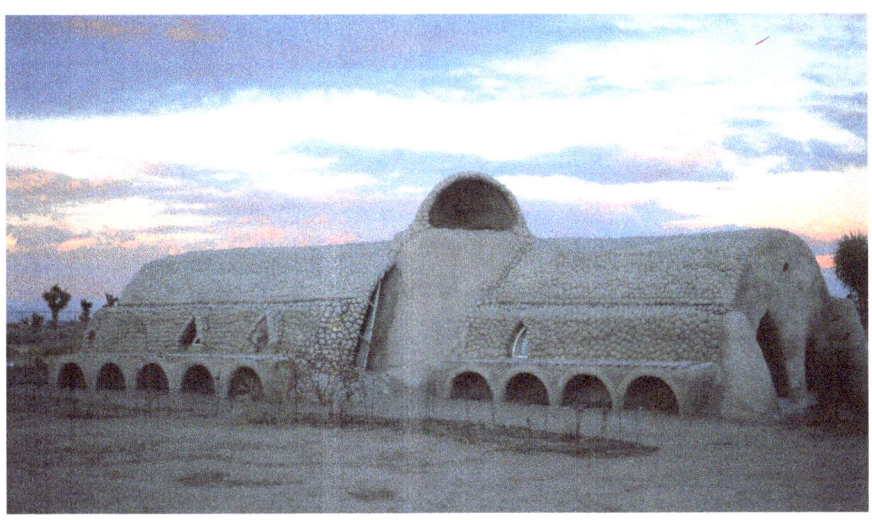

CalEarth SuperAdobe – California 1999. Photo by author

I had the great fortune to meet Nader Khalili in 2000 with two of my friends and colleagues, Bosco Büeler and Mary Cordaro. And after meeting him and visiting CalEarth, I quickly found inspiration in his work and mindset. As is posted on the CalEarth website, "Rumi, the Persian language mystic poet, was the inspiration behind Khalili's work for his wisdom concerning humanity and the elements of Earth, Water, Air, and Fire."[277]

I'd say his mindset and heart were akin to those inspiring souls such as Buckminster Fuller and Gandhi. His architecture can be seen as practical idealism in his autobiographical comment:[278]

> "Is it really sane to follow one's ideals and dreams and race alone in today's world?...
>
> Midway in my life I stopped racing with others. I picked up my dreams and started a gentle walk...
>
> I touched my dreams in reality by racing and competing with no one but myself."
>
> — Nader Khalili

While those such as Nader Khalili have visions of humans living on exoplanets successfully, I do think that the wisdom of Buckminster Fuller and Nader Khalili originates in humans seeking these exoplanets as an exploration, and not based on an urgency to find a new planet as a new home.

Obviously, these are my words and not theirs, so please note this appropriately. I still believe they would echo these sentiments equally with the determination to find solutions here on planet earth before needing or being forced to find another planet for survival.

The fact remains that on planet earth, nature is the most advanced technology, and our current technology is still no match for what Nature can provide.

Unfortunately, many humans disagree or haven't thought this through, and as a result, they do not take the care and consideration necessary to keep nature in the balance right now. Instead, in human's egotistical state, many disobey the laws of nature and do so with the premise that they are above the natural laws of this planet. As we should have all learned from the failures of the Biosphere 2 experiments, there is no other Biosphere I, and Biosphere 3 does not exist.

As such, we need to ensure that we take care of Biosphere I as global citizens and recognize the importance of conserving that which we already have.

Unfortunately, we are witnessing and have historically witnessed what happens when humans and political movements disobey the natural laws and venture beyond the common day law of life on planet Earth. The result of this is the unnecessary suffering of fellow humans and the many other creatures that inhabit this planet along with humanity.

The Global Citizen and Global Citizenship

Obviously, this book is focused on health and wellness in the built environment, yet to ignore the topics of health and wellness on a planetary level is to ignore the big picture. And as stated throughout this book and the *Architectural Medicine* book, you cannot separate the topics of health in buildings from the topics of sustainability and the energy topics of green building. These all relate to the health of the environment, as well as the built environment.

The DNA of Cities is created from the DNA of a single structure, and as such, the individual building's impact on the surrounding environment needs to be factored into this big picture equation.

So, what this means is that the future of health in the built environment requires consideration of the health of the ecological systems, otherwise, the built environment cannot exist. At least it cannot exist in a healthy format.

And so, what is required is a mindset that considers planetary health, which in turn requires an overview of the entire planet. This means that one needs to be acting locally, yet considering the entire globe in one's actions. This can be defined as a *global citizen*, and as such, means that the local mentality is transformed to embrace the global mindset.

This is not easy for many humans to achieve, as we can see over the past several centuries of war between locals around the world. The global citizen is not something that will happen overnight, but that said, it is required for us as humanity to move forward. And just to be clear and not to be overly pessimistic, the natural world does not depend upon humanity to survive. In time if we do not recognize the laws of nature, we will no longer be welcomed here, and nature can easily achieve this: [279]

> "Nature is trying very hard to make us succeed, but nature does not depend on us. We are not the only experiment."[280]
>
> — R. Buckminster Fuller

And if this is too depressing, then this should at least encourage humans to make changes, because not only would we as humans be eliminated, but most other sentient beings on this planet would go extinct as well.

And ask yourself this question. Is this fair for all other sentient beings to endure this detriment because human animals chose to do so?

Again, not to be pessimistic and dark, yet don't you think this is an unfair scenario to create for all humans and all sentient beings?

A global citizen is one who is concerned about the health of the planet and all of its sentient beings. Even if you're not going to go out and hug and have as pets those creatures that may be harmful to humans, that is very different than recognizing that they live on this planet too and deserve to have what the planet has provided to them all.

Whether it be a furry, friendly fox or a venomous creature dangerous to humans, it is not our choice to make as to what exists on this planet. We can certainly create built environments that protect us from nature's elements.

We can also protect ourselves from the creatures that may cause us harm, yet to eliminate all of these creatures by destroying the very nature of the planet's ecological systems is neither wise nor a sign of an intelligent animal as so-called humans.

We all have a choice, and that choice can be to provide a healthy environment in which all creatures on this planet can exist within, or we can choose to not change and not alter our ways and suffer the consequences. In turn, this will also negatively impact all other creatures on this planet.

This mindset of thriving cannot include this form of destructive behavior at the same time. And so, as mentioned throughout this book, the premise of Architectural Medicine and the Architectural Doctor is to provide a thriving environment, mostly focused on the built environment, yet factoring into the equation the health of the entire planet. There is no other planet.

I wanted to select one of the following quotes to evoke the sentiment of important topics of the global citizen, yet I found the best quote was several of them together. Perhaps a reflection of this book and my thinking that many facets working together achieve a cohesive solution.

The following quotes, to me, seem even more prescient than when Buckminster Fuller stated them many decades ago:[281]

Chapter: 18 — Some Thoughts on the Future

"Man now enters the phase of meager yet conscious participation in the anticipatory design undertakings of nature. This conscious participation itself is changing from an awkward, arbitrary, trial and error ignorance to an intuitively conceived, yet rigorously serviced, disciplined elegance..."

"Pollution is nothing but the resources we are not harvesting. We allow them to disperse because we've been ignorant of their value."

"We are now entered into Earthian's most critical moment, that of imminent, technically feasible economic success for all humanity. This however, is frustrated by the large and prosperous minority's fearful procrastination at the entrance into the unknown, epochal changes, obviously essential to realization of comprehensive human success and total planetary freedoms and enjoyment."

"Never forget that you are one of a kind. Never forget that if there weren't any need for you in all your uniqueness to be on this earth, you wouldn't be here in the first place. And never forget, no matter how overwhelming life's challenges and problems seem to be, that one person can make a difference in the world. In fact, it is always because of one person that all the changes that matter in the world come about. So be that one person. "

"To make the world work for 100% of humanity in the shortest possible time through spontaneous cooperation without ecological damage or disadvantage to anyone."

Outer Space and Inner Space – Why a Focus on Mindfulness?

While the global citizen approach can help to provide a better mindset for global health, much of this begins with the individual. And while humanity is just now beginning to set its sights into outer space and the potential for traveling to other worlds, there is no time better than now to focus on "inner space."

What's meant by this is that, while William Shatner's character Captain James T. Kirk, is renowned for his statement "where no man has gone before," there is another facet of this statement that must also be addressed. The full quote, updated after the initial series, spoken by Sir Patrick Stewart as Captain Jean-Luc Picard at the beginning of each episode, is as follows:

> "Space: the final frontier. These are the voyages of the starship Enterprise. Its continuing mission: to explore strange new worlds. To seek out new life and new civilizations. To boldly go where no one has gone before!"[282]

And what does any of this have to do with the Architectural Doctor and Architectural Medicine?

If the global citizen is to explore space as in outer space, then what's required for this to be achieved in an honest and healthy manner is to ensure that "inner space" is also explored.

This is not just about the inner spaces as architecture, but also the inner spaces of humans. The frontier of emotional and psychological space, in terms of mindfulness and being aware and honest with our inside processes, can have a tremendous impact on how we create or destroy our external environments.

Whether this is the external environments on this planet or the many external spaces and places that we may venture into "outer space." As Socrates is known for stating, "to know thyself is the beginning of wisdom"[283] and "the unexamined life is not worth living,"[284] each of these quotes provides deep insights into internal and inner development and wisdom.

If we are to have true health and wellness in our spaces, either inner or outer, there must be awareness and mindfulness of how our actions impact ourselves and all the other creatures and beings that we exist with. And this wisdom includes not only our stewardship of this planet, but the way in which we will impact all the many beings that we might eventually meet in outer space.

This diving into personal psychology is critical for both personal health, as well as planetary health. And as a global citizen, this approach to personal responsibility requires that we think in both the big picture views of our life on planet Earth, as well as our internal processes towards wellness.

For if we do not address and accept this responsibility for personal health, then when we venture outside of this planet, we may not do so with the intention of caring for the other beings that exist external to our planet. And this is neither a healthy nor responsible approach to living. With the advent of human developments in technology that have increased capabilities for large impacts on the planet, this requires a responsibility that everyone will need to consider into the future. Ensuring that technological advancements are balanced with personal mindfulness in how these technologies are utilized is critical.

The Architectural Doctor Conclusion – Final Thoughts on a Realistic, Honest, Yet Hopeful Future

This last section of the book has been a bit gloomier and, as such, perhaps requires more personal reflection on serious topics. Yet it's not meant to infer a lack of positivity or good vibes toward a utopic future.

In these words, I hear my father's viewpoints, which is to state that I'm being honest with the current scenario, even if dark and depressing. Yet I also hear my mother's voice, stating there is hope if we are honest with our current scenario and take necessary steps for positive change.

Both my father and mother taught me lessons and a way of looking at life that I've pondered during my lifetime, and these thoughts have continued beyond their time on this planet.

It is my hope that my words may provide some solace and pondering for others, as my parents' words have provided for me. While I don't have children, I care a lot about this planet, sometimes to a fault. But if this is a fault of mine, then I happily embrace this fault of myself.

It is my hope that we can wake up to become more aware of these problems and be more adept at facing these challenging problems for what they are — problems that have solutions.

In having this mindset for myself, I have been provided the lessons from my father to view the truth in honesty, even if negative, dystopic, and survival based. And yet I also see the potential of thriving for humanity through the eyes of my mother.

My mother reminded me, through her actions in supporting my dreams and visions, oftentimes without words, that there is hope. It is my hope that the future of humanity, through the silent but powerful words of architecture and designs of the built environment, may also provide effective support for human thriving.

May this book find you on this journey of an honest and hopeful future, where human thriving may be a focus and goal. And just as my mother supported me, it is my hope that mother earth, in providing for her the proper care and attention, can support humanity's thriving.

Timothy D. Rossi

Chapter: 18 Some Thoughts on the Future

"We each pay a fabulous price for our visions of paradise, but a spirit with a vision is a dream with a mission."

— **Neil Peart**

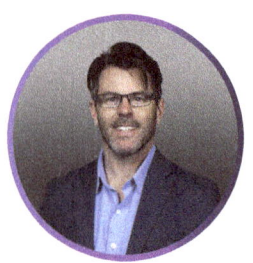

ABOUT THE AUTHOR

My journey through life has brought me on many paths. From my early childhood days to my adult years, as I've viewed my life in retrospect, there has been a strong element of opposites. My childhood home was located in the suburbs of Long Island, just 15 minutes away from the origins of suburbia — Levittown, New York. Growing up between one of the biggest cities in the world, New York City, and the rural, natural environments spent during summers at my grandmother's house, provided me with a wide range of scenarios and environments to experience in my early and formative years. This juxtaposition of nature and the built environment was very dynamic, and the older I become, the more I see the importance of finding a balance between these two worlds.

Another example of this apposition was growing up a mile away from Walt Whitman's home, which is across the street from one of the biggest malls in the metro NY region, the Walt Whitman mall. I've often thought of what Whitman, this great poet of nature, would have thought of this scenario.

An antithesis of "Leaves of Grass," the poetry of nature, sucked away by asphalt and the glistening, shiny materiality of commerce. This is not to say that commerce is negative, but in contrast to the poetry of Whitman's world of nature, the world I grew up experiencing as a young person was quite the contradiction to Whitman's literature as art.

I also grew up near the famous Cold Spring Harbor Laboratory, "one of a handful of institutions that played a central role in the development of molecular genetics and molecular biology."[285] And just down the road from Cold Spring Harbor is the town of Greenlawn, often stated as the origin of planned obsolescence. Eastern Long Island is also the home of the famous Wardenclyffe, a structure built by Tesla to experiment with global wireless communications.

This wide range of urban, rural, and suburban exposures, with bustling businesses combined with the natural beauty of New York, brought up many questions about experiencing these different worlds.

A Note About This Segment of the Book

This section about myself is a bit long for a reason, and I'd like to take a moment to comment on this. During the editing of this book, it became apparent that many comments that I was making in the book relating to the origins of the Architectural Doctor and my story of these experiences through the years did not seem to fit into the chapters in which they were initially written. I have worked to keep the book professional, yet also personal in terms of these topics being meaningful to me in my life. This work has been a lifelong process, and while the book is focused on the professional processes, I also think it's important for people to tell their story. This story is an important part of my life, and as such, I didn't want to leave it out of this book relating to the content for context.

So, as I was editing the book, I recognized that it might be better to remove them from the parts of the introduction or in chapters throughout the book, and instead place them in this section as part of the story of the Architectural Doctor. I also realized that I could define the parameters of how long this segment would be, and as such, I have decided to leave in some of these extended details as part of my professional and personal timeline.

In commenting about the extended length, I've decided to just call it what it is and recognize this as a reality of my journey. While it increases the page length in a perhaps, verbose fashion, I have added this writing as an important part of my life's journey. The guidelines of this about page may be unorthodox, yet perhaps this is fitting as my journey in the development of these topics can reflect my unusual path.

The Influence of Human Developments and Nature's Role as Part of My Story

Spending my summers in rural Long Island, surrounded by nature and spending most of my time by myself, was another facet of development which was more introspective. The population of this small town, with only several hundred people, few of them children, led to a contemplative quality of my life growing up during the summertime. This was in strong contrast with the larger populations of people in the suburban and urban environments that I experienced during the rest of the year.

These dichotomies of time and place were in contradiction to each other in many ways, from the poetic words of Whitman and the natural worlds of ecology to the marvels of genetics and the complicated wonders of the architecture and skyscrapers of New York.

I grew up, literally, between the worlds of nature and the "Big Apple" of these skyscrapers of concrete and steel.

These worlds of opposites brought up many contemplative moments in my life, and have led to a life filled with questioning. My inquisitiveness was either embraced by those I was around or rejected as too much thinking. Yet the older I became, the more relevant these questions came to be in my professional and personal life. Over the years, it has merged into a striving for balance, and a process of defining how this balance can be achieved.

I grew up wanting to be an architect since a young child, and I spent many of my younger days building and making things with whatever I could find in which to build.

After studying architectural engineering in college, I went into the building and construction fields (AEC) and learned a tremendous amount of "on the job" training that information in textbooks could not provide.

However, it was also a window into a world of building that I felt was unhealthy in both materials and methods, and had little focus on ecological awareness nor energy efficiency, not to mention health. But perhaps even more influential was my interest in architecture as a nurturing component for humanity instead of just the colossal expressions of human ego and exponential development.

I had always felt the impacts of the built environment, and as someone who was sensitive to these often harsh environments, I could not understand how others in construction could constantly be around the toxic substances and materials used to build these structures. As time went on, I learned that my sensitivity to these environments was a positive facet of my life, and it provided me with greater insights into how the built environment impacts human health and well-being. This, in turn, has been a reflection of my own reflections of this world of construction and the lack of empathy and compassion that is sometimes seen in the building and healthcare fields. If these ideas, words, systems, and developments can create a more harmonious, healing, and healthier built environment for others in the world for wellness, then I view this work as a great success.

A lot of the ideas as seeds of Architectural Medicine began in the early 90s for me, yet I didn't know it at the time. The question of how my journey would unfold and develop took decades to evolve into an interconnected whole.

In my early to late 20s, I was involved in the fields of architecture and health in very nontraditional formats. During my early 20s, I spent several years working at a health center, learning about traditional methodologies of health and wellness, often focused on the whole person and not just the human as a conglomeration of parts and pieces put together like a car. During this time, I learned of the many centuries-old methodologies and traditions still practiced all around the world today. It was also the beginning of big changes in the field of medicine, and today, these changes have become known as Integrative Medicine. These experiences inspired and provided a baseline for reference to the creation and development in what I've defined as Integrative Architecture.

This health center provided a tremendous education on eastern thoughts involving body-mind connections, including traditional Chinese medicine (TCM), and traditional Indian medicine (TIM) Ayurveda, which remain some of the most ancient living traditions for health. These discoveries about health consist of all facets of one's life, including architecture and both the built environment and the importance of connections with the natural world. This included education about natural foods and the many healing modalities that have become more commonplace in today's 21st century.

Applying these principles of viewing the whole person, and implementing modalities such as yoga, meditation, tai chi, chi gong, and the benefits of traditional medicinals, provided insights into the whole person and seeing the whole picture. This education provided an understanding of whole system solutions and expanded my view of how the built environment impacts health. All of these subjects expanded my range of knowledge on physiology, and the connection with the natural and built environments. This experience planted the seeds of explorations between physiology, psychology, and the built environment and eventually built into the ideas of Architectural Medicine and the Architectural Doctor.

One of the benefits of working at this health center was that I learned about a conference that was held in New York City in 1993, which I jumped on the opportunity to attend. The event, called the Eco-Design Conference, was filled with pioneers in the green, sustainable, and healthy building fields. From James Wines and William McDonough to Paul Bierman-Lytle, Mary Cordaro, and Katherine Metz, it was a who's who before they were known in these emerging fields. It was a tremendous learning experience and influential in my path toward weaving together many concepts and topics into, hopefully, a cohesive whole. Each of these teachers provided a piece of the big jigsaw puzzle to form a cohesive whole in supporting more energy-efficient, environmentally friendly, and healthy built environments.

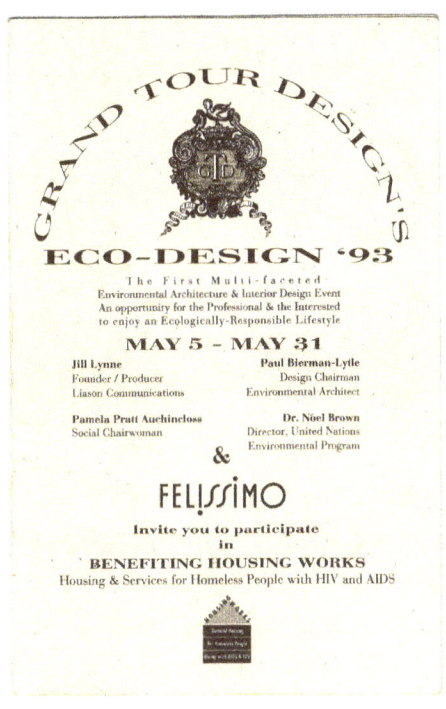

The Eco-Design Conference, New York City – 1993

In retrospect, it's probably not so strange that Architectural Medicine came into being, with a lifetime surrounded by visions of architecture, attending architecture school, a young adult life in construction, and several years working at a health center in my 20s.

In the mid-90s, I began my journey back into the fields of architecture, building, and construction when I attended the inaugural sustainable building course at the Yestermorrow design/build school in the summer of 1995. This, combined with attending the Yestermorrow professional design/build program, led to my learning about many of the hands-on processes of sustainable building in a professional context. It was the first time in my adult life that I was surrounded by others seeking solutions of this nature, and interested in the world of building.

It was also my introduction to James Hubble, an amazing soul whose

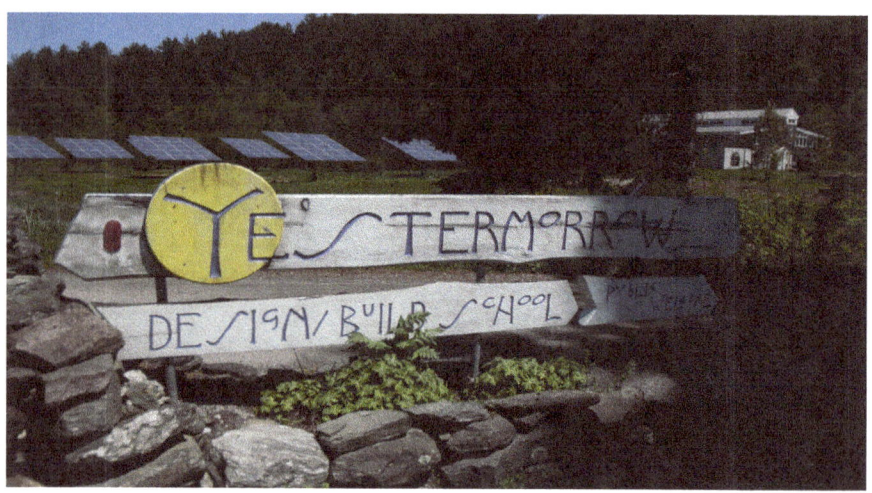

Yestermorrow Design/Build School, Vermont – 2010. Photo by author

"architecture as poetry" is embedded into his buildings. I was so inspired by his course "soil and soul" at Yestermorrow that I attended his organic architecture course that same summer held in Mexico and southern California. This is where I first had hands-on experience with organic architecture and topics such as permaculture, taught by James Hubble, Bill Roley, and Penny Livingston. That summer's experience included the architectural wisdom of Kyle Bergman, the creator of the well-known Architecture & Design Film Festival (ADFF), who taught this course alongside James Hubble.

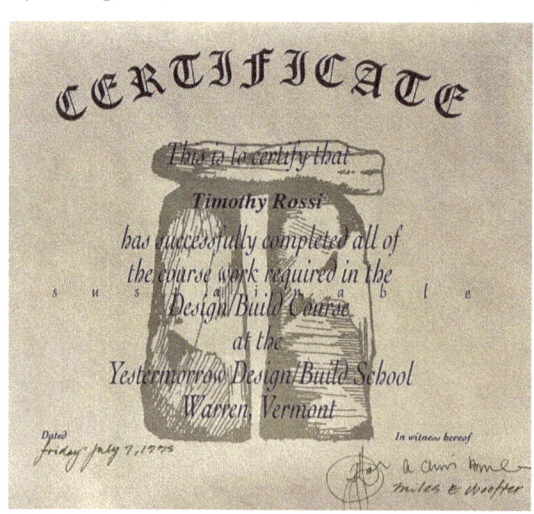

Certificate of author's attendance at the Inaugural Sustainable Design/Build Course at Yestermorrow – 1995

James Hubble's focus on "architecture for the soul" provided an education on the importance of landscape architecture as an integral part of the entire built environment. His ideas supported my initial beliefs on this topic as an architecture student, and

Mr. Hubble's spirit kept my flame of interest alive. After not finding this in my architecture studies and work in the construction fields, his enthusiasm and interest in the many facets of the human experience rekindled my own interest in this pathway in architecture.

After this '95 summer's experience, I began taking the German Bau Biologie (Building Biology) course after revisiting this topic during that summer, which I originally learned from the '93 event in NYC. Originally, the course was transcribed by Helmet Ziehe and brought to the USA. The content was taught as a distance learning course with several in person classes. Several years ago, the main location in Germany, the IBN – Institut für Baubiologie + Nachhaltigkeit, began to provide an English version of the course, yet before this was established, the US version provided by Helmet was the main source of this content. The course provided a deeper look into how buildings impact the ecology and biological health, and connected me to many consultants in the United States striving to provide healthier built environments.

I then had the unique opportunity to work in Arizona with the architect Paolo Soleri, a student of Frank Lloyd Wright. Mr. Soleri's designs and writings were inspirational, and I immersed myself in his concepts for a future more in alignment with the natural world, while embracing the technological capabilities of humanity. It was a time when I recognized the value of dreaming big, and while I worked at Soleri's residence and workplace of Cosanti, his visions of a city called Arcosanti were in full experimental mode just north of Phoenix.

Later that year, I had the chance to learn and work with a group of natural building experts led by the mastery of Cedar Rose Guelberth. I didn't hesitate at the opportunity to work with her and her amazing team in Carbondale, Colorado. The hands-on experiences utilizing timber frame, straw bale building, earthen floors, and natural plasters was invaluable. I was also fortunate to attend Cedar Rose's teachings during her workshops at the Solar Energy Institute (SEI), as it provided access to courses on passive and active solar energy. This exposure to multiple concepts being developed in the natural, sustainable, and green building fields set a strong foundation for my knowledge of these topics. While many of these subjects today have become more commonplace and important in creating sustainable solutions in the built environment, at the time, they were considered very strange materials and methods and foreign to many in the fields of architecture and construction.

It was here that I attended the first ever "Building for Health" conference, held in Aspen, Colorado, which was a great privilege. It was the first time meeting pioneers Paula Baker-Laporte and Carol Venolia. This set the foundation for focusing on health in the built environment and led me on a journey on this topic that has continued to this day.

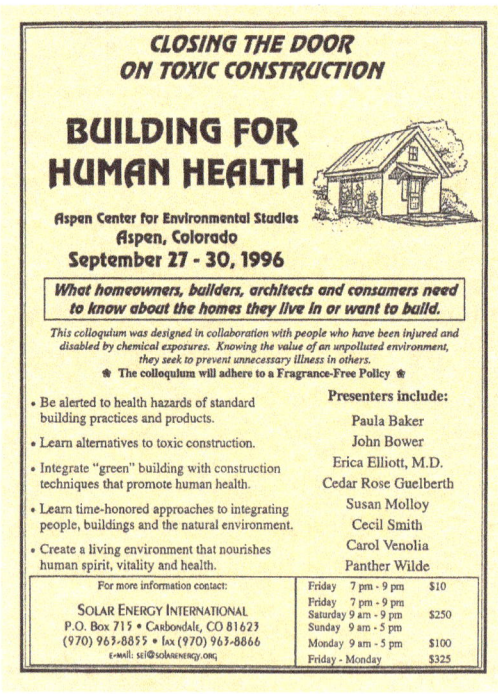

The Building for Human Health Conference, Colorado – 1996

Years later, I learned it was the first time Paula presented, and while her name may not be familiar, if you know anything about healthy building, you know she wrote one of the best books providing solutions for health in the built environment titled *Prescriptions for a Healthy House.*

A few years later, during a trip to Europe to learn more about Bau Biologie facilitated by Helmet Ziehe, I first met the architect, engineer, and bau biologist in Switzerland, Bosco Büeler. He became an important mentor and has been a good friend to this day. It was on this trip that I reconnected with Mary Cordaro, a teacher at the initial Eco-Design conference I attended in NYC in 1993. Soon after this meeting, we co-formed the company Integrated Environmental Solutions with a few other individuals striving to provide positive solutions in the built environment. We then merged with other professionals to form H3Environmental, providing education and training for professionals striving to create greener,

About the Author

more sustainable, and healthier built environments.

It was an enormously exciting time in my life, and while we might have been a bit ahead of the curve in terms of business timing, the lessons learned provided experiences beyond what I could have learned in any other format, both personally and professionally.

This experience led to working and learning from other great environmental consultants, such as the late Will Spates, and a great building inspector and mentor, Richard Scarborough, as well as meeting other influential professionals, such as Peter Sierk. The lessons learned during this time allowed me to recognize that business practices in this field needed more development, and I set out on another professional journey that has lasted to this very day.

From a process and a business standpoint, I recognized the value and benefits of technology, which at that time of the late 90s into the early 2000s, was focused on the internet, websites, and the emerging world of consumer technology. My visions for the company, Integrated Environmental Solutions and H3Environmental, included databases, applications, technological support, websites, and online training, all of which were either extremely expensive to provide or out of reach for the small or even medium-sized businesses at that time. To provide context, YouTube did not exist, and broadband was the exception, with dial-up still the modern form of internet connectivity.

My professional time in the first decade of the 2000s was focused on providing support to groups for green, sustainable, and healthy building solutions while immersed in learning about the worlds of technology, which most define today as Information Technology or the IT world.

In the mid-2000s, I began to reflect on my time traveling around the United States in the late 90s into the early 2000s, working and learning from pioneers in the healthy, green, and sustainable building worlds. I began to recognize the challenge of this concept of one person as a healthy building consultant and inspector to make changes in the built environment. This, combined with the huge amount of information and education required to be both professional and helpful, was enormous in scope. Having been directly involved in this work, I realized three important factors that, in my opinion, have led to much of the development of Architectural Medicine. The first was a lack of support in the architecture and building fields doing this work to investigate, inspect, and provide useful solutions to clients seeking healthier building environments. The second was the recognition that doctors and healthcare professionals have a limited understanding of the built environment in how buildings can impact patient health. The third was a complete lack of systems in place to help support those who were striving to provide information and consultations for these healthier building solutions.

The disconnect between the architecture and the medical fields added to this challenge, and without proper education and integration in how health is impacted by the built environment, it led to a lack of serious responses and an absence of working together within these two professions. In addition, almost all building inspectors are not trained nor educated to evaluate building issues related to human health. The average building inspector is trained and hired to provide structural inspections to ensure the structural integrity of the engineering aspects of the building. They provide limited focus on inspecting issues related to human health.

A big part of this work was realizing the amount of time spent educating and informing the client, who would often then strive for confirmation of this information from their architect, building professional or doctor and health professional. And often, these two professional groups did not know much about health in the built environment, so either the healthy building consultant was ignored, or the healthy building consultant would have to spend time educating and informing these professionals as well as the client. The amount of work to achieve this was a never-ending process, and eventually, many consultants would stop providing these helpful services.

The other major challenge is that the building and construction professionals often not wanting to change their use of materials and methods, even if it negatively impacts their own health in the construction process. In all fairness, these professionals have good reasons to be wary of changes, as they depend on materials and methods to both last and provide proven results.

So, the combination of those in the architecture and building trades not having much interest in healthy materials and designs, combined with the doctors and medical health professionals not having much knowledge of how the built environment impacts health, has left a large gap in the public's ability to receive and confirm these health topics in their built environments. In the late 90s, I was struggling to achieve these goals of healthier architecture. And while my past experiences showed the positive potential for these integrations, achieving them was a daunting task, if not a constant uphill battle.

During this time, I discussed these challenges with my mentor in Switzerland, architect Bosco Büeler. He advised me to recognize that often in life, you cannot simply go from point A directly to point Z to achieve your goals. His advice was to navigate life as in sailing, where you tack back and forth to get to a destination. And so began my journey in this tacking back and forth for the past 20-plus years.

In retrospect, this tacking back and forth from point to point not only provided a

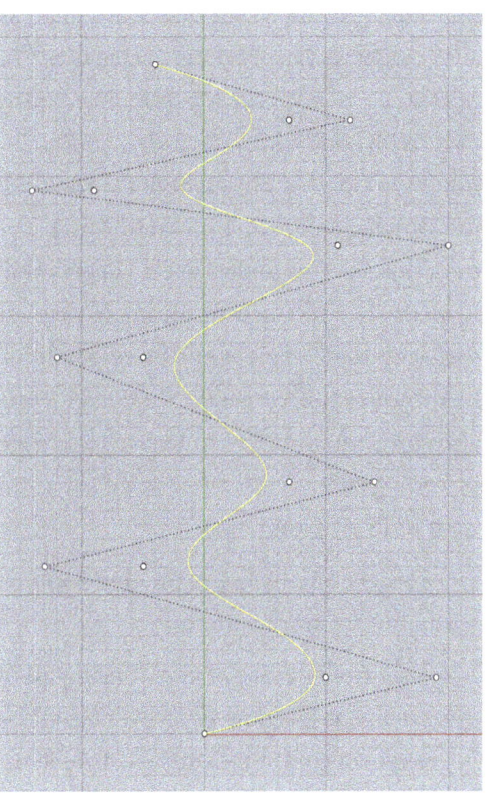

Control points creating a parametric form in Rhino3D emulating the patterns of tacking in sailing

wealth of knowledge from many fields, yet if I were to plot this pattern of sailing movements as multiple points into a CAD application, it would also actually create a parametric curving pattern. This, interestingly, mimics the parametric design focus of more nurturing forms and shapes that I discuss in chapter 16 as well as in the Architectural Medicine book.

Continuing With Goals and Staying the Course

My goal during this timeframe was to follow through on an idea I had when traveling cross country to learn more about these green, eco, healthy, sustainable modalities in building. In the late 90s, I was in Tucson, Arizona, on my way to attend a lime and natural plasters course in southern Arizona. On the way from my travels through Texas to Tucson, just nearby the airport on route 10, I saw a huge billboard of an inspector with a clipboard of some sort. A few weeks previous to this trip, I had spent time thinking about the next steps on my path. My thoughts of providing more interconnected solutions with technology were on my mind. As I viewed that billboard, it was at that moment that I thought of the idea called "The Electronic Clip Board or the Datalog software approach." Quite a mouth full, yet the concept was to have this electronic clip board that worked as software for a healthy building inspection, consultation, and database solution. It would incorporate all of the facets that I knew would be very helpful as I participated in this process of healthy building consulting and inspections. In my mind, this type of device and software solution would provide a process for inspecting, recording, and providing clients with valuable information that they could utilize to improve their built environments.

This eventually led to the development of ARxMD — the Architectural Medicine Software Solution.

After many years of considering all of the facets and then developing this system, it has now become a functioning software application that can be used on a computer and tablet, such as an iPad, instead of the electronic clipboard. I'm sure Steve Jobs and Apple are happy they used the iPad as a name and not the Electronic Clip Board.

There are a few reasons why it has taken so long for this to become a reality from those late 90s as my focus on healthy building became more palpable. As I began to surround myself with others involved and interested in this emerging field considering health and wellness in the built environment, it was the absence of systems that stood out as a gap that prevented a scaled-up version for these solutions.

Much of this process has been in an embryonic stage over several decades, yet as my mentor and friend Bosco put it, I have needed to tack from point to point to get to my destination. And in some ways, this is both a destination and a beginning. I state this because as I set out years prior to learn more about how to achieve the goals of these concepts that eventually became Architectural Medicine and the Architectural Doctor, it required a large range of multi-disciplinary topics I have had to learn and comprehend.

My initial vision was to see this training done through the internet and online learning, as well as developing databases of information utilizing video production to achieve all of this. Yet in 2000, when we began to approach this process, as I mentioned, YouTube was not even in existence, and video services, as well as internet bandwidth, were at a premium. As well, the ability to create software, databases, online learning and video production were all extremely expensive and out of reach for a small business.

The World of Information Technology

Fortunately, my experience through the 80s and 90s included computers and technology. In those days, I had the ability to learn to use computers, from the commodore 64 and the IBM PC to the use of the Macintosh SE in college. These early days of word processing, AutoCAD, and graphics, along with basic networking, set the stage for my role as CTO for both Integrated Environmental Solutions and H3Environmental. This set the foundation for work in the Information Technology world, and I have continued to navigate on this development path.

With an interest in developing more business computing solutions, after spending time with Bosco traveling with him during his presentations in the US, I decided to purchase the software he developed called the BauBio-DataBank. He created this to support a healthier and sustainable building approach for European professionals. Yet there were two big challenges in using this software in the USA. One was that it was based on mostly European materials, and the second was it was written mostly in German. While these challenges prevented common use in the USA, I learned the software and began my education in software and database development. These software developments provided the education that has led to the development of ARxMD.

It was a challenging time because the cost of software development was huge at that time, and the online world was still in its infancy. As well, the concept of the iPad and smartphone was still a concept, not a reality – at least not a usable reality. I was working with a laptop and a palm pilot, which was not quite at the development potential of the iPad and iPhone.

But this was the beginning of my process to create software and database solutions to support these integrative approaches, and moving forward, I provided software solutions to help individuals run a business and achieve their work. Back in those days, I wrote that software could "bridge the architecture and medical fields," yet I wasn't sure how it would unfold into the interoperability solutions available today. My work in IT has also provided the necessary skills to understand the complex code integrations and medical and building taxonomies for this interoperability to conform to the appropriate standards.

These developments were the origin of the Healthy Building Inspector and Building Informaticist concepts and developed into the foundation of the Architectural Doctor. It has come a long way, and I've put many, many years into the ways of how it would all function. There is still much work to be done, yet the foundation of these goals is in process.

While the journey has been long and challenging, I kept with it and learned a huge amount about software development, digital media, video production, database systems, coding, computers, technology, and the many facets of this digital frontier that we live in today.

However, technology was, for me, a tool to be utilized for a better way of life and a better quality of life to achieve. My deep roots in ecology and nature, merged with technological developments, reminded me of the quintessential purpose of creating a better world. Having a constant reminder of the importance of the health of the natural world has provided a good balance between technological development and the natural, ecological world. This ongoing balance ensures that these developments will not harm the very natural world that we depend upon for life. I write about the importance of this interconnected balance in the forthcoming book *Symbiosis Global – Nature is the Most Advanced Technology.*

Moving Forward With Purpose and Goals

When I began to focus on Architectural Medicine, I knew that if I didn't produce something of value in a production format, then the results might be ideal, yet not usable.

During this time, I began to think about the topic of a book, and so began my venture into the world of writing and publishing.

Fortunately, over the years, I have been learning many Adobe applications, starting with Illustrator, and Adobe PageMaker, along with the extinct GoLive for developing websites. I took courses at the original Lynda.com location in Ojai, California, and then began taking online courses in the early 2000s at Lynda.com. This became an online learning hub for an enormous number of professionals, which is now merged into LinkedIn learning.

Throughout the past 20 years, I've taken courses on everything digital, from photoshop, video editing, and production, to database and software development, along with a huge amount of IT courses that have provided extensive technical skills for my consulting work today. It provided a foundation to create the many facets of this work, from the Architectural Medicine website and the creation and publishing of these books to the ARxMD application and development.

After developing Architectural Medicine, it became clear that the Architectural Doctor was a critical part of this process. And as I was writing Architectural Medicine, I also began writing more robust sections detailing the Architectural Doctor. These two books go hand in hand, and it is my hope that they can both bring more clarity to these integrative approaches as well as "why" this is important and meaningful.

These writings and the projects that I've been working on recognize that nothing exists in a vacuum, and therefore the integration between other professions and fields is required, not just recommended. It is with this mindset and viewpoint that there are overlaps between many other fields that need to be included if a successful whole systems approach is to be developed. The goal is not to create another subfield of a field or to become a form of a separate entity, but instead to help provide a foundation as well as an umbrella to pull together many fields and, with wisdom, to support the goal of health and wellness in the built environment.

And so it is that overlap and integration between these fields are required to support and strengthen the role of the Architectural Doctor. It provides a supportive entity for both professions and offers a liaison between different groups to achieve these goals of health and wellness.

This, in turn, provides better quality of life, and that is what these writings, books, and projects are all about. To achieve the goal of optimum living, even if that definition may differ between people. While health and wellness as a goal can be achieved in many ways and can appear in different formats, there are similar core processes that can achieve these goals. And this is part of the focus of the Architectural Doctor and the aim of Architectural Medicine.

Big Life Moments and the Origins of Architectural Medicine

The late portion of the first decade of the 2000s found me in a challenging time personally, with the passing of my parents and an unknown professional future and direction. It was a time of deep soul-searching and contemplation in my life and led to a bit of a eureka moment in 2011. After spending time thinking about how to put together the many facets of my life that had occurred up until that time, the idea of Architectural Medicine came into vision and was born.

From that moment onwards, I began putting together 25-plus years of what might seem to be disparate facets of my life experiences in ways that would be integrated together. As a fabric of many concepts woven together into a tapestry of hopeful solutions and viewpoints, this became defined as Architectural Medicine.

About the Author

At first, I had no initial thought of writing books, as the ideas were more about utilizing previous concepts of training and education and putting that together. Yet once again, I took heed of a mentor Bosco Büeler's recommendations that in life, you need to sail back and forth from place to place instead of going in a simple, straight line. I recognized that I would once again need to zig-zag in motions to learn new topics, eventually becoming a curving path and gathering all of these concepts and forming them into a cohesive whole. In some ways, I can view these zig-zag paths as parametric pathways in my life. And just as curving materials often provide a stronger structure, I can view these curving, parametric pathways of learning as strengthening the structure of my ideas.

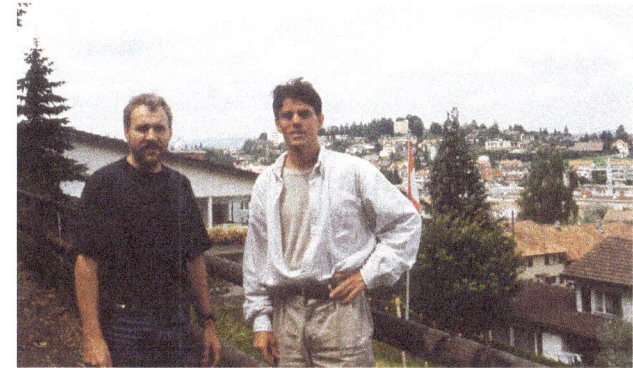

Bosco Büeler on left, with author on right – Switzerland 1998

The destination of Architectural Medicine is another point on this map, yet when I arrived at the goal and destination of achieving this initial step, it soon became clear that writing books along with developing the software I had thought about all those years ago were the best route.

Some Great Experiences of My Journey

My experiences have led me on a journey of both highs and lows. Part of those high points was during the fall and winter of 1999. I was traveling with Bosco Büeler while he was teaching courses and providing talks here in the United States.

We met in Los Angeles and then traveled up the coast to San Francisco, where I met up with my friend Christi Graham, who had set up Bosco to talk at an ADPSR meeting.

If you aren't aware of the ADPSR group – Architects, Designers, and

Developers for Social Responsibility – I highly recommend you find them online and review some of the great work they have been doing for decades:

https://www.adpsr.org/

This was my introduction to tremendous leaders in the eco, green, and healthy building fields in northern California and on the west coast, who have been at the forefront of these progressive building developments for decades. A huge benefit of my exposure to these topics has been the ability to see the big picture and recognize the importance of cohesive solutions. This understanding provided the foundation of the concept I discuss in chapter 4 focused on Integrative Architecture. As this chapter was only a brief summary of this topic and it is an important issue by itself, I plan to publish the book Integrative Architecture in the near future.

A Positive and Hopeful View of the Future

During the past 20-plus years, I have spent my time working in the worlds of IT while providing solutions for the green, sustainable, and healthy built environment, in tandem. This path has led to the writings of this book, as well as the Architectural Medicine book and the ARxMD software development and offerings.

It is my intention to continue to provide resources and value-added solutions for these developments, and to contribute to a better world in which I hope to co-create. With this intention, it is my hope that these resources may provide value for you on your journey. It is my wish that by working together in collaboration, humanity can benefit from creating and living in healthier built environments for wellness, well-being, and a better quality of life.

Thank you for your interest in these topics and in co-creating a better future.

Best wishes to you on your journey in this realm,

Tim

About the Author

Chapter Quote Citations

Chapter 1: "Never doubt that a small group of thoughtful, committed citizens can change the world; indeed, it's the only thing that ever has."[286] — Margaret Mead

Chapter 2: "Unless someone like you cares a whole awful lot, nothing is going to get better. It's not."[287] — Dr. Seuss

Chapter 3: "When a flower doesn't bloom, you fix the environment in which it grows, not the flower."[288] — Alexander Den Heijer

Chapter 4: "We need to treat the planet as a system, and up until now, we've operated more as if the world were made of separate parts - this part is environment, this part is economy. But everything is connected. You can't fix global warming with a Ph.D. in thermodynamics!"[289] — Neri Oxman

Chapter 5: "You never change things by fighting the existing reality. To change something, build a new model that makes the existing model obsolete."[290] — R. Buckminster Fuller

Chapter 6: "My main task has been to show that there is a deep and important underlying structural correspondence between the pattern of a problem and the process of designing a physical form which answers that problem."[291] — Christopher Alexander

Chapter 7: "The things to do are: the things that need doing, that you see need to be done, and that no one else seems to see need to be done."[292] — R. Buckminster Fuller

Chapter 8: "The reward for work well done is the opportunity to do more."[293] — Jonas Salk

Chapter 9: "Cure sometimes, treat often, comfort always."[294] — Hippocrates

Chapter 10: "The architect should also have a knowledge of the study of medicine on account of the questions of climates, air, the healthiness and unhealthiness of sites...for without these considerations the healthiness of a dwelling cannot be assured."[295] — Vitruvius

Chapter 11: "If you have built castles in the air, your work need not be lost; that is where they should be. Now put the foundations under them."[296] — Henry David Thoreau

Chapter 12: "What I do is the opposite of building walls. I build bridges. A bridge is something that connects instead of separating."[297] – Santiago Calatrava

Chapter 13: "We shape our buildings; thereafter they shape us."[298] — Winston Churchill

Chapter 14: "Without standards, there can be no improvement."[299] — Taiichi Ohno

Chapter 15: "Knowing is not enough; we must apply. Willing is not enough; we must do."[300] — Johann Wolfgang von Goethe

Chapter 16: "If I were asked to name the chief benefit of the house, I should say: the house shelters day-dreaming, the house protects the dreamer, the house allows one to dream in peace."[301] — Gaston Bachelard

Chapter 17: "I will not follow where the path may lead, but I will go where there is no path, and I will leave a trail."[302] — Muriel Strode

Chapter 18: "A profound design process eventually makes the patron, the architect, and every occasional visitor in the building a slightly better human being."[303] — Juhani Pallasmaa

About the Author: "We each pay a fabulous price for our visions of paradise, but a spirit with a vision is a dream with a mission."[304] — Neil Peart

NOTES

"1. Introduction - REST API Design Rulebook [Book]." Accessed November 3, 2022. https://www.oreilly.com/library/view/rest-api-design/9781449317904/ch01.html.

8 weeks to optimum health: spontaneous healing, 2004.

14:00-17:00. "ISO 16739-1:2018." ISO. Accessed January 16, 2021. https://www.iso.org/cms/render/live/en/sites/isoorg/contents/data/standard/07/03/70303.html.

"1918 Pandemic (H1N1 Virus) | Pandemic Influenza (Flu) | CDC," June 16, 2020. https://www.cdc.gov/flu/pandemic-resources/1918-pandemic-h1n1.html.

"2023 ICD-10-CM | CMS." Accessed November 20, 2022. https://www.cms.gov/medicare/icd-10/2023-icd-10-cm.

"A Quote by Alexander Den Heijer." Accessed October 30, 2022. https://www.goodreads.com/quotes/8708203-when-a-flower-doesn-t-bloom-you-fix-the-environment-in.

"A Quote by Neil Peart." Accessed November 17, 2022. https://www.goodreads.com/quotes/88721-a-spirit-with-a-vision-is-a-dream-with-a.

"A Quote by R. Buckminster Fuller-To Change Something." Accessed October 30, 2022. https://www.goodreads.com/quotes/13119-you-never-change-things-by-fighting-the-existing-reality-to.

"A Quote by Socrates." Accessed January 30, 2022. https://www.goodreads.com/quotes/452128-to-know-thyself-is-the-beginning-of-wisdom.

"About - The Long Now." Accessed March 18, 2021. https://longnow.org/about/.

Warner Babcock Institute. "About Green Chemistry." Accessed November 22, 2022. https://www.warnerbabcock.com/green-chemistry/about-green-chemistry/.

"About Health Level Seven International | HL7 International." Accessed October 24, 2022. http://www.hl7.org/about/index.cfm?ref=nav.

"About Legionnaires Disease and Pontiac Fever | Legionella | CDC," October 31, 2019. https://www.cdc.gov/legionella/about/index.html.

"About OSHA | Occupational Safety and Health Administration." Accessed December 12, 2020. https://www.osha.gov/aboutosha.

"About Us." Accessed November 21, 2022. https://www.cochrane.org/about-us.

X12. "About X12." Accessed November 21, 2022. https://x12.org/about/about-x12.

"Aetiology | Etiology, n." In OED Online. Oxford University Press. Accessed January 10, 2022. https://www.oed.com/view/Entry/3268.

Notes

"AMIA-UNDERSTANDING WHY (AND HOW) Informatics Is Accelerating Healthcare's Transformation," n.d.

Rocky Mountain Institute. "Amory Lovins." Accessed January 24, 2021. https://rmi.org/people/amory-lovins/.

"Analemma Fishburn." In Wikipedia, August 26, 2022. https://en.wikipedia.org/w/index.php?title=Analemma&oldid=1106732441.

"Analemma_Earth." In Wikipedia, August 26, 2022. https://en.wikipedia.org/w/index.php?title=Analemma&oldid=1106732441.

"Architect | Origin and Meaning of Architect by Online Etymology Dictionary." Accessed January 2, 2021. https://www.etymonline.com/word/architect.

"Architecture | Origin and Meaning of Architecture by Online Etymology Dictionary." Accessed January 2, 2021. https://www.etymonline.com/word/architecture.

"Architecture, n." In OED Online. Oxford University Press. Accessed October 31, 2020. https://www.oed.com/view/Entry/10408.

"BACnet." In Wikipedia, November 16, 2022. https://en.wikipedia.org/w/index.php?title=BACnet&oldid=1122199887.

Bar, Moshe, and Maital Neta. "Humans Prefer Curved Visual Objects." Psychological Science 17, no. 8 (August 1, 2006): 645–48. https://doi.org/10.1111/j.1467-9280.2006.01759.x.

Bar-Cohen, Yoseph. "Biomimetics: Biologically Inspired Technology," January 1, 2006.

"Bio- | Origin and Meaning of Prefix Bio- by Online Etymology Dictionary." Accessed June 27, 2021. https://www.etymonline.com/word/bio-.

"Biomimetics." In Wikipedia, October 18, 2022. https://en.wikipedia.org/w/index.php?title=Biomimetics&oldid=1116741650.

"Biophilia Hypothesis." In Wikipedia, June 3, 2021. https://en.wikipedia.org/w/index.php?title=Biophilia_hypothesis&oldid=1026562060.

Biophilic Design: The Architecture of Life. "Biophilic Design: The Architecture of Life." Accessed April 2, 2014. http://www.biophilicdesign.net/.

"Biosphere 2." In Wikipedia, December 12, 2021. https://en.wikipedia.org/w/index.php?title=Biosphere_2&oldid=1059870393.

"Bisphenol A (BPA) Factsheet | National Biomonitoring Program | CDC," September 2, 2021. https://www.cdc.gov/biomonitoring/BisphenolA_FactSheet.html.

"Bisphenol-a-in-Building-Materials-High-Performance-Paint-Coatings.Pdf," 2009.

https://healthybuilding.net/uploads/files/bisphenol-a-in-building-materials-high-performance-paint-coatings.pdf.

"Blueprint, n." In OED Online. Oxford University Press. Accessed January 15, 2022. https://www.oed.com/view/Entry/20610.

"Blueprint, v." In OED Online. Oxford University Press. Accessed January 15, 2022. https://www.oed.com/view/Entry/353123.

Boissoneault, Lorraine. "The Cuyahoga River Caught Fire at Least a Dozen Times, but No One Cared Until 1969." Smithsonian Magazine. Accessed January 24, 2021. https://www.smithsonianmag.com/history/cuyahoga-river-caught-fire-least-dozen-times-no-one-cared-until-1969-180972444/.

Braungart, Michael, and William McDonough. Cradle to Cradle: Remaking the Way We Make Things, 2019.

"Buckminster Fuller - Wikiquote." Accessed October 30, 2022. https://en.wikiquote.org/wiki/Buckminster_Fuller.

Alliance to Save Energy. "Buildings," July 22, 2013. https://www.ase.org/initiatives/buildings.

Carson, R. Silent Spring. 40th Anniversary ed. Boston: A Mariner Books, 2002.

"Circular Economy Schools Of Thought." Accessed January 11, 2021. https://www.ellenmacarthurfoundation.org/circular-economy/concept/schools-of-thought.

"COBie." In Wikipedia, July 2, 2021. https://en.wikipedia.org/w/index.php?title=COBie&oldid=1031643285.

"Cold Spring Harbor Laboratory." In Wikipedia, August 29, 2022. https://en.wikipedia.org/w/index.php?title=Cold_Spring_Harbor_Laboratory&oldid=1107284074#cite_note-4.

"Committee E31 on Healthcare Informatics." Accessed November 14, 2021. https://www.astm.org/COMMITTEE/E31.htm.

"Coronavirus Disease (COVID-19) – World Health Organization." Accessed October 11, 2022. https://www.who.int/emergencies/diseases/novel-coronavirus-2019.

"Cyanotype." In Wikipedia, October 5, 2021. https://en.wikipedia.org/w/index.php?title=Cyanotype&oldid=1048332161.

Davenhall, Bill. "Geomedicine: Geography and Personal Health," 2012, 33.

Gartner. "Definition of Clinical Data Repository (CDR) - Gartner Information Technology Glossary." Accessed January 23, 2022. https://www.gartner.com/en/information-tech-

nology/glossary/cdr-clinical-data-repository.

"Definition of DETERMINANT." Accessed February 5, 2022. https://www.merriam-webster.com/dictionary/determinant.

"Detailed Overview - Overview - About Us." Accessed November 21, 2022. https://www.astm.org/about/overview/detailed-overview.html.

"Determinant, Adj. and n." In OED Online. Oxford University Press. Accessed October 23, 2022. https://www.oed.com/view/Entry/51232.

"Determinants of Health Visualized." Accessed December 12, 2020. https://www.goinvo.com/vision/determinants-of-health/.

"Diagnosis vs. Prognosis: What's The Difference? | Merriam-Webster." Accessed April 9, 2022. https://www.merriam-webster.com/words-at-play/usage-of-diagnosis-and-prognosis-difference.

"Digital Twin." In Wikipedia, June 18, 2022. https://en.wikipedia.org/w/index.php?title=Digital_twin&oldid=1093732352.

AIHA. "Discover IH." Accessed February 13, 2021. https://www.aiha.org/ih-careers/discover-industrial-hygiene.

"Document Display | NEPIS | US EPA," 1989. https://nepis.epa.gov/Exe/ZyNET.exe/9100LMBU.TXT?ZyActionD=ZyDocument&Client=EPA&Index=1986+Thru+1990&Docs=&Query=&Time=&EndTime=&SearchMethod=1&TocRestrict=n&Toc=&TocEntry=&QField=&QFieldYear=&QFieldMonth=&QFieldDay=&IntQFieldOp=0&ExtQFieldOp=0&XmlQuery=&File=D%3A%5Czyfiles%5CIndex%20Data%5C86thru90%5CTxt%5C00000022%5C9100LMBU.txt&User=ANONYMOUS&Password=anonymous

BrainyQuote. "Dr. Seuss Quotes." Accessed October 30, 2022. https://www.brainyquote.com/quotes/dr_seuss_105646.

Duncombe, Jenessa. "Aerosol Scientists Try to Clear the Air About COVID-19 Transmission." Eos, March 31, 2021. http://eos.org/articles/aerosol-scientists-try-to-clear-the-air-about-covid-19-transmission.

"Eco- | Origin and Meaning of Prefix Eco- by Online Etymology Dictionary." Accessed February 14, 2021. https://www.etymonline.com/word/eco-.

"Ecology | Origin and Meaning of Ecology by Online Etymology Dictionary." Accessed November 19, 2020. https://www.etymonline.com/word/ecology.

"Edifice, n." In OED Online. Oxford University Press. Accessed October 31, 2020. https://

www.oed.com/view/Entry/59535.

"Endocrine Diseases." Text. National Library of Medicine. Accessed January 9, 2022. https://medlineplus.gov/endocrinediseases.html.

The Andrew Weil Center for Integrative Medicine. "Environmental Health: An Integrative Approach - Andrew Weil Center for Integrative Medicine." Accessed January 3, 2021. https://integrativemedicine.arizona.edu/education/online_courses/enviro-med.html.

"Fast Healthcare Interoperability Resources." In Wikipedia, September 27, 2022. https://en.wikipedia.org/w/index.php?title=Fast_Healthcare_Interoperability_Resources&oldid=1112729939.

"Fiscal Year (FY) 2019 Medicare Hospital Inpatient Prospective Payment System (IPPS) and Long Term Acute Care Hospital (LTCH) Prospective Payment System Proposed Rule, and Request for Information | CMS." Accessed July 16, 2022. https://www.cms.gov/newsroom/fact-sheets/fiscal-year-fy-2019-medicare-hospital-inpatient-prospective-payment-system-ipps-and-long-term-acute.

BrainyQuote. "Florence Nightingale Quotes-752511." Accessed October 21, 2022. https://www.brainyquote.com/quotes/florence_nightingale_752511.

BrainyQuote. "Florence Nightingale Quotes-752512." Accessed October 21, 2022. https://www.brainyquote.com/quotes/florence_nightingale_752512.

RMI. "Gas Stoves: Health and Air Quality Impacts and Solutions." Accessed November 10, 2022. https://rmi.org/insight/gas-stoves-pollution-health/.

BrainyQuote. "Gaston Bachelard Quotes." Accessed October 30, 2022. https://www.brainyquote.com/quotes/gaston_bachelard_149802.

"Geomedicine Definition & Meaning | Merriam-Webster Medical." Accessed October 24, 2022. https://www.merriam-webster.com/medical/geomedicine.

"Glaze, v.1." In OED Online. Oxford University Press. Accessed January 11, 2021. https://www.oed.com/view/Entry/78821.

"Goinvo/HealthDeterminants." HTML. 2016. Reprint, GoInvo, October 17, 2020. https://github.com/goinvo/HealthDeterminants.

Grammaticos, Philip C., and Aristidis Diamantis. "Useful Known and Unknown Views of the Father of Modern Medicine, Hippocrates and His Teacher Democritus." Hellenic Journal of Nuclear Medicine 11, no. 1 (April 2008): 2–4.

Gravity Project. "Gravity Project." Accessed November 20, 2022. https://thegravityproject.

Notes

net/.

"Greenhouse Effect | C-SPAN.Org." Accessed August 4, 2022. https://www.c-span.org/video/?125856-1/greenhouse-effect.

Harkness, Jon. "A Lifetime of Connections: Otto Herbert Schmitt, 1913-1998." Physics in Perspective (PIP) 4 (January 12, 2002): 456–90. https://doi.org/10.1007/s000160200005.

"Heal | Origin and Meaning of Heal by Online Etymology Dictionary." Accessed December 2, 2020. https://www.etymonline.com/word/heal.

"Healing | Origin and Meaning of Healing by Online Etymology Dictionary." Accessed December 2, 2020. https://www.etymonline.com/word/healing.

"Health | Origin and Meaning of Health by Online Etymology Dictionary." Accessed December 2, 2020. https://www.etymonline.com/word/health.

HHS.gov. "Health Information Privacy." Text, August 26, 2015. https://www.hhs.gov/hipaa/index.html.

"Health Information Technology for Economic and Clinical Health Act." In Wikipedia, January 26, 2022. https://en.wikipedia.org/w/index.php?title=Health_Information_Technology_for_Economic_and_Clinical_Health_Act&oldid=1068109800.

"Healthcare Standards Training for Interoperability | HL7 International." Accessed November 21, 2022. https://www.hl7.org/training/index.cfm?ref=nav.

BrainyQuote. "Henry David Thoreau Quotes." Accessed October 30, 2022. https://www.brainyquote.com/quotes/henry_david_thoreau_105332.

Hersh, William. "A Stimulus to Define Informatics and Health Information Technology." BMC Medical Informatics and Decision Making 9, no. 1 (December 2009): 24. https://doi.org/10.1186/1472-6947-9-24.

"Hippocrates | Biography, Works, & Facts | Britannica." Accessed October 10, 2022. https://www.britannica.com/biography/Hippocrates.

BrainyQuote. "Hippocrates Quotes." Accessed October 30, 2022. https://www.brainyquote.com/quotes/hippocrates_379317.

"HL7.FHIR.US.SDOH-CLINICALCARE\Home Page - FHIR v4.0.1." Accessed November 20, 2022. http://hl7.org/fhir/us/sdoh-clinicalcare/.

"Home (2020 TV Series)." In Wikipedia, October 19, 2022. https://en.wikipedia.org/w/index.php?title=Home_(2020_TV_series)&oldid=1117100290#Episodes.

"Household Air Pollution and Health." Accessed November 10, 2022. https://www.who.int/news-room/fact-sheets/detail/household-air-pollution-and-health.

buildingSMART International. "Industry Foundation Classes (IFC)." Accessed December 14, 2020. https://www.buildingsmart.org/standards/bsi-standards/industry-foundation-classes/.

AMIA - American Medical Informatics Association. "Informatics: Research and Practice." Accessed August 2, 2022. https://amia.org/about-amia/why-informatics/informatics-research-and-practice.

"Integration | Origin and Meaning of Integration by Online Etymology Dictionary." Accessed January 1, 2021. https://www.etymonline.com/word/integration.

Health IT Buzz. "Interoperability vs Health Information Exchange: Setting the Record Straight," January 9, 2013. https://www.healthit.gov/buzz-blog/meaningful-use/interoperability-health-information-exchange-setting-record-straight.

"Introduction | Meaningful Use | CDC," September 17, 2020. https://www.cdc.gov/ehrmeaningfuluse/introduction.html.

ioha-admin. "Our Vision & Mission." IOHA (blog). Accessed February 13, 2021. https://www.ioha.net/about/vision-mission/.

BrainyQuote. "Jiddu Krishnamurti Quotes." Accessed April 10, 2022. https://www.brainyquote.com/quotes/jiddu_krishnamurti_107856.

BrainyQuote. "Johann Wolfgang von Goethe Quotes." Accessed October 30, 2022. https://www.brainyquote.com/quotes/johann_wolfgang_von_goeth_161315.

BrainyQuote. "Jonas Salk Quotes." Accessed October 30, 2022. https://www.brainyquote.com/quotes/jonas_salk_129207.

A-Z Quotes. "Juhani Pallasmaa Quote." Accessed October 30, 2022. https://www.azquotes.com/quote/550123.

Kharnagy. English: Illustration Showing Stages in a DevOps Toolchain. September 7, 2016. Own work. https://commons.wikimedia.org/wiki/File:Devops-toolchain.svg.

Klepeis, Neil E., William C. Nelson, Wayne R. Ott, John P. Robinson, Andy M. Tsang, Paul Switzer, Joseph V. Behar, Stephen C. Hern, and William H. Engelmann. "The National Human Activity Pattern Survey (NHAPS): A Resource for Assessing Exposure to Environmental Pollutants." Journal of Exposure Science & Environmental Epidemiology 11, no. 3 (July 2001): 231–52. https://doi.org/10.1038/sj.jea.7500165.

Klepeis, Neil, William Nelson, Wayne Ott, and John Robinson. "The National Human Activity Pattern Survey (NHAPS): A Resource for Assessing Exposure to Environmental Pollutants," January 1, 2001.

Kühn, Shafreena, Robert Sader, and Ulrich M. Rieger. "'Without Standards, There Can Be No Improvement'—Taiichi Ohno." *Gland Surgery* 8, no. 6 (December 2019): 591–92. https://doi.org/10.21037/gs.2019.11.23.

"Legionnaire Disease | Britannica." Accessed January 11, 2021. https://www.britannica.com/science/Legionnaire-disease.

LOINC. "LOINC License." Accessed November 20, 2022. https://loinc.org/kb/.

LOINC. "LOINC-PhenX-Environmental Exposures Archives." Accessed November 20, 2022. https://loinc.org/panels/category/clinical-assessments-scales-measures/phenx-domains-consensus-measures-for-phenotypes-and-exposures/environmental-exposures-phenx-domains-consensus-measures-for-phenotypes-and-exposures/.

Lowry, S. "Housing." *BMJ : British Medical Journal* 303, no. 6806 (October 5, 1991): 838-40.

Mandavilli, Apoorva. "239 Experts With One Big Claim: The Coronavirus Is Airborne." *The New York Times*, July 4, 2020, sec. Health. https://www.nytimes.com/2020/07/04/health/239-experts-with-one-big-claim-the-coronavirus-is-airborne.html.

BrainyQuote. "Margaret Mead Quotes." Accessed December 26, 2021. https://www.brainyquote.com/quotes/margaret_mead_100502.

mars.nasa.gov. "Trip to Mars." Accessed December 26, 2021. https://mars.nasa.gov/mars2020/timeline/cruise/.

BrainyQuote. "Maya Lin Quotes." Accessed October 30, 2022. https://www.brainyquote.com/quotes/maya_lin_344886.

"Medicine | Origin and Meaning of Medicine by Online Etymology Dictionary." Accessed December 2, 2020. https://www.etymonline.com/word/medicine.

"Medicine, n.1." In *OED Online*. Oxford University Press. Accessed November 1, 2020. https://www.oed.com/view/Entry/115715.

Monteiro, L. A. "Florence Nightingale on Public Health Nursing." *American Journal of Public Health* 75, no. 2 (February 1985): 181–86. https://doi.org/10.2105/ajph.75.2.181.

Morawska, Lidia, and Donald K Milton. "It Is Time to Address Airborne Transmission of Coronavirus Disease 2019 (COVID-19)." *Clinical Infectious Diseases* 71, no. 9 (November 1, 2020): 2311–13. https://doi.org/10.1093/cid/ciaa939.

BrainyQuote. "Muriel Strode Quotes." Accessed October 30, 2022. https://www.brainyquote.com/quotes/muriel_strode_101322.

"National COVID-19 Aerosol Workplace Standard Urged." Accessed October 22, 2022.

http://www.workerscompensation.com/news_read.php?id=38064&type=7.

National Geographic Society (U.S.). *Energy: Facing up to the Problem, Getting down to Solutions : A Special Report in the Public Interest*. Washington, D.C.: National Geographic Society, 1981.

Nations, United. "World Population to Reach 8 Billion on 15 November 2022." United Nations. United Nations. Accessed October 21, 2022. https://www.un.org/en/desa/world-population-reach-8-billion-15-november-2022.

Negri, Elisa, Luca Fumagalli, and Marco Macchi. "A Review of the Roles of Digital Twin in CPS-Based Production Systems." Procedia Manufacturing, 27th International Conference on Flexible Automation and Intelligent Manufacturing, FAIM2017, 27-30 June 2017, Modena, Italy, 11 (January 1, 2017): 939–48. https://doi.org/10.1016/j.promfg.2017.07.198.

"Neighborhood and Built Environment - Healthy People 2030 | Health.Gov." Accessed February 12, 2021. https://health.gov/healthypeople/objectives-and-data/browse-objectives/neighborhood-and-built-environment.

"Notes on the Synthesis of Form." In Wikipedia, November 19, 2021. https://en.wikipedia.org/w/index.php?title=Notes_on_the_Synthesis_of_Form&oldid=1056124266.

"Nourish | Etymology, Origin and Meaning of Nourish by Etymonline." Accessed November 22, 2022. https://www.etymonline.com/word/nourish.

"Nurture | Etymology, Origin and Meaning of Nurture by Etymonline." Accessed December 30, 2021. https://www.etymonline.com/word/nurture.

"Nurture Definition & Meaning - Merriam-Webster." Accessed November 22, 2022. https://www.merriam-webster.com/dictionary/nurture.

"Nurture, n." In OED Online. Oxford University Press. Accessed December 30, 2021. https://www.oed.com/view/Entry/129243.

on behalf of the Swedish Digital Twin Consortium, Bergthor Björnsson, Carl Borrebaeck, Nils Elander, Thomas Gasslander, Danuta R. Gawel, Mika Gustafsson, et al. "Digital Twins to Personalize Medicine." Genome Medicine 12, no. 1 (December 2020): 4. https://doi.org/10.1186/s13073-019-0701-3.

"Ontology (Information Science)." In Wikipedia, July 12, 2022. https://en.wikipedia.org/w/index.php?title=Ontology_(information_science)&oldid=1097810148.

DrWeil.com. "Optimum Health - Dr. Andrew Weil," September 8, 2006. https://www.drweil.com/diet-nutrition/nutrition/optimum-health/.

Notes

"Otto H. Schmitt - Como History." Accessed November 22, 2022. https://sites.google.com/a/comogreenvillage.info/como-history/home/people-of-the-past-documents/como-people-of-the-past/otto-h-schmitt.

CalEarth. "Our Founder." Accessed December 26, 2021. https://www.calearth.org/our-founder.

"Overview-Dev - FHIR v4.0.1." Accessed January 16, 2021. https://www.hl7.org/fhir/overview-dev.html.

"Overview-Dev - FHIR v4.3.0." Accessed October 23, 2022. http://hl7.org/fhir/overview-dev.html.

Oxman, Neri. "Neri Oxman Quotes-I Approach the World." BrainyQuote. Accessed October 28, 2022. https://www.brainyquote.com/quotes/neri_oxman_906502.

———. "Neri Oxman Quotes-We Need to Treat the Planet as a System." BrainyQuote. Accessed October 28, 2022. https://www.brainyquote.com/quotes/neri_oxman_906488.

"PhenX Toolkit: About." Accessed April 5, 2022. https://www.phenxtoolkit.org/about.

"Philo- | Meaning of Suffix Philo- by Etymonline." Accessed November 22, 2022. https://www.etymonline.com/word/philo-.

Podder, Vivek, Valerie Lew, and Sassan Ghassemzadeh. "SOAP Notes." In StatPearls. Treasure Island (FL): StatPearls Publishing, 2021. http://www.ncbi.nlm.nih.gov/books/NBK482263/.

"Precision Health: Improving Health for Each of Us and All of Us | CDC." Accessed January 2, 2022. https://www.cdc.gov/genomics/about/precision_med.htm.

"Public Health | Definition, History, & Facts | Britannica." Accessed October 10, 2022. https://www.britannica.com/topic/public-health.

"Public Health - National Developments in the 18th and 19th Centuries | Britannica." Accessed November 19, 2022. https://www.britannica.com/topic/public-health/National-developments-in-the-18th-and-19th-centuries.

"Q2811-How Long Would a Trip to Mars Take?" Accessed August 4, 2022. https://image.gsfc.nasa.gov/poetry/venus/q2811.html.

Quinn, Caroline, Ali Zargar Shabestari, Tony Misic, Sara Gilani, Marin Litoiu, and J. J. McArthur. "Building Automation System - BIM Integration Using a Linked Data Structure." Automation in Construction 118 (October 1, 2020): 103257. https://doi.org/10.1016/j.autcon.2020.103257.

BrainyQuote. "R. Buckminster Fuller Quotes-Main." Accessed December 26, 2021. https://

www.brainyquote.com/authors/r-buckminster-fuller-quotes.

BrainyQuote. "R. Buckminster Fuller Quotes-Nature Is Trying Very Hard to Make Us Succeed." Accessed August 4, 2022. https://www.brainyquote.com/quotes/r_buckminster_fuller_151697.

Rasmussen, Mads Holten, Pieter Pauwels, Maxime Lefrançois, Georg Ferdinand Schneider, Christian Anker Hviid, and Jan Karlshøj. "Recent Changes in the Building Topology Ontology," 2017. https://doi.org/10.13140/RG.2.2.32365.28647.

Rees, William E. "Ecological Footprints and Appropriated Carrying Capacity: What Urban Economics Leaves Out." Environment and Urbanization 4, no. 2 (October 1, 1992): 121–30. https://doi.org/10.1177/095624789200400212.

Rose, Stephanie. "Social Determinants of Health PRAPARE Tool Training," n.d., 57.

"Rx | Search Online Etymology Dictionary." Accessed December 2, 2020. https://www.etymonline.com/search?q=Rx.

BrainyQuote. "Santiago Calatrava Quotes." Accessed November 17, 2022. https://www.brainyquote.com/quotes/santiago_calatrava_1061471.

Schroeder, Greyce N., Charles Steinmetz, Carlos E. Pereira, and Danubia B. Espindola. "Digital Twin Data Modeling with AutomationML and a Communication Methodology for Data Exchange." IFAC-PapersOnLine, 4th IFAC Symposium on Telematics Applications TA 2016, 49, no. 30 (January 1, 2016): 12–17. https://doi.org/10.1016/j.ifacol.2016.11.115.

"Sick Building Syndrome and the Problem of Uncertainty : Environmental Politics, Technoscience, and Women Workers (Book, 2006) [WorldCat.Org]." Accessed January 11, 2021. https://www.worldcat.org/title/sick-building-syndrome-and-the-problem-of-uncertainty-environmental-politics-technoscience-and-women-workers/oclc/1064988081&referer=brief_results.

"SNOMED CT - Environment or Geographical Location - Classes | NCBO BioPortal." Accessed November 21, 2022. https://bioportal.bioontology.org/ontologies/SNOMEDCT?p=classes&conceptid=308916002.

"SOAP Note." In Wikipedia, September 20, 2022. https://en.wikipedia.org/w/index.php?title=SOAP_note&oldid=1111249751.

"Social Determinants of Health." In Wikipedia, December 7, 2020. https://en.wikipedia.org/w/index.php?title=Social_determinants_of_health&oldid=992923740.

"Social Determinants of Health." Accessed January 2, 2022. https://www.who.int/

Notes

health-topics/social-determinants-of-health#tab=tab_1.

"Social Determinants of Health | CDC," January 26, 2021. https://www.cdc.gov/socialdeterminants/index.htm.

"Social Determinants of Health - Healthy People 2030 | Health.Gov." Accessed February 12, 2021. https://health.gov/healthypeople/objectives-and-data/social-determinants-health.

BrainyQuote. "Socrates Quotes." Accessed January 30, 2022. https://www.brainyquote.com/quotes/socrates_101168.

Söder, Mathias. "INTRODUCTION." RealEstateCore (blog). Accessed November 18, 2022. https://www.realestatecore.io/introduction/.

———. "RECcon22." RealEstateCore (blog). Accessed November 18, 2022. https://www.realestatecore.io/reccon22/.

Söderlund, Jana, Peter Newman, Jana Söderlund, and Peter Newman. "Biophilic Architecture: A Review of the Rationale and Outcomes." AIMS Environmental Science 2, no. 4 (2015): 950–69. https://doi.org/10.3934/environsci.2015.4.950.

"Spanish Flu." In Wikipedia, June 21, 2022. https://en.wikipedia.org/w/index.php?title=Spanish_flu&oldid=1094318174.

https://buildingbiology.com/. "Standard of Building Biology Testing Methods SBM - Buildingbiology.Com." Accessed November 7, 2022. https://buildingbiology.com/building-biology-standard/.

https://www.apa.org. "Stressed in America." Accessed July 17, 2022. https://www.apa.org/monitor/2011/01/stressed-america.

"Summary - FHIR v4.0.1." Accessed January 23, 2022. http://hl7.org/fhir/summary.html.

"System | Origin and Meaning of System by Online Etymology Dictionary." Accessed February 14, 2021. https://www.etymonline.com/word/system.

"System, n." In OED Online. Oxford University Press. Accessed November 19, 2020. https://www.oed.com/view/Entry/196665.

Biomedical Informatics. "The History of BMI." Accessed August 3, 2022. https://med.stanford.edu/bmi/biomedical-informatics/history-program.html.

"The Project Gutenberg EBook of Ten Books on Architecture, by Vitruvius." Accessed December 26, 2020. https://www.gutenberg.org/files/20239/20239-h/20239-h.htm.

"The Radiologist," November 19, 2019. https://www.hopkinsmedicine.org/health/treatment-tests-and-therapies/the-radiologist.

Mayo Clinic. "Tips to Reduce BPA Exposure." Accessed November 10, 2022. https://www.mayoclinic.org/healthy-lifestyle/nutrition-and-healthy-eating/expert-answers/bpa/faq-20058331.

Towell, Colin., DK Publishing, Inc.,. *Essential Survival Skills : Key Tips and Techniques for the Great Outdoors.* London; New York: DK Pub., 2011.

Ulrich, R. S. "View Through a Window May Influence Recovery from Surgery." Text. The Center for Health Design. The Center for Health Design, October 16, 2012. https://www.healthdesign.org/knowledge-repository/view-through-window-may-influence-recovery-surgery.

———. "View through a Window May Influence Recovery from Surgery." Science (New York, N.Y.) 224, no. 4647 (April 27, 1984): 420–21. https://doi.org/10.1126/science.6143402.

"UMLS Metathesaurus Browser." Accessed October 23, 2022. https://uts.nlm.nih.gov/uts/umls.

"UMLS Quick Start Guide." Training Material and Manuals. U.S. National Library of Medicine. Accessed January 9, 2022. https://www.nlm.nih.gov/research/umls/quickstart.html.

"Understanding Brick - BrickSchema." Accessed November 18, 2022. https://brickschema.org/concepts/.

Urbina, Ian. "Think Those Chemicals Have Been Tested?" The New York Times, April 13, 2013, sec. Sunday Review. https://www.nytimes.com/2013/04/14/sunday-review/think-those-chemicals-have-been-tested.html.

US EPA, OA. "The Origins of EPA." Collections and Lists. US EPA, January 29, 2013. https://www.epa.gov/history/origins-epa.

US EPA, ORD. "Indoor Air Quality." Reports and Assessments. US EPA, November 2, 2017. https://www.epa.gov/report-environment/indoor-air-quality.

Vergano, Dan. "Brave New World of Biosphere 2?" Science News Science News 150, no. 20 (1996): 312.

Vitruvius. "Vitruvius Quote #1879894." Quotepark.com. Accessed February 6, 2022. http://quotepark.com/quotes/1879894-vitruvius-the-architect-should-also-have-a-knowledge-of-the/.

Lib Quotes. "Vitruvius Quote." Accessed October 10, 2022. https://libquotes.com/vitruvius/quote/lbx6g6s.

Wall Street (1987) - IMDb. Accessed October 28, 2022. http://www.imdb.com/title/tt0094291/characters/nm0000140.

"Welcome | Yestermorrow Design/Build School." Accessed February 21, 2021. https://yestermorrow.org/about/welcome.

"What Are CI/CD and the CI/CD Pipeline?," April 8, 2022. https://www.ibm.com/cloud/blog/ci-cd-pipeline.

"What Is a REST API?" Accessed January 23, 2022. https://www.redhat.com/en/topics/api/what-is-a-rest-api.

Biomimicry Institute. "What Is Biomimicry?" Accessed June 27, 2021. https://biomimicry.org/what-is-biomimicry/.

"What Is Computerized Provider Order Entry? | HealthIT.Gov." Accessed November 13, 2021. https://www.healthit.gov/faq/what-computerized-provider-order-entry.

"What Is DevOps? DevOps Explained | Microsoft Azure." Accessed August 28, 2022. https://azure.microsoft.com/en-us/resources/cloud-computing-dictionary/what-is-devops/.

"What Is GIS? | Geographic Information System Mapping Technology." Accessed October 23, 2022. https://www.esri.com/en-us/what-is-gis/overview.

The Andrew Weil Center for Integrative Medicine. "What Is Integrative Medicine?" Accessed January 3, 2021. https://integrativemedicine.arizona.edu/about/definition.html.

What Is Integrative Medicine? | Andrew Weil, M.D., 2010. https://www.youtube.com/watch?v=4pXsm3qaFIk&feature=youtu.be.

"What Is Integrative Medicine? - Andrew Weil, M.D." Accessed April 2, 2014. http://www.drweil.com/drw/u/ART02054/Andrew-Weil-Integrative-Medicine.html.

PRAPARE. "What Is PRAPARE." Accessed October 23, 2022. https://prapare.org/what-is-prapare/.

"What Is Single Pane of Glass? - Definition from Techopedia." Accessed November 18, 2022. https://www.techopedia.com/definition/32235/single-pane-of-glass.

"What Is the Precision Medicine Initiative?: MedlinePlus Genetics." Accessed January 2, 2022. https://medlineplus.gov/genetics/understanding/precisionmedicine/initiative/.

"Where No Man Has Gone Before." In Wikipedia, November 6, 2021. https://en.wikipedia.org/w/index.php?title=Where_no_man_has_gone_before&oldid=1053907150.

WHO. "WHO | Social Determinants of Health." World Health Organization. Accessed December 11, 2020. https://www.who.int/gender-equity-rights/understanding/sdh-definition/en/.

PRAPARE. "Who We Are." Accessed May 8, 2022. https://prapare.org/who-we-are/.

AMIA - American Medical Informatics Association. "Why Informatics?" Accessed August 3, 2022. https://amia.org/about-amia/why-informatics.

"Wilderness Survival Rules of 3 - Air, Shelter, Water & Food," May 29, 2012. https://www.backcountrychronicles.com/wilderness-survival-rules-of-3/.

Wilson, Edward O. Biophilia: Cambridge, MA: Harvard University Press, 1986.

Winkelstein, Warren Jr. "Florence Nightingale: Founder of Modern Nursing and Hospital Epidemiology." Epidemiology 20, no. 2 (March 2009): 311. https://doi.org/10.1097/EDE.0b013e3181935ad6.

BrainyQuote. "Winston Churchill Quotes." Accessed October 30, 2022. https://www.brainyquote.com/quotes/winston_churchill_111316.

Notes

ENDNOTES

1. "Aetiology | Etiology, n.," in OED Online (Oxford University Press), accessed January 10, 2022, https://www.oed.com/view/Entry/3268.
2. "Health Information Technology for Economic and Clinical Health Act," in Wikipedia, January 26, 2022, https://en.wikipedia.org/w/index.php?title=Health_Information_Technology_for_Economic_and_Clinical_Health_Act&oldid=1068109800.
3. "Fiscal Year (FY) 2019 Medicare Hospital Inpatient Prospective Payment System (IPPS) and Long Term Acute Care Hospital (LTCH) Prospective Payment System Proposed Rule, and Request for Information | CMS," accessed July 16, 2022, https://www.cms.gov/newsroom/fact-sheets/fiscal-year-fy-2019-medicare-hospital-inpatient-prospective-payment-system-ipps-and-long-term-acute.
4. "What Is the Precision Medicine Initiative?: MedlinePlus Genetics," accessed January 2, 2022, https://medlineplus.gov/genetics/understanding/precisionmedicine/initiative/.
5. "Digital Twin," in Wikipedia, June 18, 2022, https://en.wikipedia.org/w/index.php?title=Digital_twin&oldid=1093732352.
6. Elisa Negri, Luca Fumagalli, and Marco Macchi, "A Review of the Roles of Digital Twin in CPS-Based Production Systems," Procedia Manufacturing, 27th International Conference on Flexible Automation and Intelligent Manufacturing, FAIM2017, 27-30 June 2017, Modena, Italy, 11 (January 1, 2017): 939–48, https://doi.org/10.1016/j.promfg.2017.07.198.
7. "What Is the Precision Medicine Initiative?"
8. "Social Determinants of Health," accessed January 2, 2022, https://www.who.int/health-topics/social-determinants-of-health#tab=tab_1.
9. "Geomedicine Definition & Meaning | Merriam-Webster Medical," accessed October 24, 2022, https://www.merriam-webster.com/medical/geomedicine.
10. "Fiscal Year (FY) 2019 Medicare Hospital Inpatient Prospective Payment System (IPPS) and Long Term Acute Care Hospital (LTCH) Prospective Payment System Proposed Rule, and Request for Information | CMS."
11. "Document Display | NEPIS | US EPA," 1989, https://nepis.epa.gov/Exe/ZyNET.exe/9100LMBU.TXT?ZyActionD=ZyDocument&Client=EPA&Index=1986+Thru+1990&Docs=&Query=&Time=&EndTime=&SearchMethod=1&To-

cRestrict=n&Toc=&TocEntry=&QField=&QFieldYear=&QFieldMonth=&QFieldDay=&IntQFieldOp=0&ExtQFieldOp=0&XmlQuery=&File=D%3A%5Czyfiles%5CIndex%20Data%5C86thru90%5CTxt%5C00000022%5C9100LMBU.txt&User=ANONYMOUS&Password=anonymous&SortMethod=h%7C-&MaximumDocuments=1&FuzzyDegree=0&ImageQuality=r75g8/r75g8/x150y150g16/i425&Display=hpfr&DefSeekPage=x&SearchBack=ZyActionL&Back=ZyActionS&BackDesc=Results%20page&MaximumPages=1&ZyEntry=1&SeekPage=x&ZyPURL.

12. "Hippocrates | Biography, Works, & Facts | Britannica," accessed October 10, 2022, https://www.britannica.com/biography/Hippocrates.
13. Philip C. Grammaticos and Aristidis Diamantis, "Useful Known and Unknown Views of the Father of Modern Medicine, Hippocrates and His Teacher Democritus.," *Hellenic Journal of Nuclear Medicine* 11, no. 1 (April 2008): 2–4.
14. "Public Health | Definition, History, & Facts | Britannica," accessed October 10, 2022, https://www.britannica.com/topic/public-health.
15. "Vitruvius Quote," Lib Quotes, accessed October 10, 2022, https://libquotes.com/vitruvius/quote/lbx6g6s.
16. L. A. Monteiro, "Florence Nightingale on Public Health Nursing," *American Journal of Public Health* 75, no. 2 (February 1985): 181–86, https://doi.org/10.2105/ajph.75.2.181.
17. Warren Jr Winkelstein, "Florence Nightingale: Founder of Modern Nursing and Hospital Epidemiology," *Epidemiology* 20, no. 2 (March 2009): 311, https://doi.org/10.1097/EDE.0b013e3181935ad6.
18. R. Carson, *Silent Spring*, 40th Anniversary ed (Boston: A Mariner Books, 2002).
19. "Coronavirus Disease (COVID-19) – World Health Organization," accessed October 11, 2022, https://www.who.int/emergencies/diseases/novel-coronavirus-2019.
20. Jenessa Duncombe, "Aerosol Scientists Try to Clear the Air About COVID-19 Transmission," *Eos*, March 31, 2021, http://eos.org/articles/aerosol-scientists-try-to-clear-the-air-about-covid-19-transmission.
21. "National COVID-19 Aerosol Workplace Standard Urged," accessed October 22, 2022, http://www.workerscompensation.com/news_read.php?id=38064&type=7.
22. Lidia Morawska and Donald K Milton, "It Is Time to Address Airborne Transmission of Coronavirus Disease 2019 (COVID-19)," *Clinical Infectious Diseases* 71, no. 9 (November 1, 2020): 2311–13, https://doi.org/10.1093/cid/ciaa939.

23 *Vivek Podder, Valerie Lew, and Sassan Ghassemzadeh, "SOAP Notes," in StatPearls (Treasure Island (FL): StatPearls Publishing, 2021), http://www.ncbi.nlm.nih.gov/books/NBK482263/.*

24 *"SOAP Note," in Wikipedia, September 20, 2022, https://en.wikipedia.org/w/index.php?title=SOAP_note&oldid=1111249751.*

25 *"Coronavirus Disease (COVID-19) – World Health Organization."*

26 *"1918 Pandemic (H1N1 Virus) | Pandemic Influenza (Flu) | CDC," June 16, 2020, https://www.cdc.gov/flu/pandemic-resources/1918-pandemic-h1n1.html.*

27 *Duncombe, "Aerosol Scientists Try to Clear the Air About COVID-19 Transmission."*

28 *Neil E. Klepeis, William C. Nelson, Wayne R. Ott, John P. Robinson, et al., "The National Human Activity Pattern Survey (NHAPS): A Resource for Assessing Exposure to Environmental Pollutants," Journal of Exposure Science & Environmental Epidemiology 11, no. 3 (July 2001): 231–52, https://doi.org/10.1038/sj.jea.7500165.*

29 *Neil Klepeis, William Nelson, Wayne Ott, and John Robinson, "The National Human Activity Pattern Survey (NHAPS): A Resource for Assessing Exposure to Environmental Pollutants," January 1, 2001.*

30 *"Stressed in America," https://www.apa.org, accessed July 17, 2022, https://www.apa.org/monitor/2011/01/stressed-america.*

31 *"Bisphenol A (BPA) Factsheet | National Biomonitoring Program | CDC," September 2, 2021, https://www.cdc.gov/biomonitoring/BisphenolA_FactSheet.html.*

32 *"Bisphenol-a-in-Building-Materials-High-Performance-Paint-Coatings.Pdf," 2009, https://healthybuilding.net/uploads/files/bisphenol-a-in-building-materials-high-performance-paint-coatings.pdf.*

33 *"Architecture, n.," in OED Online (Oxford University Press), accessed October 31, 2020, https://www.oed.com/view/Entry/10408.*

34 *"Edifice, n.," in OED Online (Oxford University Press), accessed October 31, 2020, https://www.oed.com/view/Entry/59535.*

35 *"Architecture | Origin and Meaning of Architecture by Online Etymology Dictionary," accessed January 2, 2021, https://www.etymonline.com/word/architecture.*

36 *"Architect | Origin and Meaning of Architect by Online Etymology Dictionary," accessed January 2, 2021, https://www.etymonline.com/word/architect.*

37 *"Medicine, n.1," in OED Online (Oxford University Press), accessed November 1, 2020, https://www.oed.com/view/Entry/115715.*

38 *"Medicine, n.1."*

39 *"Medicine | Origin and Meaning of Medicine by Online Etymology Dictionary," accessed December 2, 2020, https://www.etymonline.com/word/medicine.*

40 *"Healing | Origin and Meaning of Healing by Online Etymology Dictionary," accessed December 2, 2020, https://www.etymonline.com/word/healing.*

41 *"Heal | Origin and Meaning of Heal by Online Etymology Dictionary," accessed December 2, 2020, https://www.etymonline.com/word/heal.*

42 *"Health | Origin and Meaning of Health by Online Etymology Dictionary," accessed December 2, 2020, https://www.etymonline.com/word/health.*

43 *"Medicine | Origin and Meaning of Medicine by Online Etymology Dictionary."*

44 *"Healing | Origin and Meaning of Healing by Online Etymology Dictionary."*

45 *"Spanish Flu," in Wikipedia, June 21, 2022, https://en.wikipedia.org/w/index.php?title=Spanish_flu&oldid=1094318174.*

46 *"1918 Pandemic (H1N1 Virus) | Pandemic Influenza (Flu) | CDC."*

47 *"1918 Pandemic (H1N1 Virus) | Pandemic Influenza (Flu) | CDC."*

48 *Apoorva Mandavilli, "239 Experts With One Big Claim: The Coronavirus Is Airborne," The New York Times, July 4, 2020, sec. Health, https://www.nytimes.com/2020/07/04/health/239-experts-with-one-big-claim-the-coronavirus-is-airborne.html.*

49 *"What Is the Precision Medicine Initiative?"*

50 *Winkelstein, "Florence Nightingale."*

51 *"Florence Nightingale Quotes-752512," BrainyQuote, accessed October 21, 2022, https://www.brainyquote.com/quotes/florence_nightingale_752512.*

52 *"Florence Nightingale Quotes-752511," BrainyQuote, accessed October 21, 2022, https://www.brainyquote.com/quotes/florence_nightingale_752511.*

53 *United Nations, "World Population to Reach 8 Billion on 15 November 2022," United Nations (United Nations), accessed October 21, 2022, https://www.un.org/en/desa/world-population-reach-8-billion-15-november-2022.*

54 *S Lowry, "Housing.," BMJ : British Medical Journal 303, no. 6806 (October 5, 1991): 838–40.*

55 *"Florence Nightingale Quotes-752511."*

56 *"Florence Nightingale Quotes-752512."*

57 *8 weeks to optimum health: spontaneous healing, 2004.*

58 *Ian Urbina, "Think Those Chemicals Have Been Tested?," The New York Times, April*

13, 2013, sec. Sunday Review, https://www.nytimes.com/2013/04/14/sunday-review/think-those-chemicals-have-been-tested.html.

59 "Optimum Health - Dr. Andrew Weil," DrWeil.Com (blog), September 8, 2006, https://www.drweil.com/diet-nutrition/nutrition/optimum-health/.

60 "Welcome | Yestermorrow Design/Build School," accessed February 21, 2021, https://yestermorrow.org/about/welcome.

61 "What Is Integrative Medicine?," The Andrew Weil Center for Integrative Medicine, accessed January 3, 2021, https://integrativemedicine.arizona.edu/about/definition.html.

62 "What Is Integrative Medicine? - Andrew Weil, M.D.," accessed April 2, 2014, http://www.drweil.com/drw/u/ART02054/Andrew-Weil-Integrative-Medicine.html.

63 Neri Oxman, "Neri Oxman Quotes-I Approach the World," BrainyQuote, accessed October 28, 2022, https://www.brainyquote.com/quotes/neri_oxman_906502.

64 "Buildings," Alliance to Save Energy, July 22, 2013, https://www.ase.org/initiatives/buildings.

65 "Circular Economy Schools Of Thought," accessed January 11, 2021, https://www.ellenmacarthurfoundation.org/circular-economy/concept/schools-of-thought.

66 Michael Braungart and William McDonough, Cradle to Cradle: Remaking the Way We Make Things, 2019.

67 William E. Rees, "Ecological Footprints and Appropriated Carrying Capacity: What Urban Economics Leaves Out," Environment and Urbanization 4, no. 2 (October 1, 1992): 121–30, https://doi.org/10.1177/095624789200400212.

68 "Glaze, v.1," in OED Online (Oxford University Press), accessed January 11, 2021, https://www.oed.com/view/Entry/78821.

69 "Sick Building Syndrome and the Problem of Uncertainty : Environmental Politics, Technoscience, and Women Workers (Book, 2006) [WorldCat.Org]," accessed January 11, 2021, https://www.worldcat.org/title/sick-building-syndrome-and-the-problem-of-uncertainty-environmental-politics-technoscience-and-women-workers/oclc/1064988081&referer=brief_results.

70 "About Legionnaires Disease and Pontiac Fever | Legionella | CDC," October 31, 2019, https://www.cdc.gov/legionella/about/index.html.

71 "Legionnaire Disease | Britannica," accessed January 11, 2021, https://www.britannica.com/science/Legionnaire-disease.

72 "Integration | Origin and Meaning of Integration by Online Etymology Dictionary," accessed January 1, 2021, https://www.etymonline.com/word/integration.

73 "What Is Integrative Medicine?"

74 What Is Integrative Medicine? | Andrew Weil, M.D., 2010, https://www.youtube.com/watch?v=4pXsm3qaFIk&feature=youtu.be.

75 What Is Integrative Medicine?

76 What Is Integrative Medicine?

77 "Environmental Health: An Integrative Approach - Andrew Weil Center for Integrative Medicine," The Andrew Weil Center for Integrative Medicine, accessed January 3, 2021, https://integrativemedicine.arizona.edu/education/online_courses/enviro-med.html.

78 Lorraine Boissoneault, "The Cuyahoga River Caught Fire at Least a Dozen Times, but No One Cared Until 1969," Smithsonian Magazine, accessed January 24, 2021, https://www.smithsonianmag.com/history/cuyahoga-river-caught-fire-least-dozen-times-no-one-cared-until-1969-180972444/.

79 OA US EPA, "The Origins of EPA," Collections and Lists, US EPA, January 29, 2013, https://www.epa.gov/history/origins-epa.

80 National Geographic Society (U.S.), Energy: Facing up to the Problem, Getting down to Solutions : A Special Report in the Public Interest. (Washington, D.C.: National Geographic Society, 1981).

81 Wall Street (1987) - IMDb, accessed October 28, 2022, http://www.imdb.com/title/tt0094291/characters/nm0000140.

82 "Amory Lovins," Rocky Mountain Institute, accessed January 24, 2021, https://rmi.org/people/amory-lovins/.

83 Braungart and McDonough, Cradle to Cradle.

84 ORD US EPA, "Indoor Air Quality," Reports and Assessments, US EPA, November 2, 2017, https://www.epa.gov/report-environment/indoor-air-quality.

85 "System | Origin and Meaning of System by Online Etymology Dictionary," accessed February 14, 2021, https://www.etymonline.com/word/system.

86 "System, n.," in OED Online (Oxford University Press), accessed November 19, 2020, https://www.oed.com/view/Entry/196665.

87 "Eco- | Origin and Meaning of Prefix Eco- by Online Etymology Dictionary," accessed February 14, 2021, https://www.etymonline.com/word/eco-.

88 "Ecology | Origin and Meaning of Ecology by Online Etymology Dictionary," accessed November 19, 2020, https://www.etymonline.com/word/ecology.

89 "Ecology | Origin and Meaning of Ecology by Online Etymology Dictionary."

90 "System | Origin and Meaning of System by Online Etymology Dictionary."

91 "Rx | Search Online Etymology Dictionary," accessed December 2, 2020, https://www.etymonline.com/search?q=Rx.

92 "About Health Level Seven International | HL7 International," 7, accessed October 24, 2022, http://www.hl7.org/about/index.cfm?ref=nav.

93 "What Is a REST API?," accessed January 23, 2022, https://www.redhat.com/en/topics/api/what-is-a-rest-api.

94 "1. Introduction - REST API Design Rulebook [Book]," accessed November 3, 2022, https://www.oreilly.com/library/view/rest-api-design/9781449317904/ch01.html.

95 "Fast Healthcare Interoperability Resources," in Wikipedia, September 27, 2022, https://en.wikipedia.org/w/index.php?title=Fast_Healthcare_Interoperability_Resources&oldid=1112729939.

96 "Rx | Search Online Etymology Dictionary."

97 "Blueprint, v.," in OED Online (Oxford University Press), accessed January 15, 2022, https://www.oed.com/view/Entry/353123.

98 "Blueprint, n.," in OED Online (Oxford University Press), accessed January 15, 2022, https://www.oed.com/view/Entry/20610.

99 "Cyanotype," in Wikipedia, October 5, 2021, https://en.wikipedia.org/w/index.php?title=Cyanotype&oldid=1048332161.

100 "Introduction | Meaningful Use | CDC," September 17, 2020, https://www.cdc.gov/ehrmeaningfuluse/introduction.html.

101 "Introduction | Meaningful Use | CDC."

102 "Summary - FHIR v4.0.1," accessed January 23, 2022, http://hl7.org/fhir/summary.html.

103 "Industry Foundation Classes (IFC)," buildingSMART International, accessed December 14, 2020, https://www.buildingsmart.org/standards/bsi-standards/industry-foundation-classes/.

104 14:00-17:00, "ISO 16739-1:2018," ISO, accessed January 16, 2021, https://www.iso.org/cms/render/live/en/sites/isoorg/contents/data/standard/07/03/70303.html.

105 "Industry Foundation Classes (IFC)."

106 "Overview-Dev - FHIR v4.0.1," accessed January 16, 2021, https://www.hl7.org/fhir/overview-dev.html.

107 "Health Information Privacy," Text, HHS.gov, August 26, 2015, https://www.hhs.gov/hipaa/index.html.

108 "Discover IH," AIHA, accessed February 13, 2021, https://www.aiha.org/ih-careers/discover-industrial-hygiene.

109 ioha-admin, "Our Vision & Mission," IOHA (blog), accessed February 13, 2021, https://www.ioha.net/about/vision-mission/.

110 "About OSHA | Occupational Safety and Health Administration," accessed December 12, 2020, https://www.osha.gov/aboutosha.

111 "Standard of Building Biology Testing Methods SBM – Buildingbiology.Com," https://buildingbiology.com/, accessed November 7, 2022, https://buildingbiology.com/building-biology-standard/.

112 "Why Informatics?," AMIA - American Medical Informatics Association, accessed August 3, 2022, https://amia.org/about-amia/why-informatics.

113 "Informatics: Research and Practice," AMIA - American Medical Informatics Association, accessed August 2, 2022, https://amia.org/about-amia/why-informatics/informatics-research-and-practice.

114 "AMIA-UNDERSTANDING WHY (AND HOW) Informatics Is Accelerating Healthcare's Transformation," n.d.

115 "AMIA-UNDERSTANDING WHY (AND HOW) Informatics Is Accelerating Healthcare's Transformation."

116 "AMIA-UNDERSTANDING WHY (AND HOW) Informatics Is Accelerating Healthcare's Transformation."

117 "AMIA-UNDERSTANDING WHY (AND HOW) Informatics Is Accelerating Healthcare's Transformation."

118 "AMIA-UNDERSTANDING WHY (AND HOW) Informatics Is Accelerating Healthcare's Transformation."

119 "AMIA-UNDERSTANDING WHY (AND HOW) Informatics Is Accelerating Healthcare's Transformation."

120 "AMIA-UNDERSTANDING WHY (AND HOW) Informatics Is Accelerating Healthcare's Transformation."

121 "Informatics."

122 "Informatics."

123 "The History of BMI," Biomedical Informatics, accessed August 3, 2022, https://med.stanford.edu/bmi/biomedical-informatics/history-program.html.

124 William Hersh, "A Stimulus to Define Informatics and Health Information Technology," BMC Medical Informatics and Decision Making 9, no. 1 (December 2009): 24, https://doi.org/10.1186/1472-6947-9-24.

125 "Informatics."

126 "Informatics."

127 "Informatics."

128 "What Is DevOps? DevOps Explained | Microsoft Azure," accessed August 28, 2022, https://azure.microsoft.com/en-us/resources/cloud-computing-dictionary/what-is-devops/.

129 "What Are CI/CD and the CI/CD Pipeline?," April 8, 2022, https://www.ibm.com/cloud/blog/ci-cd-pipeline.

130 "What Are CI/CD and the CI/CD Pipeline?"

131 Podder, Lew, and Ghassemzadeh, "SOAP Notes."

132 "Household Air Pollution and Health," accessed November 10, 2022, https://www.who.int/news-room/fact-sheets/detail/household-air-pollution-and-health.

133 "Household Air Pollution and Health."

134 "Household Air Pollution and Health."

135 "Household Air Pollution and Health."

136 "Gas Stoves: Health and Air Quality Impacts and Solutions," RMI, accessed November 10, 2022, https://rmi.org/insight/gas-stoves-pollution-health/.

137 "Gas Stoves."

138 "Tips to Reduce BPA Exposure," Mayo Clinic, accessed November 10, 2022, https://www.mayoclinic.org/healthy-lifestyle/nutrition-and-healthy-eating/expert-answers/bpa/faq-20058331.

139 "Tips to Reduce BPA Exposure."

140 "The Radiologist," November 19, 2019, https://www.hopkinsmedicine.org/health/treatment-tests-and-therapies/the-radiologist.

141 Vitruvius, "Vitruvius Quote #1879894," Quotepark.com, accessed February 6, 2022, http://quotepark.com/quotes/1879894-vitruvius-the-architect-should-also-have-a-knowledge-of-the/.

142   "The Project Gutenberg EBook of Ten Books on Architecture, by Vitruvius.," accessed December 26, 2020, https://www.gutenberg.org/files/20239/20239-h/20239-h.htm.

143   "Medicine | Origin and Meaning of Medicine by Online Etymology Dictionary."

144   "Healing | Origin and Meaning of Healing by Online Etymology Dictionary."

145   "Heal | Origin and Meaning of Heal by Online Etymology Dictionary."

146   "Health | Origin and Meaning of Health by Online Etymology Dictionary."

147   "Medicine, n.1."

148   "Rx | Search Online Etymology Dictionary."

149   Mathias Söder, "INTRODUCTION," RealEstateCore (blog), accessed November 18, 2022, https://www.realestatecore.io/introduction/.

150   "Understanding Brick - BrickSchema," accessed November 18, 2022, https://brickschema.org/concepts/.

151   Mathias Söder, "RECcon22," RealEstateCore (blog), accessed November 18, 2022, https://www.realestatecore.io/reccon22/.

152   Mads Holten Rasmussen et al., "Recent Changes in the Building Topology Ontology," 2017, https://doi.org/10.13140/RG.2.2.32365.28647.

153   "What Is Single Pane of Glass? - Definition from Techopedia," accessed November 18, 2022, https://www.techopedia.com/definition/32235/single-pane-of-glass.

154   Podder, Lew, and Ghassemzadeh, "SOAP Notes."

155   "Precision Health: Improving Health for Each of Us and All of Us | CDC," accessed January 2, 2022, https://www.cdc.gov/genomics/about/precision_med.htm.

156   Greyce N. Schroeder et al., "Digital Twin Data Modeling with AutomationML and a Communication Methodology for Data Exchange," IFAC-PapersOnLine, 4th IFAC Symposium on Telematics Applications TA 2016, 49, no. 30 (January 1, 2016): 12–17, https://doi.org/10.1016/j.ifacol.2016.11.115.

157   Negri, Fumagalli, and Macchi, "A Review of the Roles of Digital Twin in CPS-Based Production Systems."

158   Caroline Quinn et al., "Building Automation System - BIM Integration Using a Linked Data Structure," Automation in Construction 118 (October 1, 2020): 103257, https://doi.org/10.1016/j.autcon.2020.103257.

159   Quinn et al.

160   on behalf of the Swedish Digital Twin Consortium et al., "Digital Twins to

Personalize Medicine," *Genome Medicine* 12, no. 1 (December 2020): 4, https://doi.org/10.1186/s13073-019-0701-3.

161 on behalf of the Swedish Digital Twin Consortium et al.

162 "About - The Long Now," accessed March 18, 2021, https://longnow.org/about/.

163 "Definition of Clinical Data Repository (CDR) - Gartner Information Technology Glossary," Gartner, accessed January 23, 2022, https://www.gartner.com/en/information-technology/glossary/cdr-clinical-data-repository.

164 "Public Health - National Developments in the 18th and 19th Centuries | Britannica," accessed November 19, 2022, https://www.britannica.com/topic/public-health/National-developments-in-the-18th-and-19th-centuries.

165 "Public Health - National Developments in the 18th and 19th Centuries | Britannica."

166 "Public Health - National Developments in the 18th and 19th Centuries | Britannica."

167 "Public Health - National Developments in the 18th and 19th Centuries | Britannica."

168 "Public Health - National Developments in the 18th and 19th Centuries | Britannica."

169 "Public Health - National Developments in the 18th and 19th Centuries | Britannica."

170 Monteiro, "Florence Nightingale on Public Health Nursing."

171 Winkelstein, "Florence Nightingale."

172 Winkelstein.

173 Monteiro, "Florence Nightingale on Public Health Nursing."

174 Monteiro.

175 "Public Health - National Developments in the 18th and 19th Centuries | Britannica."

176 "Definition of DETERMINANT," accessed February 5, 2022, https://www.merriam-webster.com/dictionary/determinant.

177 "Determinant, Adj. and n.," in OED Online (Oxford University Press), accessed October 23, 2022, https://www.oed.com/view/Entry/51232.

178 "WHO | Social Determinants of Health," WHO (World Health Organization), accessed December 11, 2020, https://www.who.int/gender-equity-rights/understand-

ing/sdh-definition/en/.

179 "Social Determinants of Health," in Wikipedia, December 7, 2020, https://en.wikipedia.org/w/index.php?title=Social_determinants_of_health&oldid=992923740.

180 "Goinvo/HealthDeterminants," HTML (2016; repr., GoInvo, October 17, 2020), https://github.com/goinvo/HealthDeterminants.

181 "Social Determinants of Health - Healthy People 2030 | Health.Gov," accessed February 12, 2021, https://health.gov/healthypeople/objectives-and-data/social-determinants-health.

182 "Social Determinants of Health | CDC," January 26, 2021, https://www.cdc.gov/socialdeterminants/index.htm.

183 "Neighborhood and Built Environment - Healthy People 2030 | Health.Gov," accessed February 12, 2021, https://health.gov/healthypeople/objectives-and-data/browse-objectives/neighborhood-and-built-environment.

184 "Overview-Dev - FHIR v4.3.0," accessed October 23, 2022, http://hl7.org/fhir/overview-dev.html.

185 "UMLS Quick Start Guide," Training Material and Manuals (U.S. National Library of Medicine), accessed January 9, 2022, https://www.nlm.nih.gov/research/umls/quickstart.html.

186 "UMLS Metathesaurus Browser," accessed October 23, 2022, https://uts.nlm.nih.gov/uts/umls.

187 "Gravity Project," Gravity Project, accessed November 20, 2022, https://thegravityproject.net/.

188 "HL7.FHIR.US.SDOH-CLINICALCARE\Home Page - FHIR v4.0.1," accessed November 20, 2022, http://hl7.org/fhir/us/sdoh-clinicalcare/.

189 "HL7.FHIR.US.SDOH-CLINICALCARE\Home Page - FHIR v4.0.1."

190 "HL7.FHIR.US.SDOH-CLINICALCARE\Home Page - FHIR v4.0.1."

191 "2023 ICD-10-CM | CMS," accessed November 20, 2022, https://www.cms.gov/medicare/icd-10/2023-icd-10-cm.

192 "PhenX Toolkit: About," accessed April 5, 2022, https://www.phenxtoolkit.org/about.

193 "PhenX Toolkit: About."

194 "LOINC License," LOINC (blog), accessed November 20, 2022, https://loinc.org/

kb/.

195   "LOINC-PhenX-Environmental Exposures Archives," LOINC (blog), accessed November 20, 2022, https://loinc.org/panels/category/clinical-assessments-scales-measures/phenx-domains-consensus-measures-for-phenotypes-and-exposures/environmental-exposures-phenx-domains-consensus-measures-for-phenotypes-and-exposures/.

196   "Who We Are," PRAPARE (blog), accessed May 8, 2022, https://prapare.org/who-we-are/.

197   "What Is PRAPARE," PRAPARE (blog), accessed October 23, 2022, https://prapare.org/what-is-prapare/.

198   Stephanie Rose, "Social Determinants of Health PRAPARE Tool Training," n.d., 57.

199   "Endocrine Diseases," Text (National Library of Medicine), accessed January 9, 2022, https://medlineplus.gov/endocrinediseases.html.

200   "Endocrine Diseases."

201   "Endocrine Diseases."

202   "Endocrine Diseases."

203   "Geomedicine Definition & Meaning | Merriam-Webster Medical."

204   "What Is GIS? | Geographic Information System Mapping Technology," accessed October 23, 2022, https://www.esri.com/en-us/what-is-gis/overview.

205   Bill Davenhall, "Geomedicine: Geography and Personal Health," 2012, 33.

206   Davenhall.

207   Davenhall.

208   Davenhall.

209   "Determinants of Health Visualized," accessed December 12, 2020, https://www.goinvo.com/vision/determinants-of-health/.

210   "Stressed in America."

211   Davenhall, "Geomedicine: Geography and Personal Health."

212   "Diagnosis vs. Prognosis: What's The Difference? | Merriam-Webster," accessed April 9, 2022, https://www.merriam-webster.com/words-at-play/usage-of-diagnosis-and-prognosis-difference.

213   Davenhall, "Geomedicine: Geography and Personal Health."

214   Davenhall.

215 Davenhall.

216 Davenhall.

217 Davenhall.

218 "Ontology (Information Science)," in Wikipedia, July 12, 2022, https://en.wikipedia.org/w/index.php?title=Ontology_(information_science)&oldid=1097810148.

219 "Ontology (Information Science)."

220 "COBie," in Wikipedia, July 2, 2021, https://en.wikipedia.org/w/index.php?title=COBie&oldid=1031643285.

221 "BACnet," in Wikipedia, November 16, 2022, https://en.wikipedia.org/w/index.php?title=BACnet&oldid=1122199887.

222 "BACnet."

223 "About X12," X12, 12, accessed November 21, 2022, https://x12.org/about/about-x12.

224 "SNOMED CT - Environment or Geographical Location - Classes | NCBO BioPortal," accessed November 21, 2022, https://bioportal.bioontology.org/ontologies/SNOMEDCT?p=classes&conceptid=308916002.

225 "About Health Level Seven International | HL7 International."

226 "Healthcare Standards Training for Interoperability | HL7 International," accessed November 21, 2022, https://www.hl7.org/training/index.cfm?ref=nav.

227 "Interoperability vs Health Information Exchange: Setting the Record Straight," Health IT Buzz, January 9, 2013, https://www.healthit.gov/buzz-blog/meaningful-use/interoperability-health-information-exchange-setting-record-straight.

228 "Healthcare Standards Training for Interoperability | HL7 International."

229 "What Is Computerized Provider Order Entry? | HealthIT.Gov," accessed November 13, 2021, https://www.healthit.gov/faq/what-computerized-provider-order-entry.

230 Podder, Lew, and Ghassemzadeh, "SOAP Notes."

231 "What Is Computerized Provider Order Entry? | HealthIT.Gov."

232 "Healthcare Standards Training for Interoperability | HL7 International."

233 "Committee E31 on Healthcare Informatics," 31, accessed November 14, 2021, https://www.astm.org/COMMITTEE/E31.htm.

234 "Detailed Overview - Overview - About Us," accessed November 21, 2022, https://www.astm.org/about/overview/detailed-overview.html.

235 "About Us," accessed November 21, 2022, https://www.cochrane.org/about-us.

236   "About Us."

237   "Home (2020 TV Series)," in Wikipedia, October 19, 2022, https://en.wikipedia.org/w/index.php?title=Home_(2020_TV_series)&oldid=1117100290#Episodes.

238   Moshe Bar and Maital Neta, "Humans Prefer Curved Visual Objects," Psychological Science 17, no. 8 (August 1, 2006): 645–48, https://doi.org/10.1111/j.1467-9280.2006.01759.x.

239   "Maya Lin Quotes," BrainyQuote, accessed October 30, 2022, https://www.brainyquote.com/quotes/maya_lin_344886.

240   "Nurture | Etymology, Origin and Meaning of Nurture by Etymonline," accessed December 30, 2021, https://www.etymonline.com/word/nurture.

241   "Nourish | Etymology, Origin and Meaning of Nourish by Etymonline," accessed November 22, 2022, https://www.etymonline.com/word/nourish.

242   "Nurture Definition & Meaning - Merriam-Webster," accessed November 22, 2022, https://www.merriam-webster.com/dictionary/nurture.

243   "Nurture, n.," in OED Online (Oxford University Press), accessed December 30, 2021, https://www.oed.com/view/Entry/129273.

244   Bar and Neta, "Humans Prefer Curved Visual Objects."

245   "Greenhouse Effect | C-SPAN.Org," accessed August 4, 2022, https://www.c-span.org/video/?125856-1/greenhouse-effect.

246   "Wilderness Survival Rules of 3 - Air, Shelter, Water & Food," May 29, 2012, 3, https://www.backcountrychronicles.com/wilderness-survival-rules-of-3/.

247   Colin. Towell DK Publishing, Inc., Essential Survival Skills : Key Tips and Techniques for the Great Outdoors. (London; New York: DK Pub., 2011).

248   "About Green Chemistry," Warner Babcock Institute, accessed November 22, 2022, https://www.warnerbabcock.com/green-chemistry/about-green-chemistry/.

249   "About Green Chemistry."

250   "About Green Chemistry."

251   "About Green Chemistry."

252   "About Green Chemistry."

253   "Biomimetics," in Wikipedia, October 18, 2022, https://en.wikipedia.org/w/index.php?title=Biomimetics&oldid=1116741650.

254   "What Is Biomimicry?," Biomimicry Institute, accessed June 27, 2021, https://biomimicry.org/what-is-biomimicry/.

255   "Biomimetics."

256   "Otto H. Schmitt - Como History," accessed November 22, 2022, https://sites.google.com/a/comogreenvillage.info/como-history/home/people-of-the-past-documents/como-people-of-the-past/otto-h-schmitt.

257   Yoseph Bar-Cohen, "Biomimetics: Biologically Inspired Technology," January 1, 2006.

258   Jon Harkness, "A Lifetime of Connections: Otto Herbert Schmitt, 1913-1998," Physics in Perspective (PIP) 4 (January 12, 2002): 456–90, https://doi.org/10.1007/s000160200005.

259   "What Is Biomimicry?"

260   "Biophilia Hypothesis," in Wikipedia, June 3, 2021, https://en.wikipedia.org/w/index.php?title=Biophilia_hypothesis&oldid=1026562060.

261   Edward O. Wilson, Biophilia: (Cambridge, MA: Harvard University Press, 1986).

262   "Bio- | Origin and Meaning of Prefix Bio- by Online Etymology Dictionary," accessed June 27, 2021, https://www.etymonline.com/word/bio-.

263   "Philo- | Meaning of Suffix Philo- by Etymonline," accessed November 22, 2022, https://www.etymonline.com/word/philo-.

264   "Biophilia Hypothesis."

265   Jana Söderlund et al., "Biophilic Architecture: A Review of the Rationale and Outcomes," AIMS Environmental Science 2, no. 4 (2015): 950–69, https://doi.org/10.3934/environsci.2015.4.950.

266   "Biophilic Design: The Architecture of Life," Biophilic Design: The Architecture of Life, accessed April 2, 2014, http://www.biophilicdesign.net/.

267   "Biophilia Hypothesis."

268   R. S. Ulrich, "View through a Window May Influence Recovery from Surgery," Science (New York, N.Y.) 224, no. 4647 (April 27, 1984): 420–21, https://doi.org/10.1126/science.6143402.

269   R. S. Ulrich, "View Through a Window May Influence Recovery from Surgery," Text, The Center for Health Design (The Center for Health Design, October 16, 2012), https://www.healthdesign.org/knowledge-repository/view-through-window-may-influence-recovery-surgery.

270   Dan Vergano, "Brave New World of Biosphere 2?," Science News Science News 150, no. 20 (1996): 312.

271 "Biosphere 2," in Wikipedia, December 12, 2021, https://en.wikipedia.org/w/index.php?title=Biosphere_2&oldid=1059870393.

272 mars.nasa.gov, "Trip to Mars," accessed December 26, 2021, https://mars.nasa.gov/mars2020/timeline/cruise/.

273 "Q2811-How Long Would a Trip to Mars Take?," accessed August 4, 2022, https://image.gsfc.nasa.gov/poetry/venus/q2811.html.

274 "Jiddu Krishnamurti Quotes," BrainyQuote, accessed April 10, 2022, https://www.brainyquote.com/quotes/jiddu_krishnamurti_107856.

275 "Our Founder," CalEarth, accessed December 26, 2021, https://www.calearth.org/our-founder.

276 "Our Founder."

277 "Our Founder."

278 "Our Founder."

279 "R. Buckminster Fuller Quotes-Nature Is Trying Very Hard to Make Us Succeed," BrainyQuote, accessed August 4, 2022, https://www.brainyquote.com/quotes/r_buckminster_fuller_151697.

280 "R. Buckminster Fuller Quotes-Nature Is Trying Very Hard to Make Us Succeed."

281 "R. Buckminster Fuller Quotes-Main," BrainyQuote, accessed December 26, 2021, https://www.brainyquote.com/authors/r-buckminster-fuller-quotes.

282 "Where No Man Has Gone Before," in Wikipedia, November 6, 2021, https://en.wikipedia.org/w/index.php?title=Where_no_man_has_gone_before&oldid=1053907150.

283 "A Quote by Socrates," accessed January 30, 2022, https://www.goodreads.com/quotes/452128-to-know-thyself-is-the-beginning-of-wisdom.

284 "Socrates Quotes," BrainyQuote, accessed January 30, 2022, https://www.brainyquote.com/quotes/socrates_101168.

285 "Cold Spring Harbor Laboratory," in Wikipedia, August 29, 2022, https://en.wikipedia.org/w/index.php?title=Cold_Spring_Harbor_Laboratory&oldid=1107284074#cite_note-4.

286 "Margaret Mead Quotes," BrainyQuote, accessed December 26, 2021, https://www.brainyquote.com/quotes/margaret_mead_100502.

287 "Dr. Seuss Quotes," BrainyQuote, accessed October 30, 2022, https://www.brainyquote.com/quotes/dr_seuss_105646.

288   "A Quote by Alexander Den Heijer," accessed October 30, 2022, https://www.goodreads.com/quotes/8708203-when-a-flower-doesn-t-bloom-you-fix-the-environment-in.

289   Neri Oxman, "Neri Oxman Quotes-We Need to Treat the Planet as a System," BrainyQuote, accessed October 28, 2022, https://www.brainyquote.com/quotes/neri_oxman_906488.

290   "A Quote by R. Buckminster Fuller-To Change Something," accessed October 30, 2022, https://www.goodreads.com/quotes/13119-you-never-change-things-by-fighting-the-existing-reality-to.

291   "Notes on the Synthesis of Form," in Wikipedia, November 19, 2021, https://en.wikipedia.org/w/index.php?title=Notes_on_the_Synthesis_of_Form&oldid=1056124266.

292   "Buckminster Fuller - Wikiquote," accessed October 30, 2022, https://en.wikiquote.org/wiki/Buckminster_Fuller.

293   "Jonas Salk Quotes," BrainyQuote, accessed October 30, 2022, https://www.brainyquote.com/quotes/jonas_salk_129207.

294   "Hippocrates Quotes," BrainyQuote, accessed October 30, 2022, https://www.brainyquote.com/quotes/hippocrates_379317.

295   Vitruvius, "Vitruvius Quote #1879894."

296   "Henry David Thoreau Quotes," BrainyQuote, accessed October 30, 2022, https://www.brainyquote.com/quotes/henry_david_thoreau_105332.

297   "Santiago Calatrava Quotes," BrainyQuote, accessed November 17, 2022, https://www.brainyquote.com/quotes/santiago_calatrava_1061471.

298   "Winston Churchill Quotes," BrainyQuote, accessed October 30, 2022, https://www.brainyquote.com/quotes/winston_churchill_111316.

299   Shafreena Kühn, Robert Sader, and Ulrich M. Rieger, "'Without Standards, There Can Be No Improvement'—Taiichi Ohno," Gland Surgery 8, no. 6 (December 2019): 591–92, https://doi.org/10.21037/gs.2019.11.23.

300   "Johann Wolfgang von Goethe Quotes," BrainyQuote, accessed October 30, 2022, https://www.brainyquote.com/quotes/johann_wolfgang_von_goeth_161315.

301   "Gaston Bachelard Quotes," BrainyQuote, accessed October 30, 2022, https://www.brainyquote.com/quotes/gaston_bachelard_149802.

302   "Muriel Strode Quotes," BrainyQuote, accessed October 30, 2022, https://www.

brainyquote.com/quotes/muriel_strode_101322.

303   "Juhani Pallasmaa Quote," A-Z Quotes, accessed October 30, 2022, https://www.azquotes.com/quote/550123.

304   "A Quote by Neil Peart," accessed November 17, 2022, https://www.goodreads.com/quotes/88721-a-spirit-with-a-vision-is-a-dream-with-a.

305   Kharnagy, English: Illustration Showing Stages in a DevOps Toolchain, September 7, 2016, September 7, 2016, Own work, https://commons.wikimedia.org/wiki/File:Devops-toolchain.svg.

306   Kharnagy, English: Illustration Showing Stages in a DevOps Toolchain, September 7, 2016, September 7, 2016, Own work, https://commons.wikimedia.org/wiki/File:Devops-toolchain.svg.

307   "Analemma_Earth," in Wikipedia, August 26, 2022, https://en.wikipedia.org/w/index.php?title=Analemma&oldid=1106732441.

308   "Analemma Fishburn," in Wikipedia, August 26, 2022, https://en.wikipedia.org/w/index.php?title=Analemma&oldid=1106732441.

v.1.1.6

THE ARCHITECTURAL DOCTOR®

AN Rx FOR HEALTH & WELLNESS IN BUILDINGS

INTEGRATING THE FIELDS OF
ARCHITECTURE & MEDICINE

Timothy D. Rossi

OTHER BOOKS BY THE AUTHOR

ARCHITECTURAL MEDICINE®
BUILDING THE BRIDGE TO WELLNESS

Are you wanting a better world in which to live, work, and play for both yourself and future generations? The focus of this book is to discuss how these two fields of Architecture and Medicine have a potential to overlap for a better built environment to live within.

(Published December 2020)

INTEGRATIVE ARCHITECTURE

Integrating the processes between green, healthy, and sustainable Architecture methodologies for energy efficient, ecologically aware, and healthier built environments.

(Forthcoming)

SYMBIOSIS GLOBAL
NATURE IS THE MOST ADVANCED TECHNOLOGY
TECHNOLOGY & ECOLOGY: LIVING TOGETHER

How can we navigate the challenges of humanity while also striving for progress in the world of Technology? How can we create a future more aligned to the planet's Ecological systems? Symbiosis Global outlines these topics with a focus on the premise "Nature is the Most Advanced Technology."

(Forthcoming)

THE ARCHITECTURAL DOCTOR®

AN Rx FOR HEALTH & WELLNESS IN BUILDINGS

INTEGRATING THE FIELDS OF
ARCHITECTURE & MEDICINE

TIMOTHY D. ROSSI

OTHER BOOKS BY THE AUTHOR

ARCHITECTURAL MEDICINE®
BUILDING THE BRIDGE TO WELLNESS

Are you wanting a better world in which to live, work, and play for both yourself and future generations? The focus of this book is to discuss how these two fields of Architecture and Medicine have a potential to overlap for a better built environment to live within.

(Published December 2020)

INTEGRATIVE ARCHITECTURE

Integrating the processes between green, healthy, and sustainable Architecture methodologies for energy efficient, ecologically aware, and healthier built environments.

(Forthcoming)

SYMBIOSIS GLOBAL
NATURE IS THE MOST ADVANCED TECHNOLOGY
TECHNOLOGY & ECOLOGY : LIVING TOGETHER

How can we navigate the challenges of humanity while also striving for progress in the world of Technology? How can we create a future more aligned to the planet's Ecological systems? Symbiosis Global outlines these topics with a focus on the premise "Nature is the Most Advanced Technology."

(Forthcoming)

www.ingramcontent.com/pod-product-compliance
Lightning Source LLC
Chambersburg PA
CBHW071114080526
44587CB00013B/1333